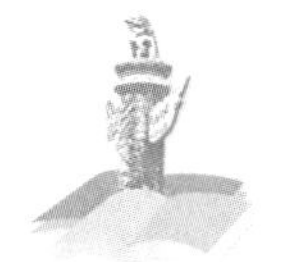

国家出版基金项目
NATIONAL PUBLICATION FOUNDATION

An Intensively Compiled Practical English-Chinese Library of Traditional Chinese Medicine
(英汉对照)精编实用中医文库

Chief General Compilers CHEN Kaixian LI Qizhong(Executive) HE Xinghai
总主编 陈凯先 李其忠(执行) 何星海
Chief General Translators SHI Jianrong HU Hongyi XU Yao(Executive)
总主译 施建蓉 胡鸿毅 徐 瑶(执行)

Health Preservation and Rehabilitation of Traditional Chinese Medicine

中医养生康复学

Chief Compiler MA Lieguang
Chief Translator YANG Yu
主编 马烈光
主译 杨 渝

上海浦江教育出版社(原上海中医药大学出版社)
Shanghai Pujiang Education Press (Former Shanghai University of TCM Press)

An Intensively Compiled Practical English-Chinese Library of Traditional Chinese Medicine

Compilation Board of the Library

Compilation and Translation Committee of the Library

Health Preservation and Rehabilitation of Traditional Chinese Medicine

《(英汉对照)精编实用中医文库》

编纂委员会

总　主　编　陈凯先　李其忠(执行)　何星海
编　　　委　(按姓氏笔画为序)
马烈光　何建成　余小萍　沈雪勇
张婷婷　陈红风　陈德兴　赵　毅
郭　忻　黄　平　虞坚尔　詹红生
缪晚虹

编译委员会

总　主　译　施建蓉　胡鸿毅　徐　瑶(执行)
编　译　者　(按姓氏笔画为序)
朱爱秀　杨　渝　肖元春　张亿萍
诸建民　黄国琪　董　晶　韩丑萍

《中医养生康复学》

主　　　编　马烈光
副　主　编　刘达平　传　鹏　张　伟　秦　源
编　　　委　(按姓氏笔画为序)
尹　巧　杨　蕻　赵羚妤　秦凯华
主　　　译　杨　渝
副　主　译　叶晓英　兰　蕾

Foreword
前　言

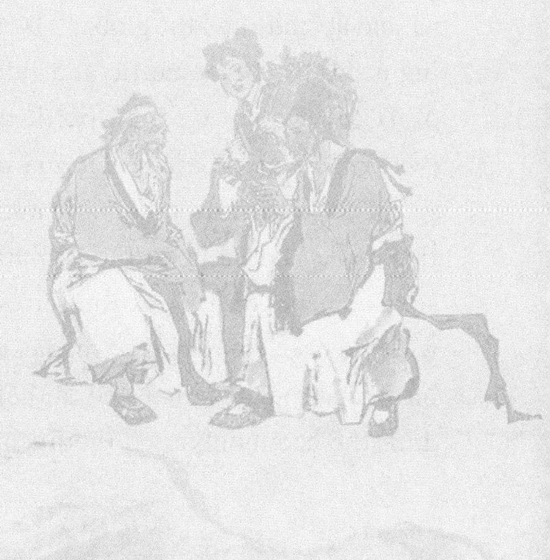

With the traditional medical philosophy and clinical experience as the principal body, the science of Traditional Chinese Medicine (TCM) is a comprehensive subject to study the rules of life activities and the disease prevention, diagnosis, treatment, rehabilitation as well as healthcare. The science of TCM has a long history of development and belongs to a summary of experiences that Chinese nation has fought against diseases for over several thousand years, is also an important component part of Chinese outstanding traditional culture and has contributed greatly to the healthcare undertaking and development of Chinese nation.

By increasing enhancement of modern living standard, change of living modes and acceleration of ageing process, the chronic diseases represented by tumors, cardiovascular diseases and diabetes become gradually the important factors in impacting the health of mankind, but TCM presents the better therapeutic effects. Nowadays, the modern medical mode of "society-psychology-biology" has been advocated in medical science, changing from the medical idea of "disease treatment" to "health promotion". The more and more patients in China and abroad have chosen natural and low side-effect Chinese herbal medicine for their problems. With the changes in medicine modes and in spectrum of diseases in the recent several dozens of years, TCM has increasingly been concerned by the medical experts and ordinary people in China and abroad, and the global "TCM upsurge" keeps rising. In order to meet the growing needs of the domestic and international professionals in learning the knowledge of TCM, we have edited particularly the series books of *An Intensively Compiled Practical English-Chinese Library of Traditional Chinese Medicine*.

The scientific, systematic and practical features have been emphasized in the series books. Based upon the full absorption of new progress in teaching and research achievements of TCM, the series books highlight the academic essentials of TCM, with precise exposition of medical philosophy and down-to-earth clinical practice, to introduce the "original and authentic" TCM to the readers. The series books introduce the commonly used therapeutic methods and clinical skills in Chinese medicine, by the clinically encountered and frequently seen diseases and the relevant ailments predominantly effective by Chinese medical therapies.By studying the series books, the readers can learn the knowledge and techniques of TCM on gradual progress and become proficient gradually in TCM.

The series books highlight "the precise features in three aspects"—capable in authors, refined in contents and accurate in translation. The majority of the authors of the series books are senior experts from the related faculties of Shanghai University of Traditional Chinese Medicine. The translator team is composed of the senior teachers with plentiful expertise in translation of TCM from international education college and foreign language center of Shanghai University of Traditional Chinese Medicine. In order to meet the needs of the readers in China and abroad, the basic and clinical core contents are selected and the latest research achievements are consulted based upon the principle "to seek its essentials but its completion" in the series books.

The series books can satisfy the beginners with certain knowledge of English language in studying TCM systematically and can also be used as the textbooks for education of TCM and pharmacy for foreign students. We sincerely hope the publication of the series books plays its promoting role for TCM going to the world.

Editors

June, 2017

中医学是以传统医学理论与实践经验为主体，研究人体生命活动规律和疾病预防、诊断、治疗、康复以及保健的一门综合性学科。中医学历史悠久，源远流长，是中华民族几千年来同疾病作斗争的经验总结，也是中国传统文化的重要组成部分，长期以来为中国人民的健康保健事业和民族繁衍作出了巨大的贡献。

随着现代生活水平的不断提高、生活方式的改变以及老龄化进程的加快，以肿瘤、心血管疾病和糖尿病等为代表的慢性病日渐成为影响人类健康的重要因素，而中医药显示了良好的治疗效果。当今的医学倡导"社会—心理—生物"的现代医学模式，医学理念从"疾病治疗"向"健康促进"转变，国内外越来越多的患者选择天然、毒副作用低的中医药治疗疾病。近几十年来，随着医学模式的转变和疾病谱的改变，中医学日益引起越来越多的海内外医学专家和普通民众的关注，全球性的"中医热"正在持续升温。为了满足海内外人士日益高涨的学习中医学知识的需求，我们特地编撰了《(英汉对照)精编实用中医文库》丛书。

本丛书注重"三性"——科学性、系统性、实用性。丛书在充分吸取近年中医教学、科研进展的基础上，突出中医学术精华，理论阐述准确、临床切合实际，向读者介绍"原汁原味"的中医学；丛书介绍中医学常用的治疗方法和临床技能，所涉及的病证均为临床常见病、多发病和中医优势病种。丛书的 13 个分册涵盖了中医基础与临床的主干课程，通过阅读本丛书，读者可以由浅入深、循序渐进地学习中医药知识和技能。

本丛书突出"三精"——作者精干、内容精炼、翻译精准。丛书的中文作者绝大部分为上海中医药大学各相关教研室的资深专家，翻译团队由上海中医药大学国际教育学院和外语中心具有丰富的中医药学翻译经验的骨干教师组成。为了适合海内外读者的需求，丛书本着"求其精而不求其全"的原则，选取了基础和临床的核心内容，翻译上参考了最新的研究成果。

本丛书既可满足具有一定英语水平的初学中医者系统学习中医所用，也可供中医药留学生教育作为教材使用，衷心希望本丛书的出版在中医药走向海外进程中发挥应有的推动作用。

编者

2017 年 6 月

Note for Compilation
编写说明

Health preservation of traditional Chinese medicine, a discipline of traditional Chinese medicine, studies and illustrates the theories, methodologies and applications of the emergence and development of human life, prevention of diseases, building up body and prolonging life. Rehabilitation of traditional Chinese medicine, another discipline of traditional Chinese medicine, focuses on the basic theories, methodologies and applications of rehabilitation. Though partially different, the two disciplines share some distinctive features of traditional Chinese medicine, hence they are combined into one science for exposition: health preservation and rehabilitation of traditional Chinese medicine.

In order to inherit the essence of traditional Chinese medicine as well as choicely absorb the modern achievements in this field, the compilation of the book adhers to the principle of practicability, abbreviates theories while details methods. There are two parts in this book. Part I is dedicated for health preservation. The introduction of this part emphasizes the basic theories, concepts and features, as well as the purpose and meanings of health preservation. Subsequently, detailed methods including the health preservation approaches of spirit, daily life, refined tastes, Qigong techniques, acupuncture and medicine, along with those in different regions and seasons, for different groups of people and for five viscera specifically are introduced; similar to the style and layout of Part I, Part II is dedicated for rehabilitation. The introduction covers the basic concept of rehabilitation and the related theories, followed by three chapters elucidating the methods respectively: rehabilitation for physical impairment and disabilities, diseases of internal medicine and exogenous febrile diseases after recovery.

It is necessary to point out that, due to some historical problems in the development of traditional Chinese medicine and the stagnation of the differentiation of disciplines, Health preservation develops in the company of rehabilitation, hence they are combined into one discipline. However, though they share some similarities, more differences lie in their contents, systems and applications respectively. Based on the relative independence of the two disciplines, this book illustrates them successively in two parts so as to clarify the two systems and ensure the applicability.

中医养生学，是研究和阐释人类生命发生发展规律、预防疾病、增强体质、益寿延年的理论、方法和应用的中医分支学科；中医康复学是在中医学理论指导下，研究中医康复学基本理论、方法及其应用的一门学科。二者虽然有所不同，但均为中医学之独具特色的分支学科，故将其合称为中医养生康复学。

本书的编写，本着继承传统精髓、择优吸收现代研究成果的态度，坚持实用性原则，略于理论，详于方法。上篇为中医养生学，概论部分着重介绍中医养生学的基本概念、基本特征及养生的目的、意义等理论知识，其后分别介绍中医养生学的精神养生、饮食养生、起居养生、雅趣养生、功法养生、针灸推拿养生、药物养生及不同地区养生、不同时令养生、不同人群养生、五脏保养等具体内容；下篇为中医康复学，其体例与上篇相同，以概论介绍中医康复学定义及相关理论知识，将中医康复学方法体系分为三章介绍，分别为中医伤残诸症康复、中医内科诸症康复、中医外感热病瘥后诸症康复等。

需要说明的是，由于中医学发展的历史原因及学科分化的滞后，中医养生学与中医康复学近年来偕同发展，统称中医养生康复学。但二者的研究内容、学科体系、应用范围等虽同中有异，且异多同少，各自具有相对的独立性。因此，本书尝试将其分篇介绍，以使其学科体系更加清晰和实用。

Contents

目　录

Part One Health Preservation of Traditional Chinese Medicine

上篇　中医养生学

Part Two Rehabilitation of Traditional Chinese Medicine

下篇 中医康复学

Part One
Health Preservation of Traditional Chinese Medicine

上篇
中医养生学

Introduction

概　论

The health preservation of traditional Chinese medicine (TCM) is both a treasure of Chinese culture and a bright pearl of TCM. It is of long history, peculiar theory, rich methods, effective practical experience, strong oriental trait and distinctive national feature. Embedded in the profound knowledge of sky, earth, human being, literature, history and philosophy of ancient China, based on the theory of TCM, the health preservation of TCM develops an extensive and profound theoretical system with accumulative wisdom of different Chinese peoples down the history as well as the comprehensive absorption of both the thoughts of Daoism, Confucianism and Buddhism, and the experience and achievement of experts on health preservation and TCM.

中医养生学是中国传统文化中的瑰宝，也是中医学宝库中的一颗璀璨明珠。她具有悠久的历史、独特的理论知识、丰富多彩的方法、卓有成效的实践经验、鲜明的东方色彩和浓郁的民族风格；她以中国古代的天、地、生、文、史、哲为深厚底蕴，以中医理论为坚实基础，集中国古今各地各族人民养生智慧为一体，融会道、儒、释及历代养生家、医学家的养生体验和研究成果，形成了博大精深的理论体系。

1　Basic Concepts of Health Preservation of TCM

In a conclusion, health preservation is to preserve life. To be more specific, health preservation refers to a variety of activities for physical and mental health on a conscious basis of principles of growing, developing and aging. To obtain better survival and development, human beings should perform these activities all through their lives.

1　中医养生学的基本概念

养生，古时也称之为摄生、道生、卫生、保生等。养生之养，含有保养、修养、培养、调养、补养、护养等意；生，就是指人的生命。概言之，养生就是保养人的生命。具体而言，养生是人类为了自身良好的生存与发展，有意识地根据人体生长衰老不可逆的量、质变化规律，所进行的一切物质和精神的身心养护活动。这种行为活动应贯穿人的一生。

Health preservation, a branch of TCM, is dedicated to the theory and methods of maintaining mental and physical health, preventing diseases and prolonging life according to the laws of nature. As a vast system, health preservation contains a variety of disciplines as astronomy, meteorology, philosophy, religion, sociology, psychology and prevention and health care and so on, many of which lately have become hot issues of multi-disciplinary study.

中医养生学是在中医理论指导下，根据人体生命活动变化规律，研究调摄身心、养护生命、却病延年的理论和方法的中医分支学科。隶属于中医学的中医养生学是一个开放的体系，其学术广泛涉及天文气象、哲学宗教、人文社会、心理行为、预防保健等诸多领域，其中的许多内容已成为当今多学科研究的热点。

2 Objective and Significance of Health Preservation

2 养生的目的和意义

2.1 Objective

The ultimate goal of health preservation is to ward off disease and prolong life span, which is deemed to be 110-120 years as the target of health preservation. Such a grand achievement takes the combination of three things: a fine social environment, medical science that can give counsel and guidance of health, and the individual's initiative to cultivate his own health and help others.

2.1 养生的目的

养生的根本目的就是保持健康、却病延命。对于人的寿限，目前认为是 110～120 岁，养生应以健康地达到寿命上限为目的。为达到这一目的，要依靠三方面的有机结合：一是依靠社会，尽量创造一个良好的生存环境；二是依靠医学，发挥健康咨询、养生指导和防治疾病的作用；三是依靠每一社会成员，发挥个人主观能动性，做好自我养生和帮助他人养生。

Specific goals consist of things as follows: to lay the healthy foundation in the embryo period; to stay fit by every means of health-preservation as a grown-up; to be active in finding the corresponding healthy methods to ward off or cure diseases; to be active in discerning, diagnosing and treating the disease when it occurs through the combination of clinic treatment and daily care, so as to minimize the effects of disease on health; in the case of incurable diseases such as diabetes, hypertension and chronic obstructive pulmonary disease, the goal supposed to be set in slowing down the development of the disease and guaranteeing the quality of life and prolonging it.

养生的具体目标：孕胎产子即应作好养生，打好生命健康的基础；出生后，常人应以保持健康为目的，通过各种养生方法强身健体，保持健康状态；当形体稍有不适、情志微有失常，出现亚健康时，应积极地选择有针对性的养生调摄方法防治临床疾病的发生，及早恢复身心健康状态；临床疾病发生后，以祛病康复为目的，应早发现、早诊断、早治疗，通过临床诊治与养生调理的综合干预，尽量将疾病对健康的影响降低；若所患疾病属暂不可治愈的，如糖尿病、高血压、慢性阻塞性肺疾病等，以延缓疾病发展、提高生存质量为目的，应临床治疗与日常养生相结合，带病延年，尽量延缓疾病的发展进程，提高生活质量，延长生存时限。

2.2 Significance

The significance of health-preservation is not to be ignored, as it is closely related to the individual's health and longevity and humanity's adaptation to environment as well as steady development.

Traditional Chinese Medicine sparkles more in the world of today, where medical science in general has made great strides under the slogan of "returning to nature".

2.2 养生的意义

养生的意义重大，不可忽视。小而言之，个人要想身心健康、益寿延年就必须养生；大而言之，人类要想与环境协调适应、持续稳定地发展进步而不致消亡也必须养生。尤其在世界医学科学有了飞速发展的今天，在人类"返璞归真，回归自然"的潮流推动下，中医养生学更加熠熠生辉，璀璨夺目，显示出强大的生命力和科学价值。

3 Characteristics of Health Preservation of TCM

Distinguishing academic characteristics have been developed in the thousands of years.

3 中医养生学的基本特征

中医养生学历经数千年，在漫长的历史发展过程中，形成了鲜明的学术特征。

3.1 Wholeness and Mobility

Rooted in fundamental theories, health preservation of TCM has developed the features of holistic concept and syndrome differentiation. In terms of wholeness, the subject takes as its core "echo between nature and man" and "oneness of body and spirit", around which unfold all perceptions, methodology and technology. In terms of mobility, the subject takes as the fundamental law "dynamic equilibrium" and "nourishing in accord with personal condition".

3.1 整体动态

中医养生理论根植于中医基础理论，中医学基本特点的整体观念和辨证论治，在中医养生学中则深化为整体动态的特征。从整体出发，中医养生学以"天人相应""形神合一"为其整个学术的核心，其所有的认识论、方法论和技术都围绕这一核心展开。从动态出发，中医养生学则以"权衡以平""审因施养"为最根本的养生法则，一切养生理法均遵从这一原则。

3.2 Harmony and Moderation

Health preservation of TCM emphasizes not going to extremes and values harmony, both in theory and methods. Health preservation consists in all aspects of life, such as clothing, dieting, housing, walking, sitting, and sleeping, emphasizing an overall harmony between man and man, man and society, man and nature. Only a harmonic moderation in all things, such as diet, rest, labour, thought, sex intercourse and emotions, can ensure equilibri-

3.2 和谐适度

"和谐适度"是中医养生学另一个突出的特征。无论在理论上还是在方法上，中医养生学都强调不偏不倚、以和为贵。例如：养生贯穿于衣、食、住、行、坐、卧各个方面，寓养生于日常生活之中，强调整体和谐，人与人之间、人与社会之间，人与自然

um and peace between yin (negative) and yang(positive), qi and blood, and preserve neutralization, thus health and longevity.

之间都要和谐;各方面和谐适度,才能保证体内阴阳平和、气血和调,守其中正、保其冲和,方可健康长寿。饮食要节制,静养休息要适度,形劳、房劳、神劳不可太过,七情调和不可过亢等等,都具体体现了这一特征。

3.3 Integrated Practicality

Health preservation of TCM holds that life activities are complex and natural elements and human organic conditions influencing health are capricious; therefore, longevity can be achieved not by a single method in a single mode, but by integrated dialectic ways with certain targets, judged in the light of personal condition and environment.

Health preservation is a lifetime project that takes constant and combined efforts, which explains why the subject values the practicality of the methods, including efficiency and operation friendliness, especially the latter being an important basis for people to persist.

3.3 综合实用

中医养生学在长期的实践中,认识到生命活动是复杂的,影响人体健康的因素在不断变化,人体的机能状态也在不断地变化。因此,健康长寿不是一功一法、一个模式所能实现的,而应该从个体和周围环境的具体情况出发,根据各方面的实际状态,采取有针对性的多种调养方法综合的辨证调摄。

在强调综合施养的同时,中医养生学也清楚地认识到养生是一生的工程,健康长寿是一个长期的目标,非一朝一夕可以实现,需要持之以恒地进行杂合以养。因此,中医养生学非常重视各种养生方法的实用性,这种实用性包括实效性和可操作性,特别是可操作性是人们能持之以恒的重要基础。

3.4 Wide Application

Health preservation is not the priority of the aged, but is supposed to run through the whole life-

3.4 适应广泛

养生不只是老年人的事,而是与每个人一生相伴。

time, from the embryo to the old. Neither is it necessary only in disease, but in fitness. Different health care methods correspond to different types of physical condition, gender, and people in different areas of the earth.

生命自妊娠于母体之始，直至耄耋老年，每个年龄阶段都存在着养生的内容。养生实践也不只在无病之时，人在未病之时、患病之中、病愈之后，都有养生的必要。人的每一个想法，每一步动作及每一句话都涉及养生的问题。不同体质、不同性别、不同地区的人也都有各自适宜的养生方法。

Health preservation of Traditional Chinese Medicine boasts a wide application. With the development of society, people are pursuing a longer life span as well as a higher quality of life. The subject with a wide application lays claim to full attention.

由此而言，中医养生学具有非常广泛的适应范围。随着社会的发展、人类的进步，人们在追求生命延长的同时，也在不断追求更高的生存质量，具有广泛适应性的中医养生应引起人们高度重视。

Chapter 1 Spirit Approach to Health Preservation

第1章 精神养生

Spirit approach to health preservation means protecting and promoting mental health under the guidance of TCM theories, by means of cultivating morals and regulating jing (essence), qi and shen (spirit), resisting bad moods and restoring psychological balance through moderating, channeling, reasoning, empathy and suggestion, so as to achieve longevity in a fine psychological and mental condition.

The spirit is an inner phenomenon, including various psychological activities such as thought, will, emotion and the like. TCM classifies it into the category of shen, deeming that the human body is the material foundation of shen, while shen expresses the body, and emphasizing the dominance of shen, that is, shen, as the master, controls the body in its functions of metabolism, adjustment and adaptation, and defense of the organs; shen, as a material, can ensure the relative balance of inner and outer environment of the body, and life activity can run with its overall characteristics, functions and rules. Therefore, TCM lays much emphasis on spirit cultivation, which guarantees harmony of seven emotions, coordination of inner organs, smooth flow of qi and blood, and balance between yin and yang, thereby warding off disease.

精神养生是指在中医理论指导下，通过主动修养品德、调养精气神，保护和增强人的精神心理健康；通过节制、疏泄、移情、开导、暗示等措施及时排解不良情绪，恢复心理平衡，从而达到形与神俱、尽终天年的养生方法。

精神，是指人的内心世界现象，包括思维、意志、情感及其他各种心理活动。中医学将其统一归属“神”的范畴，认为形是神的物质基础，神是形的生命表现；强调神的主导地位，认为神为形之主，神可驭形。神不仅主导着人体的精神活动，也主宰着物质能量代谢、调节适应、卫外抗邪等脏腑组织的功能活动；只有在神的统帅下，才能保持机体内外环境的相对平衡，生命活动才表现出整体特性、整体功能、整体规律。因此中医养生学既重视养形，更强调养神，养神得当，则人体七情调和，脏腑协调，气顺血充，阴平阳秘，健康少病。

Section 1 Moral Cultivation

第 1 节 修德怡神

Moral cultivation has an ulterior link with health of organs, and most people of high morals can also enjoy longevity. The secret lies in the fact that good morals bless the person with a peaceful mind and balance and harmony between yin and yang, like a wall protecting him from harassment from the outside, hence health and longevity. So moral cultivation is supposed to be the prime concern, which centres on heart cultivation. The process is that of spirit coming into peace and mood adaptation in the harmonic interaction between man and society. It falls into the five aspects below.

道德修养与脏腑阴阳协调具有内在联系，德行高尚的人多享长寿，其秘诀在于拥有高尚的道德品质，能使人身心安详舒泰，阴阳之气平秘调和，且不易受外界的扰动，如此则体健寿长。因此养生调神应以修德为首务，修德则以修心为中心，修德养神的过程是人与社会和谐互动过程中精神、情绪平适、安适的过程。具体宜从以下 5 个方面注意修德。

1 Kindness and Benevolence

Confucius said in *the Analects* that kind and benevolent people tend to live a long life. What is benevolence? Benevolence in Confucianism refers to a kind heart, or high moral pursuit, in a larger degree. A loving heart can help maintain a harmonic interpersonal relationship which naturally keeps worry away, with pleasure contributing to good health. Benevolence is closely associated with good morals. Moral cultivation has benevolence as its consummation. Confucius and Mencius with their benevolence lived to be 73 and 84 years old respec-

1 仁德常驻 爱心永存

孔子在《论语 · 雍也》中指出具有仁爱之心的人会长寿。何谓“仁”？孔子及孟子均总结为“爱人”。儒家的“仁”即指人的爱心，或完美的道德修养。重视道德修养，长存仁爱之心，能使人始终与他人保持和谐的人际关系，自然心神无忧，精神愉悦而有益于健康长寿。仁与德有着重要的联系，修身与养

tively, as longevity stars of their times.

德都是为了追求仁,有着非常高尚的境界。孔子、孟子的仁德思想让他们分别以73岁和84岁的高龄,成为他们所在时代的长寿之星。

2 Frankness and Open-heartedness

People of good morals are those with an open heart who do not harm others' interest in their own, neither desire wealth from unjustified source, nor do wicked things against reason. Frankness and an open heart keep a clear conscience and a calm mind, thus a fine inner operation of organs conducive to health.

2 胸怀坦荡　光明磊落

道德品质高尚之人总是心胸豁达宽广,心怀坦荡,不做损人利己之事,不贪不义之财,不做伤天害理的勾当。胸怀坦荡,光明磊落,自然心安理得,心神安宁,生活在舒心如意的气氛中,其乐融融。如此则内环境始终保持良好的状态,有利于人的健康长寿。

3 Charity and Generosity

Sun Simiao pointed out in his renowned work *Thousand Ducat Prescriptions* (Qian Jin Yao Fang) that character cultivation is moral cultivation featured by "kindness". One who is charitable and helpful can receive friendliness and gratitude from others, which warms his heart and assuages his daily anxiety, and keeps the balance between yin and yang in his viscera, hence health in the body and spirit. Generosity refers to a grand tolerance in dealing with people. A generous person must have an open and broad mind, wearing pleasure on the face, unlike one who looks ever grim, weighing his trivial gains and losses.

3 乐善好施　豁达开朗

孙思邈在《千金要方》中指出,养性就是以"善"为特征的道德修养。一个人性善好施,以奉献为荣,乐于助人,可以激发人们对他的友爱感激之情,他从中获得的内心温暖缓解了他在日常生活中常有的焦急,从而能很好地维持其脏腑阴阳的协调与平衡,有益于维护其身心健康。豁达则是一个人在为人处世中所表现出来的宏大度量。豁达之人必是开朗之人,也是胸怀博大之人,这样的人喜悦之情常现,不会因计较个人得失而整天愁容满面。如此，则鲜有烦恼、忧愁、厌恶等不良情绪。

4 Integrity without Expediency

A healthy mind stems from rightful perception of oneself and various social relations. A man of integrity can always observe social norms, which reduces daily conflicts and frustrations, and a healthy mind results. In contrast, a lesser man cannot get a right recognition of himself and social relations, which leads to difficult adaptation to the environment. Surrounded by greed, envy and grudge, he is prone to psychological disorder and diseases. Rectitude of thought, which controls excessive desires with reason and will and even abandons some desires, can guard the spirit from stir. "Reducing desires" upheld by the ancient Chinese does not mean cutting off all desires, but reducing unnecessary ones, with the recognition of the harm of excessive desires. Harnessing wild desires with a good sense and cultivating the character with integrity guarantee an orderly spirit in harmonic equilibrium with the body and environment.

4 谨守操品 德全不危

健康的心理来源于个体对自身以及各种社会关系的正确认识和把握。道德高尚的人往往能遵循社会规范行事，从而减少生活中的矛盾、冲突和挫折，保持心理健康。反之，道德品质低下的人，现实中总是不能正确认识自己和处理各种社会关系，导致个体对外部环境的适应困难，常常被贪婪、嫉妒和怨恨的心理包围，容易发生心理障碍和疾病。因此，纯正思想，以理性和意志控制人的过度欲望，摒弃个人私欲也就避免了精神受到的纷扰。古人所言“寡欲”绝非无欲，而是要尽量减少过多的、不必要的私欲，并充分认识过欲的危害，以理收心，以德养性，如此则可内守精神，使机体和环境保持协调平衡而不紊乱，才能有健康的精神心理。

5 Nihilism and Aloofness from Fame and Fortune

Aloofness, as a Taoist term, means a peaceful mind without wild action; nihilism, a pure heart without worldly stain. The combined meaning is abandoning worldly thoughts, smoothing out emo-

5 恬惔虚无 淡泊名利

“恬惔”乃道家之语，意谓心神宁静而不妄为；“虚无”意谓心无杂念。恬惔虚无即指摈除杂念，畅遂情志，

tions to retain a clear and calm mind. A person indulging in fantasies and busy with his unrealistic desires would end up frustrated, which must give rise to a distressed and stirring mind, the essential qi undermined and organs in disorder, hence illness and premature wane. So the key lies in "reducing desires", thus achieving aloofness, thus a calm heart and smooth qi and well-guarded spirit and orderly organs, thus cultivating full essential qi and well-built body and longevity.

神静淡泊，以使心神保持"清静"的状态。人如果整日想入非非，好高骛远，处于不切实际的幻想中，忙碌于实现不了的私欲，结果所愿总是不遂，所求总是不得，必致心情不悦，心神躁动，五脏六腑之气机紊乱，精气日益耗损，形体必因之而多病早衰。可见调神摄生，贵在对"外物"要"少欲"，少欲就能恬惔，恬惔则心清气顺，精神内守，五脏六腑气机协调，精气日渐充实，形体随之健壮，自可少病延年。

Aloofness and nihilism advocated by *Yellow Emperor's Inner Canon* (Huang Di Nei Jing) and doctors of later generations, however, does not mean for people to give up ambitions or lead a mundane life, but lays emphasis on reducing desires and standing aloof from fame and fortune, and devoting oneself to the proper work and serving society. The objective of health preservation is self-fulfillment based on fitness. So aloofness and nihilism should be interpreted in a positive sense.

《内经》及后世医家主张的恬惔虚无，并非要世人胸无大志，碌碌平生，而是要人们排除私欲，不为名利所困扰，且孜孜于事业，以期有成，造福社会。养生的目的是增进健康，也是为了更好地实现自我，因此应当从积极的意义上理解"恬惔虚无"。

Section 2 Emotion Adjustment

第 2 节 调志摄神

Emotion is a comprehensive action of the spirit and psychology when people deal with the world. Moderate and harmonic emotions benefit normal functions of the body. Normal people have proper

人的情志也称情感，它是人在接触客观事物时，精神心理的综合反映。情志活动适度，调和而有节制，则有

emotional reaction to outside stimulation, most of the time being positively open-hearted, optimistic, joyous and satisfied, which shows human love for life. But if emotions go unbridled beyond endurance of the body, up to the point of upsetting normal metabolism, physical organism goes wrong in a light case, and in a grave case diseases ensue with some being fatal. So when the emotion goes wrong, one should actively contain and adjust it, in an effort to command the spirit, so as to avoid harm done to health by strong emotions. One can follow the methods below.

利于机体各脏腑组织生理功能的进行。正常人对外界刺激能作出适度和恰当的情绪反应,且开朗、乐观、愉快、满意等积极的情绪总是占优势,这是人类热爱生活的表现。但若因内、外因素影响而导致情志放纵、偏激,超过机体的耐受程度,扰乱并影响人体脏腑气机的正常运行时,小则引起功能失调,大则导致疾病发生,甚至危及生命,对人体的健康带来危害。因此当情志过激时,应及时通过主动的控制和调节,调志以摄神,避免不良情绪对人体内环境的进一步损害。过激情志产生时,以下方法可酌情选择运用。

1 Mutual Resistance

Among the emotions exists a relation of mutual promotion and resistance of the five elements, a relation in which one emotion can be used to restrain and disperse another, so as to coordinate them and restore a peaceful mind.

1 情志相胜法

当产生不良情绪时,可根据情志之间存在的五行生克制化规律,用互相制约、互相克制的情志,转移和干扰原来对机体有害的情志,借以协调情志,恢复或重建精神平和的状态。

1.1 Fright Overcomes Ecstasy that Harms the Heart

The method applies to the excited and ecstatic type. Pleasure is linked to the heart. Causing endless laughter in a grave case, ecstasy dispels the qi of the heart, which can be collected by fright. So stim-

1.1 喜伤心者,以恐胜之

适用于神情兴奋、狂躁者。喜为心志,过喜则心气涣散,神不守舍,严重者表现为精神恍惚,嬉笑不休;恐令

ulus of terror can be applied to one who goes wildly happy to the point of perversion. This is based on the principle that water property of the kidney quenches the fire one of the heart, according to the five-element theory of TCM.

气怯,骤然令人惊恐,则能收敛涣散之气机。因此,如果遇到因高兴过度而出现身心异常的人,可以用使其恐惧的刺激加以调节。此方法利用的是中医五行理论中,肾水克制心火的原理。

1.2 Anger Overcomes Anxiety that Harms the Spleen

It applies to the ever gloomy ones whose anxiety develops into disease. Anxiety, linked to the spleen, triggers stagnation of spleen qi and upsets its function of transportation, while anger uplifts the qi of the liver that disperses the stagnation. So the stimulus of anger is applicable to those who are trapped in anxiety and who have developed some uncanny symptoms. This is based on the principle that wood property of the liver holds the soil one of the spleen.

1.2 思伤脾者,以怒胜之

适用于长期思虑不解、气结成疾、情绪异常低沉者。思为脾志,过度思虑则脾气郁结,运化失常,怒令肝气升发,郁结之气则可得宣散。因此,遇到因长期思虑不解,而出现身心异常的人,可以用使其发怒的刺激加以调节。此方法利用的是中医五行理论中,肝木克制脾土的原理。

1.3 Joy Overwhelms Sorrow that Attacks the Lungs

It applies to the sorrowfully depressed type. Sorrow is related to the lungs and grief upsets qi in the lungs and sparks disorder, and makes the qi unable to fill up what is exhaled, while joy releases the qi movement and brings down the qi in the lungs. So stimulus of joy can be resorted to for the grief-stricken. This does not evade the principle that fire property of heart contains the metal one of the lungs.

1.3 悲伤肺者,以喜胜之

适用于因神伤而表现为情绪抑郁低沉者。悲为肺志,过悲则肺气不敷、制节失职;喜令气机和缓散达,肺气得以恢复正常宣降。因此,遇到因悲伤过度而出现身心异常的人,可以用使其高兴快乐的刺激加以调节。此方法利用的是中医五行理论中,心火克制肺金的原理。

1.4 Thought Dissolves Fright that Impairs the Kidney

It applies to suspicious people readily startled

1.4 恐伤肾者,以思胜之

适用于因惊恐而致坐卧

and restless. Fright pushes qi down and shock upsets it, with the result that qi in the kidney drifts in disorder, while thought collects the wandering qi and thus the patient can ward off bad mood and restore health. So the therapy of deep thought can be used to treat those shocked to an extraordinary state. This follows the principle that the soil property of the spleen stops the water of the kidney.

不宁，多疑易惊者。恐则气下，惊则气乱，神气惮散不能敛藏；思则气结，可以收敛涣散之神气，使患者主动地排除某些不良情绪，达到康复之目的。因此，遇到因惊恐过度而出现身心异常的人，可以用使其深思的刺激加以调节。此方法利用的是中医五行理论中，脾土克制肾水的原理。

1.5 Sorrow Disperses Anger that Burns the Liver

It applies to those sullen with qi stagnation and those fuming to the extreme point of excitement, especially those who feel like weeping the anger out. Anger is associated with the liver, and fume upsets the order of qi and blood, causing impossible confusion of the mind, while sorrow drives the anger away and brings boiling qi and blood down. So the therapy of sorrow is recommended for those boiling mad or lastingly sullen to the point of perversion. This conforms to the principle that the metal property of lungs limits the wood one of the liver.

When resorting to "mutual resistance", we should give heed to the intensity of the stimulus, that is, the curing emotion must surpass the ailing one, with a sudden strong stimulation or lastingly cumulative effect. Meanwhile the patient's personality must be taken into account, that is, one can endure the shift between emotions and is free from extreme character.

1.5 怒伤肝者，以悲胜之

适用于因情志抑郁而致气机郁结或因怒而致情绪亢奋不宁者，尤其适用于自觉以痛哭为快者。怒为肝志，暴怒则气血逆乱，神迷惑而不治；悲则气消，血气得以消散下行。因此，遇到因突然大怒或持久郁怒而出现身心异常的人，可以用使其悲泣的刺激加以调节。此方法利用的是中医五行理论中，肺金对肝木的克制原理。

在运用"情志相胜"之法调节异常情志时，要注意刺激的强度，即干预的情志刺激要超过原有的情志刺激，或是采用突然强大的刺激，或是采用持续不断的强化性刺激。总之，后者要超过前者，才能达到以情制情的目的。同时还要注意对象的性格特征，要对情志的转换有一定的承受能力，并且不能具有极端性格。

2 Transference

Transference means transferring the mood and mind by some means such as changing the environment so as to bring the patient away from the negative emotion. The diverse transference ways allow for free choice depending on different psychology, environment, and specific conditions. Here are presented two common ways.

2 移情法

又称转移法，即通过一定的方法和措施改变人的情绪和意志，或改变其周围环境，使之与不良的刺激因素脱离，从而从不良情绪中解脱出来。移情的方法有很多，应用时可根据不同人的心理、环境和具体条件，采取不同的措施并加以灵活运用。这里介绍两种常用的移情法。

2.1 Transferring the Mind to Some Artistic Pursuits

Enjoying music and drama in low spirits can cheer the patient up and get rid of the tension and bitterness. Or calligraphy and painting are recommended if the patient is such inclined, with the benefit that bad moods can be melted, qi movement goes smooth and the spirit be refreshed.

2.1 琴棋书画移情

在烦闷不安、情绪不佳时欣赏音乐、戏剧等，可使精神振奋，紧张和苦闷的情绪也会随之而消。平时，可根据自己的兴趣和爱好，从事自己喜欢的活动，如书法、绘画等，可排解愁绪，寄托情怀，舒畅气机，颐养心神，有益于身心健康。

2.2 Transmitting to Sports

Not only can physical exercises build up vitality of life, but they drive away tension and bad moods and restore balance of the body. As transferring the mind to different environment, sports and moderate manual labour, for instance, means substituting physical strain for spiritual one, hence enhancing physical strength and pleasing the spirit. The tradi-

2.2 运动移情

运动不仅可以增强生命的活力，而且能有效地把不良情绪发散出去，使机体重臻平衡。因此，经常从事体育运动能显著地松弛紧张感，并能消除失望、沮丧情绪。如果遇有情绪紧张、郁

tional Chinese sports in particular, characterized by natural alternation between move and quiescence, can refresh and pacify the mind in harmony between yin and yang. When one does sports, an unrestrained atmosphere arises and pervades the air, which eliminates negative moods.

闷时，不妨转移环境，转移注意力，去参加体育活动或参加适当的体力劳动，以形体的紧张消除精神的紧张，既强健了体魄，又愉悦了心神。尤其是传统的体育运动，因其锻炼中主张动静结合，松静自然，因而能使形神舒畅，心神安和，达到阴阳协调平衡，锻炼之中自有一种浩然之气充满天地之间之感，一切不良情绪随之而消。

2.3 Elevation

Elevation means breaking away from negative moods, by resorting to the strong will and reason that motivate one to devote the mind to the career. Take Sima Qian of the Han Dynasty for instance, after receiving the torture of cutting the genital, he plunges into composition of *Record of the Grand Historian* with indomitable perseverance. In this way he turned a great trauma into an industrious action, which transfers the unbearable bitterness and drowns grief.

2.3 升华法

升华，就是用顽强的意志战胜不良情绪的干扰，用理智将其化作行动的动力，投身于事业生活中去。如中国两汉时期的司马迁虽惨受宫刑，但其以坚强不屈的精神全力投入《史记》的撰写之中，把身心创伤这一不良刺激变为奋发努力的行动，以舒志解愁，调整缓解心理矛盾，转移不幸遭遇所带来的痛苦心境。

2.4 Nonchalance

Nonchalance means taking things lightly and drifting away from the unpleasant environment. For example, facing failure in the college entrance examination, some students get despondent and even tend to commit suicide. They should calm down and reflect upon the significance of the exam. "To some end I must've been born", as the ancient poem said. College is not the only gateway into society. One

2.4 超脱法

超脱，即超然，是在思想上把事情看淡，在行动上主动脱离导致不良情绪的环境。如高考落榜后，有的考生灰心丧气，感到前途无望，更有甚者竟想轻生，这时应冷静想想考试的意义。“天生我材必有用”，上大学不是

can always accomplish something so long as he bucks up and faces music.

唯一的出路，一个人只要不气馁，振作精神，面对现实，前途总是光明的。

2. 5 Psychological Suggestion

Suggestion means indirectly inducing the patient to directly accept the suggested idea—without logical thought or judgment—to have some notion established in him, or to change his mood and activity, so as to alleviate the bad moods. Language suggestion is feasible in most cases, with such alternatives as gesture, facial expression, signal or suggestive medicine.

It should be noted that people vary in suggestion reception, depending on personality, psychology, characteristics of advanced neurotic activity, and age, yet not associated with intellectual level or educational background. The patient's trust and cooperation are priorities beforehand, and success should be ensured at every administration. Otherwise the trust in the doctor would falter, which poses greater difficulties in Fu Ture administrations, hence slim chance of success.

2. 5 暗示法

暗示是指用含蓄、间接的方法，诱导患者不经逻辑的思维和判断直接接受被灌输的观念，主动树立某种信念，或改变其情绪行为，达到缓解不良情绪的目的。一般多采用语言暗示，也可采用手势、表情，或采用暗示性药物及其他暗号来进行。

暗示时要特别注意：人的受暗示性是各不相同的，这与人的个性心理特征及高级神经活动特点密切相关，亦与年龄有关，而人的智力水平与文化程度在能否接受暗示方面并无决定性作用。施术前要取得对象的充分信任与合作，每次施术过程应尽量取得成功。如不成功，则易动摇对象的信心，影响其对施术者的信任，做第二次暗示时就会困难很多，成功的希望也就相对较小。

2. 6 Reasoning

Reasoning refers to talking with the patient, adjusting his mind to reason and bringing him into the right perspective, which drives away the negative moods. Its common methods are explaining, encouraging, consoling, and assuring. Explanation is the basic way, aiming at the patient's seeing sense

2. 6 开导法

开导，是指通过交谈，用浅显易懂的道理，经过劝说引导，使患者主动解除消极情绪的一种调畅情志方法。开导最常用的方法有解释、鼓励、安慰、保证。解释是开

and conquering emotion with reason, thus the right state of mind; while the latter three ways rid the patient of anxiety and establish trust and confidence. A frustrated person should confide in his friends and family, in order to get strength and support from their counsel and comfort.

导的基本方法，是使对方明白事理，以理制情，这样自然可保持正确的心态；鼓励、安慰和保证是帮助患者消除疑虑、建立信任和树立信心的具体方法。一个人在生活中受到挫折或遭遇不幸时，可找自己的知心朋友、亲人倾诉苦衷，以便从亲人、朋友的开导、劝告、同情和安慰中得到力量和支持。

2.7 Moderation

Moderation means moderating the seven emotions from extremes so as to reach psychological balance. This is a prime task of spirit cultivation. Letting emotions go rampant would injure the viscera, upset movement of qi and circulation of blood, impair the vital qi and self-regulation of the body. So the emotions should be moderated, without being subdued or going extreme.

Mankind is by nature happy and angry. The former should be minded not to go extreme, and the latter be avoided. To remove anger, one should "reason" with himself, "Anger can only hurtmyself"; or cultivate "tolerance" that cushions the blaze; or transfer the attention to escape it. Stay optimistic and smiling, and the inner fire can be quenched, qi run smooth and blood full.

2.7 节制法

节制即调和节制情感，防止七情过激，从而达到心理平衡的方法。重视精神修炼，首先要节制自己的情感，才能维持心理的协调平衡。七情太过，不仅可直接伤及脏腑，引起气机升降失调，气血逆乱，还可损伤人体正气，使人体的自我调节能力减退。所以情志既不可压抑，也不可过纵，贵在有节适度。

喜怒之情，人皆有之，喜贵于调和，而怒宜戒除。戒怒最重要的是能以"理"制怒，一旦发怒或将发怒，应先想到怒足以伤身；或以"忍"养性，使怒气消于缓冲中；或转移注意力，使怒失之自然。此外尽量避免忧郁、悲伤等消极情绪，使心理处于怡然自得的乐观状态，如此自然内不生火，气顺血充，健康恬愉。

2.8 Channeling

Channeling refers to giving vent to negative moods buried in the heart so as to recover psychological balance in a short time. Human life is more in adversity than in fair sailing. When emotional pressures strike, one should vent them to maintain a steady inner environment. Otherwise the pressure would affect the viscera and spark disease in the long term, accumulated by disharmony between qi and blood. Channeling can set the patient free from the negative emotions.

Channeling can be direct, such as crying, yelling, singing aloud, intensified exercises and undergoing thrill, which channel suffocated feeling out in the form of tears, perspiration and voice. There is also indirect channeling, such as confiding, composing poetry or prose, keeping a diary, chatting and playing games.

The wholesomeness and rightfulness of channeling methods must be heeded. Wholesomeness means that the methods should be positive, not transgressing the law or injuring health, as in the cases of gluttony, gambling and drug-addiction. Rightfulness means certain principles must be observed in channeling. Firstly, it should be practiced in the right time and place, without troubling others; sec-

2.8 疏泄法

疏泄法是将积聚、压抑在心中的不良情绪，通过适当的方法宣达、发泄出去，以尽快恢复心理平衡的情志调节方法。人的一生中处于逆境的时候要多于顺境的时间。当面临较大的情感压力时，及时适当地发泄情绪，可以缓解紧张，维护机体内环境的稳定。否则压力便会影响脏腑功能，日久必然使气血失和而为病患。疏泄法可使人从苦恼、郁结甚至愤怒等消极情绪中解脱出来。

疏泄可有直接疏泄，如哭泣便是一种较好的直接疏泄方法，还可以用呐喊、高歌、高强度运动、惊险刺激的娱乐等方式，令郁积的情志通过泪、汗、声音等的排出而迅速畅通。此外还有间接疏泄，如通过倾诉、赋诗作文、写日记、聊天、游戏等，也可将心中的不良情绪宣达出去。

实行疏泄法，一定要注意方法的健康和正确。疏泄方法的健康，指疏泄时使用的方式必须健康向上，不能违规、违法，也不能有损身心健康。如暴饮暴食、赌博、吸毒等，也能起到疏泄的作用，但是暴饮暴食会损害身体，

ondly, moderation should be noted. It should not be practiced beyond the endurance of the patient in terms of methods and duration; thirdly, security. It should be exercised in the safe time and place, and in the company of good friends or professionals.

引起胃肠功能的紊乱,或导致肥胖,而赌博、吸毒等,是违法行为,因此均须为疏泄法所禁忌。疏泄方法的正确,是指使用疏泄法要遵循正确的原则。首先,要注意时间和地点,不能惊扰他人;其次,要注意疏泄适度,要注意根据被疏泄者的承受能力而选择方法和时间,不能超过其身心耐受力;第三,注意安全性,直接疏泄法施行时最好有人陪同,同时不要选在危险的时间和危险的地点施行,间接疏泄法要注意选择疏泄对象,应在熟人间展开,或找专业人员进行。

Chapter 2 Diet Approach to Health Preservation

第2章 饮食养生

Diet approach to health preservation means choosing food reasonably based on its character in TCM theory, hence achieving health and longevity. Food is an indispensable part of human life. The Chinese have accumulated a wealth of experience and knowledge in their long history of food research, and come up with a unique set of food-selecting theories and methods.

饮食养生,即食养,是在中医理论的指导下,利用食物的特性,合理地摄取食物,以强身健体、延年益寿的养生方法。饮食是人体赖以生存和维持健康必不可缺的物质之一。中国人民在长期的饮食实践和探索中,积累了丰富的知识和宝贵的经验,逐步形成了一套独特的饮食养生的理论和方法。

Section 1 Fundamental Theories

第1节 饮食养生的基本理论

As the ancient saying goes, "medicine and food share the same source", the source referring to nature, so the two bear similar functions. Food, like medicine, has such attributes as "Si Qi" (four nature of drugs), "Wu Wei" (five flavors), "Sheng Jiang Fu Chen" (Upbearing, downbearing, floating and sinking), "Gui Jin" (Channel entry) and functions. Food-health approach focuses on nourishing the viscera, regulating yin and yang and warding off disease based on function of the food.

古有"药食同源"之说,药物和食物皆属天然之品,二者在性能上有相通之处。食物和中药一样也具有"四气""五味""升降浮沉""归经"和"功效"等属性。饮食养生侧重于利用食物的性能来滋养五脏六腑、调节人体阴阳和预防疾病。

Si Qi(four natures of food), refers to cold, cool, warm and hot characters of the food. Among them the former two belong to the concept of yin, so food of such characters can often clear heat and toxin, quench flaming condition of the internal organs and blood, and nourish yin; while the latter two belong to that of yang, so food of such characters can often drive away coldness, warm up meridians(Jing) and smooth collaterals(Luo) and promote yang. Besides, there is also some neutral food not too hot and not too cold, which has a mild function.

四气，又称四性，即寒、热、温、凉四种不同的食物性质。寒凉属阴，故具有寒性或凉性的食物大多具有清热、解毒、泻火、凉血、滋阴等作用。温热属阳，故具有温性或热性的食物大多具有散寒、助阳、温经、通络等作用。此外，还有一些平性食物，是指寒热之性不甚明显的食物，其作用比较缓和。

Wu Wei (five flavors) refers to five flavours of the food, that is, sour, bitter, sweet, pungent and salty. This is an abstract summary of the tastes. To be detailed, some food has a bland pleasant flavour, and other food a mild unpleasant flavour, but TCM classifies the former in the category of sweetness, and the latter in that of sourness. Generally speaking, sour food can collect and contract watery excrement; bitter food can bring down fire, nurture yin, drive away dampness and restore qi into smooth circulation; sweet food can nourish the spleen and stomach and cushion emergency; pungent food disperses and sends qi and blood going smoothly; salty food softens knot and hardness, and promotes excrement, and food of bland flavour makes dampness ooze and get out in the form of urine.

五味，即酸、苦、甘、辛、咸五种不同的食物滋味，也是对食物效用的抽象归纳。实际上有些食物还具有淡味或涩味，但中医将淡归于甘味，涩归于酸味，所以仍然称为五味。一般而言，酸（涩）味食物具有收敛、固涩的作用；苦味食物具有泻热坚阴、燥湿降逆的作用；甘味食物具有补益、和中、缓急的作用；辛味食物具有发散、行气、行血的作用；咸味食物具有软坚散结、泻下的作用；淡味食物具有渗湿、利尿作用。

In the concept of Sheng Jiang Fu Chen (ascending, descending, floating and sinking), sheng means ascending, jiang descending, fu floating and chen sinking. These functions are closely associated with characters and tastes of the food. Most of warm, hot, pungent and sweet food has the former two functions. And most of the cold, cool, sour,

食物的升降浮沉性质中，升表示上升，降表示下降，浮表示发散，沉表示泄利。食物升降浮沉的性能与食物本身的性味有不可分割的关系。具有温、热性和辛、甘味的食物，大多具有升、浮

bitter and salty food boasts the latter two.

的性能；具有寒、凉性和酸、苦、咸、涩味的食物，大多具有沉、降的性能。

Gui Jing (Channel entry) refers to targeting function of the food on certain internal organs, that is, food is more evidently effective on one or two organs. To be specific, the tonic can be divided into those for the liver, the heart, the spleen, the lungs and the kidney.

归经，指食物对于机体某一部分的选择性作用，即主要对某经或某几经发生明显的作用，而对其他经的作用较小，或没有作用。如同为补益之品，就有补肝、补心、补脾、补肺、补肾的区分。

Good effect can only be accomplished by combining the four natures of food, five flavors, ascending and descending, channel entry, and the effect and applying them comprehensively.

在饮食养生中应将食物的四性、五味、升降浮沉、归经、功效等多种性能结合起来，综合应用，才会取得良好的效果。

Section 2 Merits of Food Approach

第2节 饮食养生的作用

1 Nourishing and Regulating

Firstly, there are three elements the food nourishes and regulates, namely, jin, qi and shen, counted as three treasures forming and sustaining life activities. They have their source naturally in the food.

1 滋养调整作用

饮食养生的滋养调整作用主要体现在三个方面。首先，中医学认为构成和维系人体生命活动的基础是精、气、神，统称人身"三宝"。人体的精、气、神离不开饮食的滋养。合理的饮食能使精、气充足，神自健旺，而当人体出现精、气、神的不足时，可以通过饮食进行有目的的滋养。

Secondly, the Theory of Visceral Manifestations, core of TCM theoretical system, emphasizes

其次，中医学理论体系核心部分的藏象学说，特别

the central position of the five internal organs in human physiological and pathological activities, which also are nourished by food. Food of different tastes and targeting functions nourishes the organs differently. Besides, the food also nourishes the six hollow organs, sinew and bone, skin and hair.

强调五脏在人体生理和病理活动中的中心地位。而五脏能够正常发挥其功能,也离不开饮食的滋养。根据食物的五味不同,对五脏的营养作用有所不同,食物的归经不同,对脏腑的滋养作用也有所侧重。至于六腑、筋骨、肌肤、皮毛等皆需饮食营养。

Thirdly, according to TCM, human viscera, qi and blood must work in relative steadiness and coordination, thus a fit state with equilibrium between yin and yang. So when one part goes out of order, certain food comes in to regulate it back to norm.

第三,中医学认为人体的脏腑、气血等物质或功能必须保持相对的稳定和协调,才能达到阴阳平和的正常生理状态。当人体因阴阳失调而出现生理功能失调时,可通过饮食进行调整,从而恢复正常。

2 Postponing Aging and Promoting Longevity

2 延衰益寿作用

Doctors in history of TCM have always laid emphasis on postponing aging with food, which serves the elders particularly.

饮食养生是延衰益寿的重要环节。历代医家都十分重视通过饮食养生达到延衰防老、延年益寿的目的。特别是老年人,充分发挥饮食的延衰益寿作用尤为重要。

In the essence of the body, namely, Jing, Qi, blood and body fluid, Jing (essence) plays a good part in postponing aging. It is the most basic element that forms the life. Prenatal jin refers to the root of life, and postnatal jin nurtures the organs, tissues and body outlets and transforms qi, blood and shen. While among the organs, the kidney and the spleen & stomach are more closely linked to postponing aging. The kidney's quality traces back

在人体的精微物质精、气、血、津液中,特别强调精在延衰益寿中的作用。精是构成人体的最基本物质。先天之精是生命产生的本源;后天之精能够濡养全身的脏腑组织和关窍,并有化气、化血、化神的功能。脏腑之中特别强调肾和脾胃的功能在

to the time before birth. A weak kidney has the symptoms of frail waist and knee, urination out of order, unaccountable ringing in the ear and ill hearing, loose teeth, premature gray of the hair and beard, declining fertility, and forgetfulness, etc. And the spleen is responsible for later growth. A feeble spleen & stomach shows itself in poor appetite, fatigue, indigestion and emaciation. So food that can nurture the three organs is recommended as priority.

延衰益寿中的作用。肾乃先天之本，肾虚则会出现腰膝酸软，小便失常，耳鸣耳聋，牙齿松动，须发早白、脱落，生殖功能下降，健忘等衰老的征象；脾胃乃后天之本，脾胃虚弱则会出现食欲不振、倦怠乏力、消化不良、消瘦等身体衰弱的表现。因此，在饮食养生中应注重选用具有补精益肾、健脾益胃的食品。

Here is a list of some food than can postpone aging: royal jelly, milk, turtle, sesame, mulberry, Gou Qi Zi (*Fructus Lycii*), longan, walnut and Shan Yao (*Rhizoma Dioscoreae*).

很多食物都具有防老延衰作用。例如：蜂王浆、牛奶、甲鱼、芝麻、桑椹、枸杞子、龙眼肉、胡桃、山药等，都含有延缓衰老成分，有一定的延衰益寿作用。适当服用这些食品，有利于健康和长寿。

3 Warding off Disease

The disease is a great hazard to health. TCM maintains that the disease stems from the evil or pathogenic factor, which, from the inner cause or the outside, attacks the body and triggers disorder of physiological functions and injures organs and tissues, posing great harm to health. Many kinds of food can ward off disease, for instance, ginger and garlic can warm up the body and eliminate cold symptoms, while fermented beans and tea can cool it down and eliminate hot symptoms.

3 御邪防病作用

疾病是健康的重要危害因素。中医学认为邪气是疾病产生的重要条件。邪气或由内、或由外侵害人体，导致生理机能失调、脏腑组织的形质损害等，对健康造成极大的损害。许多食物都具有抗御邪气的功效。如生姜、大蒜等具有辛温解表的功效，豆豉、茶叶等具有辛凉解表的功效等等。

TCM has all along laid emphasis on "warding off disease before curing it", upholding "Vital Qi

中医学历来重视疾病的预防，认为正气是决定发病

(healthy qi)" as a dominant element in preventing disease. So food is emphasized as the source that cultivates the healthy qi, due to its basic function of regulating nutrition; besides, some targeting functions of food are applied to some diseases. For example, the animal liver can prevent night blindness, and the kelp swollen thyroid gland.

的主导因素,因此特别强调饮食养生在扶助正气中的作用。饮食养生首先通过其营养调整作用,达到扶助正气的目的。另外,注重在日常生活中发挥某些食物的特殊功效,直接用于疾病的预防。如食用动物的肝脏预防夜盲症;食用海带预防甲状腺肿大等。

Section 3 Principles of Diet Approach

第3节 饮食养生的原则

1 Balanced Nutrition and Sensible Proportion

Food varies in nutrition. Only a balanced food intake can meet the demand of life activities.

All nutrients should be taken in a pattern of grain as the main source, meat secondary and vegetable & fruit contributory, which can find its echo in the modern conception of "Hierarchy of Balanced Diet", both focusing on the significance of all-round food intake. Since no single food can provide all the nutrients the body needs.

1 全面膳食 合理搭配

食物的种类繁多,所含的营养成分也各不相同,只有做到全面膳食、合理搭配,才能满足生命活动和健康长寿的需求。

全面膳食就是全面摄取人体所必需的各种营养成分,主张人们的饮食以谷类为主食,肉类为副食,蔬菜、水果以辅助。这一饮食养生的原则与现代提倡的"平衡膳食宝塔"的思想是一致的,都是强调全面膳食的重要性。没有单一食物能够完全满足人体需要的全部营养,必须食用多种食物,才能保证人体的正常需要。

Sensible proportion of food should be heeded on the basis of balanced nutrition. The prime principle is to match vegetables with meat, with the former as the core. As Zhu Danxi, a renowned doctor in the Yuan Dynasty, asserted in his book *Light Flavour Puisuit* (Ru Tan Lun).

合理搭配就是在全面膳食的基础上注意各类食物所占的比例。首先，饮食的合理搭配应是荤素搭配、以素食为主。中国古代养生家一贯推崇饮食清淡、少吃油腻食物的素食主张。元代的朱丹溪还专门著有《茹淡论》，提倡荤素搭配，素食为主，少吃肉食。

Sensible proportion also means "balanced five flavours". The five flavours as are mentioned above have corresponding effect on the five solid organs. So the five tastes must be chosen in accordance with physiological needs. Otherwise a certain organ would be too much nourished to the point of being attacked by the intake of a certain taste, giving rise to disease. According to contemporary research, obesity and diabetes have a cause in sweet teeth, and preference for salty food is held responsible for hyperlipemia and atherosclerosis.

其次，合理搭配应是"谨和五味"。食物有酸、苦、甘、辛、咸五味之分，五味与五脏的生理功能密切相关。所谓谨和五味，就是根据人体的生理需要，合理地摄取食物，达到营养全身、健康长寿的目的。如果五味过偏，单一某脏长期被食物滋养或削伐，则不利于人体的健康，甚至可以导致疾病。现代研究发现，肥胖病、糖尿病等疾病的发生与偏嗜甜食有关；高血脂、动脉硬化症等疾病的发生与高盐饮食有关。

Besides, sensible proportion is also interpreted in terms of coldness and hotness. On the one hand, the cold and hot characters of the food should exist in proportion in the body. On the other hand, it refers to the mild temperature of the food. An overtake of food of warm and hot character is apt to harm the yin fluid in the spleen & stomach, while the opposite undermines their yang qi. The spleen & stomach, as is mentioned above, provided nourish-

第三，合理搭配应是寒热适宜。寒热适宜，一方面指食物的寒热属性应相互协调；另一方面指食物入口时的温度要适宜。过食温热食物，容易损伤脾胃阴液；过食寒凉食物，容易损伤脾胃阳气。脾胃乃后天之本，损伤日久则人体阴阳失调，变生

ment for postnatal growth, the harm of which would drive yin and yang out of balance and disease ensues.

各种病证。

2 Food Intake in Accordance

Food should be chosen in accordance with time, place and the individual. Time refers to the difference in season, daytime and night; place to that in altitude, latitude and accustomed area of the individual; the individual to that in age, gender and constitution type. The individual stands out among the three as the most active element, so it can also be said that the food should be chosen according to the individual, which will be discussed in detail first.

Firstly, physiological characteristics at different ages should be taken into account. For instance, children have delicate organs and grow quickly, so full and all-round nutrition easily digested should be guaranteed, especially protein, vitamins and minerals, while organ functions of the old are in decline and qi and blood do not circulate in vitality, in which case is recommended food well-cooked to be soft, digestible and nourishing, and is forbidden raw and cold food. Secondly, as regards gender, blood is vital for women, thus food nurturing qi and blood for them, while semen props men, thus food nurturing the kidney for them. Thirdly, constitution determines what one should eat. People of yang deficiency type should eatmore warm and hot food; yin deficiency, the opposite; Qi deficiency, food that nourishes Qi, and blood deficiency, food that helps produce blood.

2 审因施膳 以人为本

审因施膳是饮食养生的原则之一，即因时、因地、因人制宜地合理选择膳食。时有四季的不同，昼夜的交替等；地有地势的高低，气候的寒热，水土的不同等；人有年龄、性别、体质的差异等。在三者中，人是最积极主动的因素，所以又以人为本。

因人制宜：就是根据个人的年龄、性别、体质等生理特点进行饮食养生。首先，应根据各年龄段的生理特点进行饮食养生。例如，小儿具有脏腑娇嫩、发育迅速的生理特点，因此饮食应保证营养全面充足、易于消化，特别是要保证蛋白质的供给和丰富的维生素和矿物质；而老年人脏腑功能衰退，气血化源不足，故食宜熟软，易消化而多补益，忌食生冷和不易消化的食物。其次，性别不同，饮食有别。女子以血为用，因此应适当增加补气养血类食物的摄入，男子以精为本，因此应适当增加填精益肾类的食物。再者，人的体质有阴阳虚实的不同，故饮食养生需根据体质的不同而有所不同。阳虚之体宜食温补之品；阴虚之体宜食寒凉养阴之品；气虚者宜食补气之品；血虚者宜食补血之品等。

Speaking of time consideration, the ancient Chinese doctors accumulated rich experiences in taking food according to season. According to *Principles of Drinks and Diets* (Yin Shan Zheng Yao), in warm spring wheat and the like is suitable for its cool character, while beans of cold character can quench the steaming feeling in summer; sesame can moisturize the dry feeling in autumn, and cold winter should be fended off with such warm food as Chinese sorghum and millet.

因时制宜：主要是根据四时季节和昼夜晨昏的时序规律来进行饮食养生。古代医家在四季顺时食养方面积累了丰富的经验，如《饮膳正要》中说，春天气候温暖，应该吃麦类偏凉性的食物；夏天暑热熏蒸，应该吃豆类等寒性食物；秋天天气干燥，应该吃芝麻等滋润的食物；冬天天气寒冷，应该吃高粱、黄米等温性的食物。这就概括性地阐明了四时食养的原则。

Lastly, in the vast country of China, various altitudes and latitudes and qualities of water and soil in diverse regions should be taken into account. It is warm and damp in the southeast at a lower altitude, so the food must be sweet, cool, light and good for excretion, while warm and moisturizing food is soothing in the cold and dry northwest at a higher altitude. Some qualities of water and soil in certain places are the root of some local diseases, such as local swollen thyroid gland, Keshan Disease and Kaschin-Beck Disease. So food should be taken based on one's accustomed area.

因地制宜：主要是根据地域环境特点进行饮食养生。中国地域辽阔，地势有高下之别、气候有寒热湿燥之分、水土性质各异，因此饮食养生必须坚持因地制宜的原则。东南地势较低，气候温暖潮湿，宜食清淡通利或甘凉之品；西北地势较高，气候寒冷干燥，宜食温热滋润之品。由于各地水土性质不同，有些地方容易形成地方病，如：地方性甲状腺肿、克山病、大骨节病等,更应因地制宜进行食养以预防。食饮有节主要包括饮食要适时、适量。注意宜忌主要包括注意饮食卫生、食宜清淡、饮食禁忌。

3 Moderation and Dos and Don'ts

3.1 Moderation

Moderation means food had better be eaten regularly and in moderate amount. The Chinese have three regular meals a day, with 4-6 hours in between. Generally, breakfast is set from 6:30 to 8:30, and lunch comes in five hours later from 11:30 to 13:30, and 18:30 to 20:00 is the supper time. Such an arrangement fits in with the time of digestion and absorption. On the contrary, eating irregularly, starvation and continually eating snacks cause disorder of the digestive system, hence affecting absorption and disease strikes in the long term.

With regard to the proper quantity, breakfast focuses on full nutrition, lunch can be a little indulgent, but supper must be restricted in quantity. A sensible allocation of the calorie should follow the pattern that one takes in, at breakfast, 25%-30% of the calorie of the whole day, lunch 40% and supper 30%-35%. The proportion may be adjusted if

3 食饮有节　注意宜忌

3.1 食饮有节

食饮有节,就是饮食要有节制,适时适量的意思。饮食适时,就是按照一定的时间,有规律地进食。一般的饮食习惯是一日三餐,即早餐、午餐、晚餐,间隔时间为4~6小时。一般情况下,早餐应安排在6:30—8:30,午餐应在11:30—13:30,晚餐应在18:00—20:00进行为宜。这种时间安排与饮食物在胃肠中消化和吸收的时间比较吻合,因此符合饮食养生的要求。如果饮食不适时,或忍饥不食,或零食不断,均可导致胃肠功能紊乱,影响营养的吸收,长此以往则诸病变生。

饮食适量,就是按照一定的量进食。一日三餐中,早餐要保证其营养充足;午餐要吃好;晚餐要适量。比较合理的三餐分配是:早餐占全天总热能的25%~30%;午餐占40%;晚餐占

necessary. Moderation naturally warns against starvation and excessive fullness. Starvation cannot provide energy, and the latter overburdens the digestive system and so affects transportation and transformation of the food. A standard of moderate eating has all along been held in universal agreement in ancient China, which is, to eat to 70%-80% of fullness.

30%～35%，同时根据个人情况及习惯可适当调整比例。饮食适量还包括不要饥饱无度。过饥，则化源不足，精气匮乏；过饱，则胃肠负担过重，影响运化功能。历代养生家均认为食至七八分饱是饮食适量的标准。

3.2 Dos and Don'ts in Eating

There are things one should remember to do and not to do when eating, which is hygiene, less grease and some food taboos.

3.2 饮食宜忌

除上述饮食养生的原则外，人们在长期的饮食实践中，还发现许多与饮食有关的适宜和禁忌的事项，需要在饮食养生中加以注意。主要包括注意饮食卫生、食宜清淡和饮食禁忌。

Hygiene refers to freshness and cleanness of the food, cooking before eating and sanitary habits in eating. The raw food must be fresh and clean and cooked to be edible. TCM does not believe in long preservation of the food, and even worse if it is not appropriately preserved, when the food rots and produces harmful elements. Besides, cooking kills most of the microorganism in the food, hence preventing disease. Sanitary habits must be remembered before, in and after eating. To be specific, hands and dishes must be sterilized before one eats; a neat and cozy environment with gentle music can promote digestion and absorption; avoid eating in exhaustion, distraction, uncanny mood and talking; be patient to chew the food slowly and swallow it minutely, otherwise eating like a horse would injure the stomach. Rinse the mouth after eating, rub the stomach and take a stroll for better absorption.

注意饮食卫生主要包括食物要新鲜清洁、提倡熟食、讲究进食卫生等几个方面。选择食物要新鲜清洁，并且要经过烹饪加工变熟后再食用。如果食物放置时间过长或储存不当就会引起变质，产生对人体有害的各种物质。另外烹调加工过程是保证食物卫生的一个重要环节，高温加热能杀灭食物中的大部分微生物，防止食源性疾病。讲究进食卫生主要包括进食前、进食中和进食后应该注意的问题。进食前应注意手和餐具的消毒，防止病从口入。轻松整洁的进食环境再配合柔和的音乐，有助于脾胃的消化吸收。同时应避免劳累和情绪异常时进食。进食时应保持精神专注，尽量不要说话。进食时还要做到细嚼慢咽，否则急食暴食，易损伤肠胃。饮食后要漱口，保持口腔卫生；摩腹、散步以利于消化吸收。

Chinese cuisine boasts hundreds of cooking methods, which influence nutrition of the food. For instance, in the soup of animal material, vitamin B1 and B2 that dissolve in water, calcium, phosphorus, amino acid and sugar element have dissolving reaction, rendering it delicious and digestible, apart from that, protein, fatty acid, organic acid and inorganic salt and diverse vitamins in the material merge into the soup and make it enormously nutritious. In contrast, deep-fried food becomes too oily and indigestible, and what's worse, the high temperature spoils vitamin B group, changes the nature of protein and puts fat in chemical reaction, whereby the nutrition is undermined. And one should refrain from eating much smoked food, which may have harmful elements like benzopyrene.

中国烹饪历史源远流长，烹饪方法有几百种。不同的烹饪方法对食物的营养价值造成了不同的影响。比如：烧制过的动物性原料的汤汁中，水溶性维生素 B1 和 B2、钙、磷、氨基酸及糖类部分发生水解反应，不仅口感好而且易于消化。在煮制时，原料中所含蛋白质、脂肪酸、有机酸、无机盐和维生素浸入汤中，因此应加强汤汁的合理利用。而油炸食物可增加脂肪含量、不易消化，并且高温加热后食物中的 B 族维生素破坏较大，蛋白质严重变性，脂肪发生反应，使食物的营养价值下降。烟熏食品可能含有苯并芘等有害成分，不宜多吃。

Don't indulge in greasy food. Light and bland food is easily digested and absorbed, and excessive intake of fat and oily food injures the digestive system, bringing about abnormal food circulation, as is shown in such diseases as pediatric glycosides, obesity, ulcer, frequent drinking and urination, and tho-

饮食宜清淡，勿过食肥甘。清淡的饮食易于脾胃的消化和吸收；过食肥甘厚腻之品则易伤脾胃，导致运化失常，形成小儿疳积、肥胖、痈疽、消渴、胸痹等病。

racic obstruction, etc.

Eating taboo comes firstly in eating poisonous food, such as puffer, sprouted potato, wild mushroom, which, if not proper treated, would injure health and even be lethal. Secondly, the taboo refers to some forbidden food from certain disease. In general, pungent food should be kept away from diseases of the hot character, and raw and cold food, cold. People with a weak spleen & stomach should not be tempted by raw and cold and greasy food. Thirdly, the taboo refers to some forbidden food in the course of the patient's treatment. It is recorded in some ancient medical works that raw and cold, pungent food and meat are taboos when certain kinds of medicine are being taken. For example, the persimmon and schizonepeta cannot go with the crab; radish and tea are in conflict with ginseng. Many of such recorded taboos have been proved by modern research, though some have yet to be in the future.

饮食禁忌，首先是防止误食。河豚、发芽的土豆、野生蘑菇等，如果处理不当而误食，就会影响人体健康，甚至危及生命。其次是病证的饮食禁忌。总体而言，热证忌食辛辣之品；寒证忌食生冷之品；脾胃虚弱忌食生冷粘腻之品。第三是服药期间的饮食禁忌。古代文献中有服用某些中药时忌食生冷、辛辣、肉等，还有螃蟹忌柿、荆芥；人参忌萝卜、茶叶等记载，其中不少得到现代药物学研究证实，但也有不少内容需要继续深入研究。

Section 4 Application of Diet Approach

第4节 饮食养生的具体应用

1 Common Types of Food

The material must be processed into food before it can be conveniently consumed. The usual types consist of drink (fresh juice, tea drink, instant drink, and wine), broth, honeyed paste, porridge, grain products and cuisine.

1.1 Drink

Fresh juice, as the name suggests, is extracted

1 常见食养制剂

为了应用方便，一般将食物加工成食品。常用的膳食种类有饮料(鲜汁、茶饮、速溶饮料、酒类)、羹汤、蜜膏、粥食、米面食品、菜肴等。

1.1 饮料

鲜汁，是指直接从新鲜

from fresh food. The juice here means more than that from fruit as in the real sense of the word, also juice from vegetables. And "fresh" should also be noted, which defies storage. The cooling, freshening and nutritious fresh juice soothes people of hot constitution type or hot disease in summer. Watermelon juice, cucumber juice and five-thing juice are common choices.

的食物压榨取得的汁液。选料多为汁液丰富的水果、蔬菜。以水果为基料配成的汁称为果汁，以蔬菜为基料配成的汁称为蔬菜汁。鲜汁，多现用现取，不宜存贮。鲜汁清凉爽口，营养丰富，含汁液多，尤适宜夏天、热性体质或热证者饮用。常用的如西瓜汁、黄瓜汁、五汁饮等。

Tea drink refers to tea and other substitute drinks prepared in the same way as tea: pouring boiling water in and waiting for it to brew. The substitute material should be flimsy and fragrant, mostly flowers, leaves, fruit, peel, stem and branch, and thin root. It is prepared most instantly. Usually people take ginger drink and longevity drink, etc. And the proper tea, as is known to all, has many fortifying and curing functions, such as sobering, cooling, consuming fat, dispersing heat, furnishing digestion and diminishing greasy feeling. But please note that it is not recommended for people with insomnia.

茶饮，是指以含茶叶或不含茶叶的原料，用沸水冲泡、温浸而成的一种专供饮用的液体。原料的选择为质地轻薄，或具有芳香挥发性成分的物质，多为植物的花、叶、果实、皮、茎枝、细根等。茶饮随泡随饮，使用方便。常用的如姜茶饮、益寿饮等。以茶叶制作的茶饮具有提神醒脑、降脂减肥、清热解暑、消食解腻等多种保健治疗作用，但应注意失眠者不宜饮用浓茶。

1.2 Wine Treatment

The wine can cure disease by exuding of the elements of the material that otherwise stay inert in water. Its functions include smoothing blood circulation, nurturing qi in the spleen, fortifying the digestive system, warming up and promoting the effect of medicine.

The wine treatment can be prepared in three simple ways: a. soaking in cold wine. Soak the material in wine with a fair concentration. Shake it of-

1.2 酒剂

酒，不仅能把一些水所不能浸取出来的成分浸出，而且本身也可防治疾病。它有通血脉、养脾气、厚肠胃、润皮肤、去寒气、行药势等功效。

酒剂的简单制作方法有以下几种：其一是冷浸法，把原料浸泡在一定浓度的白酒

ten and it is ready after the storage of a month. b. soaking hotly. Boil the material with wine for some time, leave it to cool and store it. This old way can accelerate the exuding progress and draw out more elements of the material. Safety, however, is to be ensured by way of indirect heating, which means heating the wine over boiling water that comes between the wine and the fire. c. brew the wine with rice. Boil the rice with the medicinal powder or liquid, and put in distiller's yeast and ferment it.

中，经常摇动，储存一个月即可饮用。其二是热浸法，先以原料和酒同煎一定时间，然后再放冷，贮存。这是一种比较古老的药酒、食用酒浸制方法。这种方法既能加速浸取速度，又能使一些成分容易浸出。但制酒时要注意安全，可采用隔水煎炖的间接加热方法。其三是药米同酿法，把药料细粉或药汁与米同煮后，再加酒曲，经过发酵制成。

Please note that the wine treatment is only applicable to those who can drink and are free from ailments in the liver and the kidney, and the amount must be controlled. It is a taboo to the pregnant, the child, liver patients, people of yin-deficiency constitution and who are prone to disease of the hot character.

应注意，酒剂只适合能饮酒和无肝肾疾患的人饮用，并应控制用量。孕妇、小儿、阴虚体质者、肝病、热病患者忌用酒剂。

1.3 Thick Broth

This old cooking method runs in the way of boiling diced material and then adding starch to make it plaster-like. Most of the broth is from meat, egg, and milk, with a small percentage from vegetable. Common broths are broth of mutton kidney with desert cistanche and egg broth. The usual cooking ways are boiling, stewing and simmering, taking more time than is necessary for making soup. The material is usually diced, shredded or cut as small as the grain. Living material should be rid of bones, and in the case of fruit, kernel.

1.3 羹

羹是古老的烹调法之一，是指切制成丁的食物用沸汤煮后，加入湿生粉，使汤水溜成糊状的烹调方法。羹的原料有两类，一类是肉、蛋、奶等产品，此类为多；另一类是以植物性原料为主料。羹是在原料中加水烹制成汤汁稠厚的一类菜式，如肉羹、蛋羹、菜羹。常用的如羊肾苁蓉羹、鸡子羹等。羹的制作一般采用煮、炖、煨、熬等方法，其加热时间比制汤要长。制羹用的原料，多需细切，如细丁、细丝、碎粒等。动物性原料在制羹前应剔净骨、刺。果品原料应剔去皮核。

1.4 Soup

Legend has it that the age-old soup cooking was created by Yi Yin, the illustrious chef who had originally been a slave brought over by the queen of Tang, the first king of the Shang Dynasty. The decoction is widely applied since it is conveniently prepared, flexible in quantity, and easily absorbed and effective, so fitting in with the TCM principle of dialectical treating and prescribing for the individual. Common examples are ginseng & lotus seed soup, lily & yolk soup, mutton broth with Dang Gui (*Radix Angelicae Sinensis*) & ginger soup. Wine and vinegar are sometimes added into the water that boils the material.

Decoction of herbal medicine, the major prescription by the Chinese doctor, should be conducted in this way: boil it for a comparatively long time, filter the liquid and add more water for the dreg to be simmered once more(often three times), until the dreg is exhausted and deserted, then merge the liquid together and divide it for equal drink. While in the case of soup as food, just simmer it once, abandon the unpleasant herbal medicine, and eat the food material in it and drink the soup. Sugar or salt can be added to cater to different tastes. When making soup with rare medicine or that taking a longer time for hot treatment, one can steam

1.4 汤

汤液，是中医所用的较为古老的传统剂型之一，相传是商代汤的妻子所陪嫁的奴隶，当时著名的厨师伊尹所创。因为汤液制法简便，用料加减灵活，符合中医辨证施治、处方因人而异的原则，且吸收快，易发挥疗效，所以这一剂型应用较为广泛。养生常用的如人参莲肉汤、百合鸡子黄汤、当归生姜羊肉汤等。汤液一般是以水作为溶剂来蒸煮药料，有时也加一些其他液体，如酒、醋等。

药用汤剂，多煎煮一定时间，取汁留渣，加水再煎煮。最后去渣，合并煎汁，等分饮用。而食用汤液则多一煎而成，可除去不好吃的药料，喝汤并吃所煮的食料。另外，也可随口味，稍调一些糖、盐等佐料。用名贵或需较长时间热处理的药物、食料制作汤液时，可用蒸、炖药液的方法，如蒸炖人参、木耳汤液等。

or stew it, as in the case of making steamed-and-stewed ginseng, and fungus soup.

1.5 Honeyed Paste (Tonic Extract)

The extract is an improvement made on the decoction above, taking further steps of condensing it and adding honey to make the thick creamy paste. Usually there is grape paste, autumn pear paste, hair-blackening paste. The honeyed paste is characterized by high concentration, steadiness, friendliness to preservation and carrying along and drinking, with mild and lasting effect. The honey in the extract can not only sweeten it, but nourish and replenish the body, and preserve it in storage. It can be directly drunk or first diluted with a little hot water.

1.5 蜜膏

蜜膏是指原料经过加水煎煮、去渣浓缩后，加入蜂蜜制成的稠厚的、半流体状的剂型。蜂蜜有滋补的作用，所以也有人把蜜膏称为“膏滋”。常用的如葡萄蜜膏、秋梨蜜膏、乌发蜜膏等。蜜膏又叫煎膏剂，其特点是浓度高，体积小，稳定性好，利于保存，携带方便，便于服用，作用和缓、持久。蜜膏中的蜂蜜不仅有调味作用，同时也有滋润和补益的功效；蜂蜜还具有一定的防腐作用，易于保存。蜜膏服用方便，可直接食用或用热水冲化饮服。

1.6 Rice and Wheat Products

As is familiar to us, the products include steamed bread, flat bread, stuffed steamed bun, noodle, rice noodle, wonton, dumpling, cake and glutinous rice ball. They can be snacks as well as staple food.

The product of grain of rice mainly refers to porridge and rice. Porridge is often made with starch food such as rice, millet, husked sorghum, barley and wheat, which lays the foundation for medicinal porridge, to make which, we just need to add some other nutritional material such as meat, fruit and herbal medicine. The porridge is not parti-

1.6 米面食品

米面食品，又称面点、点心、糕点等，是以米、面为原料制成的一类食品，包括包子、面条、饼、馄饨、水饺、糕、粉、汤圆、馒头等。既可作主食，又可供作小吃和点心。

米制品主要是粥、饭两类。粥是以大米、小米、秫米、大麦、小麦等富含淀粉的粮食，加水煎煮成为半流体的食品。保健和医疗性质的粥食，即是以上述原料为基础，同时再添加一些具有营

cular in quantity, and well suited to people with digestive ailments. Usually there is taro porridge, lotus seed powder porridge and Shan Yao (*Rhizo ma Dioscoreae*) porridge.

养性质的食物，如肉类、果品和治疗性质的药材而制成。粥的特点是加减灵活，尤其适用于胃肠道疾病患者。常用的如芋头粥、莲子粉粥、薯蓣粉粥等。

The rice, a staple food in China known to all, is made with rice grain or millet. It can be steamed or boiled, and further processed with the steamed or boiled rice, such as rice stir-fried with egg and eight-treasured rice.

饭是指煮熟的谷类食品，多指大米或小米等煮制的干饭，是我国的主食。饭可蒸制、煮制，蒸煮熟后还可进一步加工，一般多用煮法或炒法。常用的如鸡蛋炒饭、八宝饭等。

The wheat products, as is mentioned above, suit people with a weak spleen & stomach. Usually there is spleen-furnishing flat bread, Shan Yao noodle, egg flat bread and noodle with Chinese prickly ash.

面制品主要有有饼、糕、面条、包子、饺子等。适用于脾胃虚弱者食用。常用的如益脾饼、山药面、鸡子饼、川椒面等。

1.7 Cuisine

The diversified Chinese cuisine, with its numerous features and merits that we are familiar with, also emphasizes its health-cultivating function. The Chinese cuisine boasts the global reputation of fine colour, smell, flavour, form, tableware and curing effect.

1.7 菜肴

菜肴，是指用肉类、蔬菜、水产品、果品等原料，经过切配和烹调加工制作成的一类食品。中国菜肴品种丰富，流派众多，制作精湛，具有选料讲究、刀工精细、配料合理、烹法多样、五味调和、工于火候、精于盛器、讲究食疗等特点。菜肴成品以色、香、味、形、器及食疗作用俱佳著称于世。

In cooking medicinal dishes, one should also take care with the colour, smell, flavour and form, trying to make them harmonic, not without the preserving effect, to which end, the cooking methods

养生菜肴的制作，在充分考虑养生作用的基础上，还应突出菜肴的色、香、味、形，尽量做到养生效果与色、

come best in boiling, stewing, simmering, steaming and stir-frying, while the unwholesome methods of roasting, smoking, deep-frying and pickling are to be kept at bay.

香、味、形的统一,以保证菜肴质量的完美和谐。养生菜肴制作的方法以煮、炖、煨、蒸、焖、炒较好。烤、熏、煎、炸、腌等烹调方法,不利于健康,应尽量避免。

2 Daily Medicinal Recipes

2 常用食物和食养方

2.1 Replenishing Sort

2.1 补益类

2.1.1 Breath Replenishment

2.1.1 益气类

Food: rice, glutinous rice, millet, bean, beef, chicken, quail, egg, potato, carrot, date, etc.

常用食物 粳米、糯米、小米、黄豆、牛肉、鸡肉、鹌鹑、鸡蛋、土豆、胡萝卜、大枣等。

Recipes

食养方举例

(1) Chinese yam noodle: dried Shan Yao (*Rhizoma Dioscoreae*) 30 g, Bai Zhu (*Rhizoma Atractylodis Macrocephalae*) 30 g, Ren Shen (*Radix Ginseng*) 5 g, flour 500 g.

(1) 山药面:干山药 30 克,白术 30 克,人参 5 克,面粉 500 克。

Grind the former three to powder; add flour and water; knead, roll, slice and boil it. It can be adorned with some seasonal vegetables. The noodle nourishes the spleen and replenishes qi.

将山药、白术、人参研成细粉,加入面粉、清水和面,擀切成薄片下锅煮食。可以加入一些时令蔬菜配用,具有健脾益气功效。

(2) Hen stewed with Ren Shen (*Radix Ginseng*), Dang Gui (*Radix Angelicae Sinensis*): 1 hen, Ren Shen 15 g, Dang Gui 15 g, certain amount of white part of scallion, Sheng Jiang (*Rhizoma Zingiberis Recens*), yellow wine, salt.

(2) 参归炖母鸡:母鸡 1 只,人参 15 克,当归 15 克,葱白、生姜、黄酒、食盐各适量。

Treat the hen to cleanliness and put it in the earthenware pot; add water and yellow wine; skim away the foam; turn down the fire and stew it to softness; add the two herbal medicines and salt; stew it for another hour. The broth nourishes qi and

母鸡去毛及内脏,冲洗干净,放入砂锅中,加清水、黄酒、葱白、生姜大火烧开,撇去污沫,改用小火炖至熟烂,再加入人参、当归、食盐,

blood, and replenishes marrow and essence.

2.1.2 Blood Nourishment

Food: pork, mutton, liver of the pig, the goat and the cattle, turtle, sea cucumber, spinach, carrot, fungus, mulberry.

Recipes

(1) liver broth: 1 liver, 3 eggs, white scallion, salt.

Rinse the liver, remove the tendon and membrane, soak it and change it into clean water when the previous gets tainted, for several times, and dice the liver; cut the scallion into a couple of parts; put the two into fermented bean juice and boil it thick; add eggs when it is about to be ready. The broth nourishes blood and the liver and eyes.

(2) mulberry & longan paste (folk recipe): Sang Shen (*Fructus Mori*) 1 000 g, Long Yan Rou (*Arillus Longan*) 500 g, Feng Mi (*Mel*) appropiate amount.

Wash the two fruits and simmer them to a creamy state, add Feng Mi and meanwhile stir it on weak fire for several minutes, wait for it to cool off and store it in bottles. The paste nourishes blood and yin, and replenishes the liver and the kidney.

2.1.3 Yin Nourishment

Food: yolk of chicken and duck eggs, turtle, cuttlefish, pork skin, duck, Sang Shen, Gou Qi Zi (*Fructus Lycii*), white fungus.

Recipes

(1) stewed turtle: 1 turtle, white scallion,

炖约 1 个小时即可。具有益气养血、益精填髓的功效。

2.1.2 养血类

常用食物 猪肉、羊肉、猪肝、羊肝、牛肝、甲鱼、海参、菠菜、胡萝卜、黑木耳、桑椹等。

食养方举例

(1) 猪肝羹:猪肝 1 具,鸡蛋 3 个,葱白 1 根,食盐适量。

猪肝洗净去筋膜,浸泡易水数次切成细丁,葱白切成段,以上两味原料放入豉汁中煮作羹,临熟,打入鸡蛋,待熟时即可食用。具有养血、补肝、明目的功效。

(2) 桑椹龙眼膏:桑椹 1 000 克,龙眼肉 500 克,蜂蜜适量。

将桑椹、龙眼洗净,放入锅内,加清水以小火煎煮至汁液黏稠时,调入蜂蜜,边搅拌,边小火熬,数分钟后即可停,待冷装瓶备用。具有养血滋阴、补肝益肾的功效。

2.1.3 滋阴类

常用食物 鸡蛋黄、鸭蛋黄、甲鱼、乌贼、猪皮、鸭肉、桑椹、枸杞子、银耳等。

食养方举例

(1) 清炖甲鱼:甲鱼 1

sheng Jiang, yellow wine and salt.

Treat the turtle clean and put it into the pot for steaming, together with Shan Yao; add water and steam the pot until the turtle is ready. The broth nourishes yin and diminishes heat and dryness in the body, an immensely replenishing dish.

(2) white fungus broth: dried white fungus 10 g, 1 egg, crystal rock sugar.

Soak the fungus in warm water until it spreads, clean it and boil and then stew it to softness, and add egg and sugar. Have a small bowl of the broth per day. The broth replenishes lungs and the kidney, and appeases dryness and cough.

2.1.4 Yang Promotion

Food: mutton, deer, rabbit, kidney of the goat and the pig, pigeon egg, eel, shrimp, mussel, Chinese chives, Gou Qi Zi, Dao Dou (*Semen Canavaliae*) and He Tao Ren (*Semen Juglandis*).

Recipes

(1) Chinese chives stir-fried with walnut: Chinese chives 200 g, wolfberry 50 g, sesame oil and salt.

Crack the He Tao Ren and get the kernel ready. Soak it and remove the peel, and suck extra water with the tissue; pluck out yellowish part of the chives and rinse it and cut it into inches; pour sesame oil into the frying pan and heat it to 70% of full heat, put walnut in and stir-fry it to be golden, add chives and salt and mix them. The dish replenishes the kidney and yang, and develops brains.

(2) Dang Gui broth with Chinese Dang Gui and ginger: Dang Gui 500 g, angelica 10 g, ginger 20 g,

个,葱白、生姜、黄酒、食盐适量。

将甲鱼杀死后,去除肠脏,然后连同山药,放入炖盅内,加水适量,隔水炖熟服用。具有滋阴清热、补虚润燥的功效。

(2) 银耳羹:干银耳 10 克,鸡蛋 1 个,冰糖适量。

银耳用温水泡发,去除杂质,放入锅内,加清水,大火烧沸后转用小火,炖至银耳熟软时,加入鸡蛋、冰糖。每次 1 小碗,每日 1 次。具有补肺益肾、润燥止咳的功效。

2.1.4 助阳类

常用食物 羊肉、狗肉、鹿肉、兔肉、羊肾、猪肾、鸽蛋、鳝鱼、虾、淡菜、韭菜、枸杞子、刀豆、核桃仁等。

食养方举例

(1) 韭菜炒胡桃仁:韭菜 200 克,胡桃仁 50 克,香油、食盐适量。

胡桃肉开水浸泡去皮,沥干备用;韭菜摘洗干净,切成寸段备用;香油倒入炒锅内,烧至七成热时,加入胡桃仁,炸至金黄色,再放入韭菜、食盐,翻炒至熟。具有补肾助阳,健脑益智的功效。

(2) 当归生姜羊肉汤:羊肉 500 克,当归 10 克,生姜

yellow wine and salt.

Rinse the mutton and cut it into small pieces; put them into the earthenware pot and add water, yellow wine, ginger and angelica; boil it first and then turn down the fire and stew it to softness, and add salt finally. Consume some of it for every meal. The broth warms up the body and soothes pain, a classic replenishing dish.

20 克，黄酒、食盐各适量。

羊肉冲洗干净，切成小块，放入砂锅内，加黄酒、生姜、当归、清水，大火烧开，改用小火炖至羊肉熟烂，以食盐调味。分餐食用。具有温阳补虚、祛寒止痛的功效。

2.2 Channeling Sort

2.2.1 Symptom Dispelling Sort

Food: Sheng Jiang, scallion, Yan Sui (*Herba Coriandri*), Dou Chi (*Sojae Semen Praeparatum*), Huo Xiang (*Herba Agastaches*), Bo He (*Herba Menthae*).

Recipes

(1) white scallion & coriander soup (folk recipe): half a piece of scallion, Yan Sui 20 g.

Rinse the two, shred scallion, and cut Yan Sui into inches. Boil water first and then put in the two, and boil them for a little while, and drink the soup while it is hot. The soup drives sweat out and disperses qi in the lungs, and dredges yang circulation.

(2) drink of ginger & sugar & purple perilla: Sheng Jiang 10 g, Zi Su Ye (*Folium Perillae*) 15 g, crystal rock sugar.

Clean the Sheng Jiang, slice it and put the slices and Zi Su Ye (*Folium Perillae*) into a glass; pour boiling water in and let it draw for 10-15 minutes, add sugar and the sweet drink is ready. Or they can be boiled into soup. Drink it twice a day. The drink warms up the body, smooths qi and nourishes the stomach.

2.2 泻实类

2.2.1 解表类

常用食物 生姜、大葱、芫荽、豆豉、藿香、薄荷等。

食养方举例

（1）葱白芫荽汤：大葱半根，芫荽 20 克。

把大葱、芫荽洗净，大葱切成葱花，芫荽切成段备用。锅内放入清水，上火烧开，将葱花、芫荽段放入，翻滚片刻即可，取汤趁热温饮。具有发汗解表、宣肺通阳的功效。

（2）姜糖苏叶饮：生姜 10 克，紫苏叶 15 克，冰糖适量。

先把生姜洗净切成片备用；将生姜片、紫苏叶放入茶杯中，用开水冲泡，温浸 10～15 分钟即可饮用，以冰糖调味，代茶饮。或以两味原料如常法煎汤，一日两次。具有辛温解表、理气和胃的功效。

2.2.2 Cooling Sort

Food: bitter gourd, bitter vegetable, watermelon, green bean, tofu and green tea.

Recipes

(1) semen coicis & green bean porridge: Yi Yi Ren (*Semen Coicis*) 50 g, green bean 50 g, rice 100 g.

Wash all the three and boil them together and then turn down the fire and simmer them until edible. The porridge cools the body in summer and channels the dampness out.

(2) drink of five materials: pear 1 000 g, Ou (*Nelumbinis Rhizomatis Nodus*) 500 g, fresh Lu Gen (*Rhizoma Phragmitis*) 100 g, fresh Mai Dong (*Radix Ophiopogonis*) 50 g, fresh water chestnut 500 g.

Rinse them, cut the Lu Gen (*Rhizoma Phragmitis*) into inches, boil and simmer it and get the juice ready; peel the pear and chestnut and dig out the kernel of the pear, remove joint of the Ou (*Nelumbinis Rhizomatis Nodus*); chop the Mai Dong. Extract these four materials in the juicer and pour the two kinds of juice into the glass along with some Lu Gen Juice, and the drink is ready, which cools the body and furnishes body fluid, and quenches dryness for its sweet and cold nature.

2.2.3 Cold-Dispelling Sort

Food: Gan jiang (*Rhizoma Zingiberis*), Rou Gui (*Cortex Cinnamomi*), Hua Jiao (*Zanthoxyli Pericarpium*), Xiao Hui Xiang (*Fructus Anisi Stellati*), chilli, Hujiao (*Fructus Piperis*), mutton.

Recipes

(1) pig stomach simmered with pepper: 1 stom-

2.2.2 清热类

常用食物 苦瓜、苦菜、西瓜、绿豆、豆腐、绿茶等。

食养方举例

（1）薏苡仁绿豆粥：薏苡仁 50 克，绿豆 50 克，粳米 100 克。

将薏苡仁、绿豆、粳米洗净，放入锅中，加清水以大火烧开，再改用小火，煮至豆熟米烂即可。具有清热解暑、化湿的功效。

（2）五汁饮：梨 1 000 克，鲜藕 500 克，鲜芦根 100 克，鲜麦冬 50 克，鲜荸荠 500 克。

先把五种原料洗净，然后将芦根切成段，加水煎汤取汁；梨去皮核、荸荠去皮、鲜藕去节、麦冬切碎或剪碎，将处理过的后四味原料放入榨汁机内搅拌，取榨好的汁液倒入容器中，与芦根汁混合，代茶饮。具有清热生津、甘寒润燥的功效。

2.2.3 散寒类

常用食物 干姜、肉桂、花椒、茴香、胡椒、辣椒、羊肉等。

食养方举例

（1）胡椒煲猪肚：猪肚 1

ach, Hujiao (*Fructus Piperis*) and yellow wine.

Rinse the stomach, put Hujiao (*Fructus Piperis*), wine and salt in it, tie it up with thread and simmer it to softness. Eat it once a week. The broth fortifies the spleen & stomach and dispels cold.

(2) noodle with Chinese prickly ash: Hua Jiao ash 5 g, flour 200 g, light fermented bean 10 g.

Mix the powder with flour and add water; knead, roll and cut it into noodle. Boil the noodle and fermented bean with salt. The noodle disperses cold.

2.2.4 Breath Dredging Sort

Food: Chen Pi (*Pericarpium Citri Reticulatae*), Xiang Yuan (*Fructus Citri*), Fo Shou (*Fructus Citri Sarcodactylis*), Dao Dou, Mei Gui Hua (*Flos Rosae Rugosae*).

Recipes

(1) stir-fried shredded Fo shou with spring onion: 2 Fo shou, 1 scallion, salt.

Wash the Fo shou and shred it and scallion. Pour in a little oil in the frying pan and heat it mildly, and put in the Fo shou and stir-fry it; conclude the cooking with scallion and salt. The dish smoothes the stagnation of liver and so qi circulates back to order.

(2) Xiang Yuan essence juice: 1 or 2 fresh Xiang Yuan, malt sugar.

Chop the Xiang Yuan and put it in a bowl with a lid, add malt sugar of the same amount, and steam the bowl for a couple of hours until the Xiang Yuan goes immensely soft. Take a spoon of it in the

个、胡椒、黄酒适量。

将胡椒、食盐、黄酒入洗净的猪肚内，然后用线缝好扎紧，慢火煲煮至熟烂，每周制1次。具有健脾益胃、温中散寒的功效。

（2）川椒面：川椒粉（花椒）5克，面粉200克，淡豆豉10克。

川椒粉与面粉拌匀，加适量清水，做成面条。锅中放入清水，烧开后，放入面条、淡豆豉、食盐，煮熟即可。具有温中散寒的功效。

2.2.4 行气类

常用食物 橘皮、香橼、佛手、刀豆、玫瑰花等。

食养方举例

（1）葱炒佛手丝：佛手2个，葱1根，食盐适量。

佛手洗净切成丝；葱切丝。锅内放入少量的油，烧热，即放入佛手丝炒至将熟时，投入葱丝、食盐翻炒片刻即可。具有舒肝理气、调畅气机的功效。

（2）香橼浆：鲜香橼1～2个，麦芽糖适量。

将香橼切碎，放入带盖的碗中，加入等量的麦芽糖，隔水蒸数小时，以香橼烂为度。每服1匙，早晚各1次。

morning and at night respectively. It drives qi circulation smooth and sobers up the mind.

具有行气开郁的功效。

2.2.5 Blood Invigorating Sort

Food: fungus, Shan Zha (*Fructus Crataegi*), wine, vinegar.

Recipes

(1) soup of funguses: fungus 6 g, white fungus 6 g, salt.

Soak the two funguses until they spread, and boil them and conclude the cooking with salt. It nourishes yin, invigorates blood circulation and reduces fat.

(2) Shan Zha drink: sliced Shan Zha 15 g, crystal rock sugar.

Wash the slices and put them in the glass with sugar, pour boiling water in, and wait for it to draw for 10-15 minutes. The drink invigorates blood circulation, dredges meridians and collaterals and thus kills pain.

2.2.5 活血类

常用食物　木耳、山楂、酒、醋等。

食养方举例

（1）双耳汤：黑木耳 6 克，银耳 6 克，食盐适量。

将黑木耳、银耳放入碗中，用温水泡发洗净，放入锅中，加清水上火煮，至熟时加入少量食盐。具有养阴活血降脂的功效。

（2）山楂饮：山楂片 15 克，冰糖适量。

山楂片洗净，与冰糖一起放入茶杯中，以沸水冲泡，温浸 10～15 分钟即可饮用，代茶饮。具有活血化瘀、通络止痛的功效。

2.2.6 Phlegm Reducing and Cough Appeasing Sort

Food: Hai Zao (*Sargassum*), Kun Bu (*Thallus Laminariae Eckloniae Thallus*), laver, radish, tangerine pith, Ku Xing Ren (*Semen Armeniacae Amarum*), pear, Bai Guo (*Semen Ginkgo*), loquat, Bai He (*Bulbus Lilii*).

Recipes

(1) pear stewed with almond: Ku Xing Ren 10 g, 1 pear, crystal rock sugar.

Dig out the kernel of the pear and put the pear and Ku Xing Ren in the steaming pot, and steam the pot for an hour, add sugar to sweeten it. The snack cools the body, reduces phlegm and appeases breathlessness.

2.2.6 止咳化痰平喘类

常用食物　海藻、昆布、海带、紫菜、萝卜、橘络、杏仁、梨、白果、枇杷、百合等。

食养方举例

（1）杏仁炖雪梨：杏仁 10 克，雪梨 1 个，冰糖适量。

取杏仁、雪梨放入盅内，隔水炖 1 个小时，以冰糖调味，食雪梨饮汤。具有清热、化痰、平喘的功效。

(2) Bai He & Ku Xing Ren porridge: fresh Bai He 50 g(if dried, 15 g), Ku Xing Ren 10 g, rice 50 g, crystal rock sugar.

Make rice porridge first and put in Ku Xing Ren without peel or tip, and Bai He, and keep boiling it for another 10 minutes, and sweeten it with sugar. The porridge nourishes lungs and alleviates coughing.

(2) 百合杏仁粥：鲜百合50克（干品15克），杏仁10克，粳米50克，冰糖适量。

先将粳米煮粥，再将杏仁（去皮尖）、百合放入，继续煮10分钟即可，以冰糖调味。具有润肺止咳的功效。

2.2.7 Dampness Draining Sort

Food: corn, corn beard, black bean, green bean, red bean, white gourd, Chinese cabbage, carp.

Recipes

(1) broth of carp with red bean: 1 carp alive (roughly 500 g), red bean 15 g.

Treat the carp and get it ready for use; wash the bean and boil and then stew it until edible, and then put in the carp and keep stewing until the carp is beyond readiness. Eat it without any condiments. The broth reduces oedema by channeling the water out.

(2) white gourd soup: white gourd 500 g.

Wash the gourd and slice it and boil the slices to readiness. Eat it bland. The soup has the same function as the dish above.

2.2.7 利水类

常用食物 玉米、玉米须、黑豆、绿豆、赤小豆、冬瓜、白菜、鲤鱼等。

食养方举例

(1) 鲤鱼赤小豆汤：鲜鲤鱼1条（约重500克），赤小豆15克。

鲤鱼去除鳃、鳞、头及内脏，冲洗干净备用；赤小豆洗净，放入锅内，加清水，大火烧开后改用小火，煮至豆熟时，加入鲤鱼，继续炖煮至鲤鱼熟烂即成，不加调料淡食。具有利水消肿的功效。

(2) 冬瓜汤：冬瓜500克。

冬瓜洗净，切成片，备用。锅中放入清水、冬瓜片，煮熟即可，不放盐，淡食。具有利水消肿的功效。

2.2.8 Excreting Sort

Food: banana, bamboo shoot, Feng Mi, He Tao Ren, Hei Zhi Ma (*Semen Sesami Nigum*).

Recipes

(1) black sesame porridge: Hei Zhi Ma 30 g,

2.2.8 通便类

常用食物 香蕉、竹笋、蜂蜜、核桃仁、黑芝麻等。

食养方举例

(1) 黑芝麻粥：黑芝麻

rice 100 g, sugar.

30 克,粳米 100 克,白糖适量。

Dry-fry (without oil) the Hei Zhi Ma until it gives off aroma, and keep it for later use; make rice porridge as usual and add Hei Zhi Ma when it is about to be ready, and finally sweeten it with sugar when the rice is extremely soft. The porridge nourishes the bowels so one excretes easily.

先将黑芝麻放入锅内干炒,炒出香味,倒入小盘中备用;粳米洗净,如常法煮粥,临熟时加入黑芝麻,煮至米烂即可停火,以白糖调味。具有润肠通便的功效。

(2) walnut porridge: He Tao Ren 30 g, rice 100 g.

(2) 胡桃仁粥:胡桃仁 30 克,粳米 100 克。

Cut the He Tao Ren into grain size, make rice porridge as usual and add He Tao Ren and keep boiling for another 5 minutes. The porridge fortifies the kidney and semen and nourishes lungs and appeases breathlessness.

胡桃仁切成细米粒大小备用;粳米淘洗干净,放入锅中,加入清水,以大火烧开,再改用小火煮至粥成,然后加入胡桃仁,继续煮 5 分钟即可。具有补肾固精、温肺定喘的功效。

2.2.9 Digestion-Promoting Sort

2.2.9 消导类

Food: Gu Ya (*Fructus Setariae Germinatus*), Mai Ya (*Fructus Hordei Germinatus*), Shan Zha, radish.

常用食物 谷芽、麦芽、山楂、萝卜等。

Recipes

食养方举例

(1) cake of shredded radish: radish 150 g, flour and salt.

(1) 萝卜丝饼:白萝卜 150 克,面粉适量、食盐适量。

Wash the radish and shred it, add water, flour and salt, and make pancakes with the mixture. The cake smoothes qi and promotes digestion.

将白萝卜洗净,刮成丝,调入清水、面粉、食盐,上火烙成薄饼。具有下气宽中,消食导滞的功效。

(2) spleen-furnishing cake: Bai Zhu 30 g, Gan jiang (*Rhizoma Zingiberis*) 6 g, Ji Nei Jin (*Endothelium Corneum Gigeriae Galli*) 15 g, well-made date 250 g, flour 1 000 g.

(2) 益脾饼:白术 30 克,干姜 6 克,鸡内金 15 克,熟枣肉 250 克,面粉 1 000 克。

Remove kernel of the date and chop it into paste; grind the Bai Zha, Gan jiang and Ji Nei Jin;

大枣去核取肉,捣成泥;白术、干姜、鸡内金研成细

add date paste, flour and water and knead it, roll it into little thin dough and make little pancakes with it. The cake fortifies the spleen, promotes qi and digestion.

粉,加入枣泥、面粉和清水和面,擀成小薄饼,烙熟食之。具有健脾益气、消食导滞的功效。

2.2.10 Rheumatism Dispersing Sort

Food: Yi Yi Ren, Mu Gua (*Fructus Chaenomelis*), cherry, eel.

Recipes:

(1) wine of semen coicis: ground Yi Yi Ren 500 g, yeast.

Steam the powder and let it cool, then mix it with an appropriate amount of yeast; wait for it to ferment into wine, which drives dampness and rheumatism away.

(2) cherry wine: cherry 500 g, wine.

Wash the cherry and let it dry and put it into the wine and the cherry wine is ready in a month. It drives dampness and rheumatism away.

2.2.10 祛风湿类

常用食物 薏苡仁、木瓜、樱桃、鳝鱼等。

食养方举例

(1) 薏苡仁酒:薏苡仁粉500克,酒曲适量。

薏苡仁粉500克蒸熟,摊凉,与适量的酒曲拌匀,发酵酿制成酒。具有祛风除湿的功效。

(2) 樱桃酒:樱桃500克,白酒适量。

将樱桃洗净,沥干,放入白酒中,浸泡1个月后即可饮服。具有祛风除湿的功效。

Chapter 3 Schedule Approach to Health Preservation

第3章 起居养生

The schedule approach means a series of health-cultivating measures of reasonably scheduling daily life in accordance with changes in nature. The human being, deeply influenced by nature, should actively get adapted to it. Exercises in the long term form a rule for the individual as much as that formed by his biological rhythm cultivated by the change of seasons, year in and year out. So our health-cultivating measures should go with the change of day and night, yin and yang, a theory inadvertently echoing the conception of biological clock advocated by modern medical science and time biology.

起居养生是指顺应自然变化的规律，合理安排日常生活、作息时间和运动锻炼等系列养生措施。人类在自然环境中，既受其影响制约，又积极探索适应。长时间的锻炼适应逐步固定下来形成规律；自然气候的寒来暑往的周期变化，促使人的生物节律随之产生同步现象。一般而言，每日调摄方法要顺应昼夜阴阳变化的规律，这与现代医学和时间生物学所提倡的生物钟学说不谋而合。

Section 1 Regularity in Daily Schedule

第1节 起居有常

The regularity in daily schedule falls into five aspects: regular sleep and moderate exercises, regular time and amount for three meals, a sensible match of meat and vegetables, refined and coarse grains, balance between work and repose. Only the second and the last aspects will be dealt with in this

起居有常，就是要做到按时作息，合理睡眠；适当锻炼，筋骨强健；一日三餐，定时定量；荤素粗细，配搭合理；劳逸结合，动静有度等。本节仅介绍作息劳逸，其他

episode, the others to be discussed in other chapters.

内容参见相关章节。

1 Balancebetween Work and Repose

Work and rest, seeming opposite, should actually go in balance, as alternation between strain and relaxation has always been emphasized by health pursuers. The daily exercises should advance step by step, without going to the extreme, as harmful to health is excessive leisure, in which case qi and blood run slowly, thus causing congestion, and it is also bad for tendon and bones. Regular exercise can ward off disease, even if it is mild labour just within one's reach. Mark the word, moderate labour and exercises do not tire one, only leading one in the opposite direction.

Intellectual work must go hand in hand with physical exercises that should be pursued sensibly, in the course of which repose restores the energy. "NO repose, no work", as the saying goes.

1 劳逸适度

劳和逸是既对立，又统一的关系。一动一静，有张有弛，养生家历来讲究劳逸适度。人体日常的运动，不宜过于劳累，要循序渐进，过劳于人不利；也不宜过于清闲安逸，太逸使人气血阻滞，筋骨不舒，于人同样有害。经常运动可健身防病，形体活动常可使疾病远离人体，经常做一些轻微劳动或力所能及的运动锻炼，可使人健壮少病。适度的劳动和运动锻炼并不会使人疲乏，只会使身体日益健康强壮。

养生应动静结合，劳与逸必须适度，做到脑力劳动与体力劳动相结合，量力而行，轻重相宜。劳动和运动的同时，要注意养精蓄锐，因为这是劳动锻炼中对机体消耗必不可少的休整、补充和恢复过程。所谓"不会休息就不会工作"，故劳逸适度在养生保健中是非常重要的。

2 Avoiding Excessive Labour

The ancient Chinese interprets "labour" in the three aspects of mental labour, physical labour and sex labour. Moderate labour is necessary while it is perilous to carry it too far.

2 避免过劳

古人对"劳"的理解非常全面，包括神劳、形（体）劳和房劳。正常的劳是必不可少的，而超量的劳，则是需要我们警惕的。

Lust and desire are an important aspect of mental labour. It means one likes something so much as to be obsessed, and it is also heart's desire shown in the eye, ear, nose, tongue and the whole body. Excessive desire poses a threat to the spirit. As is realized in *Chuangtse*(Zhuang Zi), the Taoist classic, to cultivate health, measures should be taken to cut desires and save spirit by removing the object of desire, shutting the five sense faculties and reducing one's desires. TCM maintains that the spirit, like the body, would be exhausted when inappropriately consumed, which would lead to shortened life span.

神劳里面一个很重要的方面是嗜欲，嗜欲是因喜好太过而致偏爱成癖，也是心之贪欲在眼、耳、鼻、舌、身上的具体反映。欲望太过，必伤心神。《庄子》很早就认识到嗜欲伤人，指出应采取措施从断嗜源、寡嗜欲、敛五官等方面断嗜欲、节精神以养生。中医学认为，心神使用太过则易衰竭，身体过度劳累则疲惫不堪。一旦人的形神早衰，必然寿命缩短。

Moderate physical labour, as is discussed above, is especially important for the middle-aged and the elders. Lust, though man's nature, should not be indulged. The ancient Chinese are not unjustifiable in practicing sex temperance for stocking energy.

戒形劳过度也是养生的基本思想之一。起居养生要从实际出发，避免过度疲劳和进行过量的运动，否则对身体有害无益，尤其是中老年人，戒过劳更显得重要。另外，性欲虽为人之天性，但不可放纵而应有所节制。

3 Avoiding Excessive Leisure

3 避免过逸

Excessive leisure, like excessive labour, does great harm to health. Staying static gives rise to pent-up energy, congested and knotted qi and blood, under-nourished organs and general frailty, and shortens life span in the long run. As the ancient book *Cultivate character and prolong life* (Yang Xing Yan Ming Lu) warns, do not indulge in sleep and leisure, which shortens life by clotting qi and blood and weakening sinew and withering muscle. Many modern civilized diseases, such as obesi-

与过劳正好相反的是过逸。静而少动甚至不动则易导致精气郁滞、气血凝结，脏腑失养，全身衰弱，久即损寿。《养性延命录》说，不要过于安逸，那会导致气血瘀滞，筋伤肉萎，从而缩短寿命。劳逸也要辨证而施，健康无病时不要过于贪睡，过逸少动。一旦长期过逸少动，现代文明病如肥胖、高脂

ty, hyperlipemia and cardio cerebral vascular disease, follow up. Additionally, do not take bed-confinement in disease absolutely, since moderate movement in many diseases or at some phases of the disease is necessary, which promotes circulation of qi and blood, otherwise the patient would contract stiff joints and withered muscle, etc, and suffer even more.

血症、心脑血管疾病等就会接踵而至。也不可一味强调病中卧床休息,有许多疾病、或在疾病的某一阶段反而确实需要一定的轻微活动,这样才有助于气血流通,不然会引起关节僵硬,肌肉萎缩等一系列不利影响,对病人危害很大。

So we should be dialectical in labour and leisure. Beware of overwork to death as well as "modern civilized disease". Moderate exercise builds up the body and prolongs life.

总之,过劳过逸都不可取。过劳,谨防走向另一个极端——过劳死;过逸,易得"现代文明病"。所以,适度劳动或运动,具有增强体质,延长寿命的作用。

Section 2 Sleep

第2节 睡眠养生

Health-cultivating sleep means forming reasonable sleeping habits based on the rule of changes of nature and of human yin and yang, aiming at full and efficient sleep, so as to restore and refresh energy, hence fortifying health and prolonging life.

睡眠养生,是指根据自然界与人体阴阳变化的规律,采用合理的睡眠方法和措施,保证充足而高质量的睡眠,以尽快恢复机体疲劳,保持充沛的精力,从而达到防病健体、延年益寿的目的。

The time in total of average individual sleep is more than 23 years, one third of human life, which is indispensable to normal physiology and replenished spirit. The quality of sleep, however, makes much difference, depending on arrangement before and during and after sleep and the bedroom and beddings.

人的一生中平均用于睡眠的时间长达23年之多,也就是说人的一生中,有1/3的时间是在睡眠中度过的,这既是生理的需要,也是健康的保证和恢复精神的必要途径。但同样是睡眠,质量的好坏却有天壤之别,这取决于睡前、入睡、醒后、卧室、卧具等相关环节的安排是否合理妥当。

1 Dos and Don’ts of Sleep

1.1 Dos and Don’ts before Sleep

Take a walk after supper or before sleep, which assists digestion, settles the mind down and brings in fresh air.

Keep the mood steady. Keep calm and mild, away from anxiety and anger. Because anger excites qi and blood, troubles and distracts the mind. All radical changes of the mood, besides anger, drive qi movement out of order, which cannot be easily collected and put to sleep.

Wash feet. Washing feet with warm water before sleep, termed “feet bath” in the ancient times, can not only remove dust, but also warm up the feet in winter, hence drawing qi and blood down and settling the mind into sleep.

Do not stuff oneself too full. It is not good to eat too much for supper, or within one hour before sleep. If one has to do so, postpone sleep. Because the digestive system does not work actively in sleep and its burden of digestion would cause a light sleep.

Do not take strong tea or coffee, because they contain caffeine that excites the brain.

1 睡眠宜忌

1.1 睡前宜忌

睡前宜散步:晚饭后,睡前出外散步,一方面有利于食物消化,还可以使情绪安定下来,并呼吸新鲜空气,十分有益。

睡前情绪应平稳:睡眠之前保持思想安静、情绪平和,切忌忧虑、恼怒。因为怒则气血上涌,情绪激动,烦躁不安,神不守舍,难于成寐。非但恼怒,任何情绪的过极变化,都会引起气机失调,导致失眠。

睡前要洗脚:上床前用温水洗脚,古称“浴足”,不仅可去足垢,冬日使足部温暖,而且能引血气下行,使心宁神安而入睡。

睡前不宜过饱:晚餐不宜过饱,睡前一小时不宜过多进餐。饱食之后不可立即寝卧,其原因是睡眠时消化功能减弱,吃多了加重消化系统负担,使睡眠不深。

此外,睡前也不要喝浓茶或咖啡,因为茶和咖啡所含咖啡因,能增强大脑皮层的兴奋性,使人不易入睡。

1.2 Taboos in Sleep

Do not sleep in draught. Sleeping with the head facing the doorway or window leads to paralysis and hemiplegia; neither can one sleep with the head near the fireplace or heater, which draws the fire in the body and sparks dried throat, red eyes and epistaxis and even headache; nor should one sleep with the quilt covering the head, which can be suffocating, especially to children.

1.3 Sleep on Time

A good sleeping habit that goes with a certain rhythm is a basic guarantee of good sleeping quality. Eight hours of sleep is advised to be ensured every day, and staying up later than 10 o'clock at night would cause great damage to health. Some rule of getting up and going to bed should be observed, that is, to coordinate them with the changes of day and night.

1.4 Ensuring Ziwu Sleep

Ziwu Sleep, one of the ancient sleeping ways to cultivate health, means one should go to sleep at Zi period (11－1 o'clock at midnight) and Wuperiod (11-1 o'clock at noon), in order to attain longevity. According to TCM, at these two periods, yin and yang in nature change shifts. So one had better lie down and await the restoration of qi. Modern researches have revealed that the function of viscera declines to the valley from 0 to 4 o'clock in the morning and the period from 12 to 1 o'clock at noon sees the greatest exhaustion of autonomic nerves; therefore, the quality of Ziwu sleep can be warranted. Statistics show that the middle-aged and the elders, in so doing, can lower the rate of cardio vertebral vascular

1.2 睡眠禁忌

睡卧时忌当风。睡卧时头对门窗风口，易造成风入脑户引起面瘫、偏瘫。卧时头对炉火、暖气，易使火攻上焦，造成咽干目赤鼻衄，甚则头痛。睡卧时还忌蒙头，以保持呼吸空气的新鲜。小儿尤应注意，以免窒息。

1.3 按时睡觉

养成良好的睡眠习惯，符合睡眠节律，是提高睡眠质量的基本保障。每天最好保证 8 小时睡眠，夜间就寝时间一般不超过 22 点，不宜睡得太晚，或者熬夜，对身体健康不利。一天之中起卧亦有规律，即要使睡眠模式符合一日昼夜晨昏的变化。

1.4 保证子午觉

子午觉是古人睡眠养生法之一，即是每天于子时、午时入睡，以达颐养天年目的。中医认为，子午之时，阴阳交接，必欲静卧，以候气复。现代研究也发现，0 点至 4 点，机体各器官功能降至最低；12 点至 13 点，是人体交感神经最疲劳的时间，因此子午睡眠的质量和效率都好，符合养生道理。据统计，中老年人睡子午觉可降低心、脑血管病的发病率，有防病保健意义。

disease.

1.5 Sleeping Gesture

Normal people should sleep on the right side. As the ancient Chinese said, "Sleeping means lying on the right side." This is confirmed by contemporary doctors.

The expectant mother should sleep on the left side. This applies even more to those in their middle and advanced pregnancy, as such a gesture provides better space for the growth of the embryo.

Some patients of heart failure and asthma should adopt a gesture in between being face up and on one side at the right angle, or sleep sitting half way up with the pillow and cushion piled higher.

2 Bedroom Environment

The bedroom does not have to be a big one, yet a neat environment should be ensured, with the requirements below:

2.1 Full Sunshine

The bedroom is the best that faces the south, which is warm in winter and cool in summer. The size should be appropriate, not too big, which is too spacious to be warm, and not to small, suffocating to the mind with its stifling air. In general, the right size should be 15 square metres. The bedroom windows should be broad so as to let in light and breeze. The windows should be opened before sleep and after getting up, for better ventilation. One should also give heed to the colour of the curtain. Light green and cream cool one in summer, and in winter, curtains of warm colours like saffron with thickness in quality are preferable.

1.5 睡觉姿势

常人宜右侧卧：古人云"卧为右侧"。古今医家都选择右侧卧为最佳卧姿。

孕妇宜左侧卧：孕妇宜取左侧卧，尤其是进入中、晚期妊娠的人，左侧卧最利于胎儿生长。

病人睡姿：对于心衰病人及咳喘发作病人宜取半侧位或半坐位，同时将枕与后背垫高。

2 卧室环境

卧室房间不一定大，但要保证良好的环境，良好的卧室环境要求具备以下条件：

2.1 阳光充足

卧室的朝向以坐北朝南为佳，这样有冬暖夏凉的优点。卧室面积要适中，太大显得空旷又不利于保暖，太小既使人郁闷又不利于空气流通。一般而言，卧室面积在 15 平方米左右为好。卧室的窗户宜宽大，以利于采光和通风，保持空气新鲜。睡前醒后应开窗换气，以免秽浊之气滞留。窗帘的色调也很重要，夏天可用浅绿、浅米色的冷色调，使人感到凉爽；冬天可选橙红等暖色调且质地厚重些的窗帘，使人感到温暖。

2.2 Tranquility

A quiet environment is prerequisite for falling asleep. Noises hinder sleep and even cause diseases such as hypertension, fast beating of the heart and neurasthenia. So the bedroom should be far from streets or be set with double-glass windows otherwise, and be sure to close the door and windows.

Less furniture in the bedroom is advised, just a few pieces to create a plain yet elegant atmosphere to soothe the mind.

2.2 恬淡宁静

安静的环境是帮助入睡的基本条件之一。嘈杂的环境使人心神烦躁，难于安眠。噪声不但可以引起许多疾病，如高血压、心动过速、神经衰弱，亦能产生睡眠障碍，因而卧室选择重在避声，窗口远离街道闹市，怕吵的人设置双层玻璃，睡觉时应关上门窗。

室内家俱越少越好，一切设置应造成简朴典雅的气氛，利于安神。

2.3 Fresh Air

Open the windows often to let in fresh air, reinforced by bonsai placed casually in the bedroom—on the floor, windowsill, table or flower stand. The species should be able to purify the air, such as monstera ceriman and dangling orchid; the latter can also absorb formaldehyde and regulate humidity in the room, in addition to other species that exude less carbon oxide and regulate temperature and humidity, such as lotus and cactus.

2.3 空气新鲜

经常开窗，可以使室外的新鲜空气与室内的污浊空气进行充分的交换，以创造良好的空气环境。室内可以放置植物盆景，摆放的位置要随意，如地上、窗台、桌角或花架上，宜选一些能净化空气的花草，如龟背竹、吊兰，这样的植物在夜间可吸收二氧化碳、释放氧气，吊兰还可以消除甲醛，同时还可调节室内的湿度，防止干燥。

2.4 Hygiene

Clean the bedroom at least once a week, without chemical detergent or germ killer. Sun the beddings once a week or every two weeks, and change

2.4 清洁卫生

卧室内要保持清洁卫生，每星期至少对卧室进行一次常规打扫，以便清除灰

them every three or four weeks.

尘，最好不要使用有化学成分的喷雾剂、除菌剂等清洁剂清理卧室。床上用品也需要定期清洗，每1～2星期至少在室外晾晒1次，每3～4星期清洗更换1次。

Place some orchid, lotus, cactus in the room for these plants can help adjust the temperature and humidity and effluent less CO at night. Do not eat or burn the coal in the bedroom, lest mosquitoes or flies should be drawn and gas poisoning occur respectively.

室内可以摆放兰花、荷花、仙人掌等植物一盆，此类植物夜间排放的一氧化碳甚少，室内植物利于温湿度调节。应注意不在卧室内用餐、烧炉子，以防蚊蝇孳生和中毒的发生。

2.5 Proper Temperature

A proper temperature is essential to falling asleep. A cozy temperature is agreed to be around 18-20 degrees Celsius. Do not put the bed close to the heater, air-conditioner or fireplace. And note great dampness also impedes sleep.

2.5 温度适宜

卧室温度适宜是入睡的重要条件。过冷、过热或潮湿，都会影响睡眠。一般认为卧室温度以18～20 ℃为宜，无条件者差几度也无妨。摆设床铺时，不要把床紧靠暖气片、空调、火炉等，尤其是不要头朝暖气装置。

2.6 Dark Light

Bright light excites people and influences sleep. Thus, close the light before sleep. If there isn't a bedroom due to limited space, bed should be placed in the dark corner with a screen to shade the light.

2.6 入睡光线幽暗

入睡环境的光线太强，易使人兴奋，影响睡眠，因此睡前必须关灯。住房面积有限，没有专用卧室者，应将床铺设在室中幽暗角落，并以屏风隔开。

3 Bedding Selection

3.1 Bed and Cotton-padded Mattress

The bed should be moderately soft, which goes with normal physiological curve of the spine and re-

3 卧具选择

3.1 床铺、褥垫

床宜软硬适中。软硬适中的床可保证脊椎维持正常

laxes muscles, thus diminishing fatigue. A standard degree of softness is a cotton-padded mattress of 0.1 metres in thickness on the board of bed, thickened or thinned with climate. The southern bamboo couch, rattan bed and coir mattress are also a good choice.

生理曲线,使肌肉放松,有利于消除疲劳。标准的软硬度以木板床上铺 0.1 米厚的棉垫为宜。其他的床,如南方的竹榻、藤床、棕绷床也较符合养生要求。

When the bed is too soft, as in the case of spring bed and inner-spring mattress, the spine's natural curve is injured, a threat to the youth's spinal and bone growth, and muscles in the sunken part of the bed would be strained and injured and thus it hurts. What's worse, the viscera would be pressed and injured. While the opposite to extreme softness would result in pain of the pressed side of the body, thus harassing sleep.

弹簧床或席梦思床垫过于柔软,睡眠时不能维持脊柱正常的生理弯曲而易导致脊柱病变,特别是对青少年而言,会影响其脊柱和四肢骨骼的正常发育,并且身体下陷部分的肌肉持续紧张会造成肌肉劳损而发生疼痛,胸腹腔内的脏器也会受到挤压而有损健康。过于坚硬平板床使人贴床的一侧压痛不舒而睡不安稳。

The height of the bed also should be considered. It is best when the bed is higher than the knee of the sleeper.

床宜高低适度。床的高度以略高于就寝者膝盖水平为好,这样的高度便于上下床。

The bed should be broad. A large bed where the sleeper can toss and turn freely makes a cozy environment for stretching tendon and bones.

床宜宽大。床铺面积较大,睡眠时便于自由翻身,宽大的床则能使人心神安逸,便于睡眠中自由转体,有利于筋骨舒展,有利于休息。婴儿床除要求一定宽长度外,宜在床周加栏杆,以防婴儿坠地。褥垫宜软宜厚。厚褥利于维持人体生理曲线。

3.2 Pillows

A right pillow relaxes the body, protects the neck and brain, furnishes sleep and wards off and cures disease. An agreed height of the pillow is that

3.2 枕头

枕头是睡眠不可缺少的用具,适宜的枕头有利于全身放松,保护颈部和大脑,促

a bit shorter than the distance between the end of the shoulder and the neck on the same side. A pillow too high hinders turning in sleep, and it is not good for patients of hypertension, cervical spondylopathy or with cervical vertebra out of place. While a low pillow is not recommended to those with problems in the lungs and the heart.

进和改善睡眠,还有防病治病效果。一般认为枕高以稍低于肩到同侧颈部距离为宜。枕头过高不便睡中翻身而影响睡眠。高血压、颈椎病及脊椎不正的病人不宜使用高枕;肺病、心脏病、哮喘病病人不宜使用低枕。

The pillow stuffing should be appropriately soft and a little elastic. A hard pillow presses the head and neck and causes discomfort, while an over-soft one cannot fully prop up the head, which grows tired by being too low.

枕芯应选质地松软之物,制成软硬适度,稍有弹性的枕头为好,枕头太硬使头颈与枕接触部位压强增加,造成头部不适;枕头太软,则头颈部得不到充分的支持,睡眠中难以维持正常高度而易疲劳。

A better choice would be medicinal pillows, which means some medicine is contained in the pillow stuffing. It balances yin and yang and cures disease. People with a hot type of constitution can use pillows with Xia Ku Cao (*Spica Prunellae*) or Can Sha (*Faeces Bombycis*), those with hearing problems Ci Shi (*Magnetitum*) pillow, and those with eye problems Ju Hua (*Flos Chrysanthemi*), tea or Jue Ming Zi (Semen Cassiae) pillows. We will discuss it in detail later.

实际养生实践中,还可选用采用不同的药物加工制成枕芯做成的枕头,称为药枕。药枕对人体既有治疗作用,又具保健作用,可以疗疾除病、协调阴阳,可酌情选用。阳热体质者宜选夏枯草枕、蚕砂枕等;耳鸣耳聋者可选磁石枕;目暗目花者可选菊花枕、茶叶枕和决明子枕等明目枕。

3.3 Quilt

The quilt should be soft with the inner side of cotton, cotton yarn or fine linen, rather than chemical fibre. Cotton, silk wadding and feather are best for warmth, among which silk wadding has to be new for the function, as the old becomes heavy and cold that traps dampness. Quilts should be light and

3.3 盖被

盖被宜软,被里可选细棉布、棉纱、细麻布等,不宜用腈纶、尼龙等带静电荷的化纤品。盖被目的在于御寒护阳,温煦内脏,故被内容物宜选棉花、丝绵、羽绒为最

broad, as heavy ones press the body and block circulation of qi and blood, and so nightmares occur. Broad quilts, just like the bed, serve greater freedom of toss and turn. That is why the popular modern sleeping bag, with three sides shut, hampers free movement of the body and metabolism of the skin, therefore not so wholesome as the traditional quilt.

好,腈纶棉次之。丝绵之物以新者为佳,陈旧棉絮既沉且冷,易积湿气,不利养生。盖被宜轻,盖被重则压迫胸腹四肢,使气血不畅,心中烦闷,易生梦惊。盖被宜宽,被子宽大利于翻身转侧,使用舒适。故现代流行的睡袋不如传统被子保健性好。睡袋上口束紧,三面封闭,影响了肢体活动和皮肤新陈代谢。

3.4 Pyjamas or Dressing Gowns

Pyjamas should be loose-fitting, cozy, sweat-absorbing and wind-shielding. A dressing gown is preferable in that it is long enough to cover all the limbs and fends off the cold better. The material should be cotton and towel cloth for autumn and winter, and silk and thin gauze for spring and summer.

3.4 睡衣

睡衣的选择总以宽长、舒适、吸汗、遮风为原则。睡衣宜宽大无领无扣,不使颈、胸、腰受束。睡衣要有一定的长度,使睡眠时四肢覆盖,不冒风寒。睡衣选料以天然织品为好,秋冬选棉绒、毛巾布为料,春夏宜选丝绸、薄纱为料。

3.5 Daily Medicinal Pillows

The medicinal pillow is one of the TCM ways of external treatment. It contains herbal medicine in the pillow stuffing, whose function is driven out by warmth of the head in sleeping, which can prevent and cure disease by stimulating the acupuncture points of the head in a mild and lasting way. There is a great diversity of them, and here is a brief introduction of the functions and making methods.

3.5 常用药枕

药枕属于中医外治法的一种。它是将中药装入枕芯中,利用睡眠时头部的温度,使药物的有效成分散发出来,以达到清心明目、健脑安神、调和阴阳的养生目的。头为精明之府,久枕药枕,可以缓慢而持久地刺激颈项部相关穴位,从而防治疾病。药枕的种类繁多,择其要者简要如下。

The chrysanthemum pillow. Medicines in the

菊花枕:选用菊花干品

stuffing: Ju Hua 1 000 g, rhizome of Chuan Xiong (*Rhizoma Ligustici Chuanxiong*) 400 g, Jue Ming Zi 200 g, Bai Zhi (*Radix Angelicae Dahuricae*) 200 g. Functions: dispersing wind-heat and refreshing eyes and mind, for such diseases as neurasthenia, hypertension and partial headache. Note that the medicinal effect is exhausted in half a year, when new medicine should substitute for the old.

1 000 克,川芎 400 克,决明子 200 克,白芷 200 克,装入枕芯内,使药物缓慢挥发,有疏风散热、清利头目之功。适用于目暗昏花之人,也可用于预防和治疗神经衰弱、高血压、偏头痛等病。因药性发散,此枕只可连续使用半年左右,如需再用可更换药物。

The granodiorite pillow. It boasts the functions of fatigue resistance, lack-of-oxygen resistance and aging resistance. The medicine can also cool and freshen the head in summer, thus facilitating sleep.

麦饭石枕:麦饭石具有抗疲劳、抗缺氧、延缓衰老的功效。麦饭石作为枕芯使用可保持头部清凉,使人在炎炎夏日能够安然入睡。

The green bean pillow. It clears heat and fire in the body, and removes troubles from mind, for the ailments of red eyes, sore throat and thirstiness, in one word, for those with yin- deficiency and fire type of constitution.

绿豆枕:取适量绿豆装入枕芯制成绿豆枕,有清热、泻火、除烦的功效。可用于目赤喉痛,口渴心烦等症,也适用于阴虚火旺体质之人。

The simple massage pillow. The pillow takes fluffy cotton as the stuffing. The fluffy cotton is a chemical synthesized fibre produced by making a number of cavities in the centre of the fibre. Such a stuffing has good permeability and elasticity, and gives the head a wonderful feel. Its thickness, however, should be heeded, since the fibre rebounds intensely (following the thickness of general pillows).

简易按摩保健枕:枕芯可选用蓬松棉作为填充物。蓬松棉是一种化学合成纤维,在生产过程中使纤维中心形成空腔,即我们所说的孔,由于工艺不同,孔的个数也不同。这种枕心透气性较好,弹性足,感觉比较舒服,但由于其纤维反弹力较大,所以必须掌握好枕芯厚度(枕高厚度参照一般要求)。

To make the massage pillow, put a thick pure cotton cloth on both sides of the stuffing, also rectangular, yet smaller than the stuffing by a margin

简易按摩保健枕的制作:在长方形的枕芯的反正面各放一块质地较厚的纯棉

of 2-3 inches, sew the four corners and the centre of the cloth to the stuffing with a thick cotton thread, thus 5 evenly protruding points on the stuffing, and finally clothe it in the pillow case. The massage pillow looks the same as other pillows. But when it is slept on, one would feel the central point pressed against the occipital bone of the head, and the lower points fit in with the physiological curve of the cervical vertebra. Therefore, the head and the neck are incidentally massaged when they lie or move on the pillow. According to TCM, the head has an assembly of important meridians and collaterals of the human body, together with 40 plus acupuncture points such as Yu Zhen (B 9), Tian Zhu (BL 10), Feng Fu (GV 16) and Ya Men (GV 15), and a dozen special stimulation zones. Massaging and stimulating such an assembly can dredge the channels, push the circulation of qi and blood, so as to refresh the mind, remove fatigue, sharpen ears and eyes and improve the quality of sleep, plus a beautifying function. It can be used in the treatment of insomnia, pain in the fifth nerve and partial headache, etc.

布，同为长方形，尺寸比枕芯的四周要缩进 2～3 英寸，然后用粗棉线把布的四个角和中心穿透缝牢，这样枕芯就形成了几个凹凸均匀的点，再把枕芯装入枕套内即可。从枕套表面看，枕头和平常的枕头无异。但人枕在上面，枕头中心的凹陷处正好是头颅枕骨粗隆的位置，而枕头下面凸起处又恰好与颈椎的生理曲度吻合，四周凹凸不平，使头在不动或不自主转动的时候，起到了按摩作用。中医学认为人体重要的经脉、四十多处大小穴位如玉枕、天柱、风府、哑门等穴、十多个特殊刺激区，均汇聚于头部。对这些穴位的按摩或刺激，能疏通经脉，促进气血运行，达到醒脑提神、消除疲劳、聪耳明目、提高睡眠质量以及美容作用，可用于治疗失眠烦躁、三叉神经痛、偏头痛等疾病。

Chapter 4 Artistic Entertainment Approach to Health Preservation

第4章 雅趣养生

Health-cultivation science is rich in content, with extraordinary methods, among which are artistic pursuits and entertainments, such as playing musical instruments, playing chess, reading and painting, raising birds, fishes and plants, fishing, traveling and aesthetics, for instance, as tea connoisseur. Such pleasant, relaxing and elegant activities give expression to the spirit and cultivate wisdom and build up physical and mental health in a graceful atmosphere.

养生学有其丰富的内容及独特的养生方法，培养自身高雅的情趣来怡养身心即是其中之一。各种富有情趣的娱乐活动，如琴棋书画、花木鸟鱼、旅游观光、艺术欣赏等，通过轻松愉快、情趣雅致的活动，在美好的生活气氛和高雅的情趣之中，使人们舒畅情志、怡养心神、增加智慧、增强体质，寓养生于娱乐之中，从而达到养神健形，益寿延年的目的。这种养生方法称之为雅趣养生。高雅的情趣活动，主要有音乐、弈棋、书画、鉴赏、垂钓、花鸟、旅游、品茗等，皆具有很重要的养生功能。

It should be noted that the term "entertaining" should also be elegant. Some pure entertainments, indulging fun and merry-making, actually harm health rather than cultivate it. So a degree must be noted in entertainment, which is easy—just remember to make it artistic.

"雅趣养生"，强调养生娱乐活动不仅要有"趣"的环节，还必须要有"雅"的取向。仅拘泥于"乐"，纵乐过度，不仅不是"养"生，还可能是"害"生。从事各种娱乐活动，必须掌握"养"和"害"之间的度,"雅"就是强调以一种高雅的情趣来规范日常的娱乐活动。

Section 1 Music

第1节 音乐养生

Listening to music improves the state of mind, organ function and yin-yang balance and circulation of qi and blood, hence nourishing the body and soul and cultivating health.

The musical instrument, chess, books and painting were grouped as "four artistic pursuits" in the ancient times, among which music comes first. Various gorgeous melodies flow out of the instrument as a powerful manna to cultivate morals and character. A vivacious melody cheers one up and stimulates passion; a serene and elegant piece expresses the heart and tranquilizes the mind; while a melancholy one in low tune drives one to tears. It shows music can adjust the balance in psychology.

音乐养生是指通过聆听音乐,使人的精神状态、脏腑机能、阴阳气血等内环境得到改善,从而调养身心、保持健康的养生方法。

琴棋书画古代称为"四雅趣",琴居四雅之首,是各种美妙乐声奔流飘逸出来的工具,说明在修身养性方面,音乐最有力量。一曲活泼欢快的乐曲能使人振奋精神,激发情趣;一首优美雅静的乐曲却让人畅志舒怀,安定情绪;而一曲悲哀低沉的音乐,能催人泪下。说明音乐可用来调节心理上的不平衡状态,对于人的心理具有重要的养生意义。

1 Mechanism

Yellow Emperor's Inner Canon (Huang Di Nei Jing) probes into the relation between music and human physiology, pathology, disease and longevity. It holds that the note 3 connects with wood quality of the liver; 5 with fire quality of the heart; 1, spleen of soil quality; 2, lungs of metal quality; 6,

1 养生机理

《黄帝内经》探讨了音乐与人体生理、病理、养生益寿及防病治病的关系,认为角为木音通于肝,徵为火音通于心,宫为土音通于脾,商为金音通于肺,羽为水音通于

kidney of water quality, and interprets the correlation among the five notes, five solid organs and exercise of the body. The human body has many rhythmic reverberations, such as the brain wave, heart beat, contraction of lungs and digesting movement of the stomach, which might be driven to disorder by disease, when appropriate music with its harmonic chord can coordinate the human reverberation back to order.

肾,阐明了五音、五脏和气的运动的内在联系。人体机能有许多规律的振动,人的脑电波运动、心脏搏动、肺的收缩、肠胃的蠕动等都有一定的节奏。当人患病时,体内节奏处于异常状态,选择适当的乐曲,借音乐产生的和谐音频,可使人体各种振频活动协调,从而有益于保持和恢复健康。

2 Essentials

The heart: music of note 5. The heart is the master of the five solid organs and spirit. A long time of strained life and work, inadequate sleep and little physical exercises would harm the qi of the heart, and cause its wild beat, stifled feeling and irritation. Music of note 5, such as *Purple Bamboo Tune* (Zi Zhu Diao), is lilting, thus good for the heart.

The liver: music of note 3. People who are long trapped in troubles and miseries would have the qi of the liver congested and knotted, with the symptoms of depression, irritation, breast pain, menalgia, and dry eyes. Music of note 3, such as 18 *Beats of Hu Jia* (Hu Jia Shi Ba Pai, an ethnic instrument), is bright and intimate, which assuages flaming qi of the liver.

The spleen: music of note 1. The spleen, as the foundation of postnatal growth, produces and transports qi and blood. Inordinate diet and anxiety at-

2 养生要领

心:徵调式乐曲　心为五脏六腑之主,精神之所舍。如果生活和工作压力大、睡眠减少以及运动过少等不良因素长期作用,就会伤害心气,引起心慌、胸闷、烦躁等症状。徵调式乐曲活泼轻松,代表曲如《紫竹调》,对调理心脏功能有较好效果。

肝:角调式乐曲　如果长期被一些烦恼的事情所困扰,会逐渐引起肝气郁结,产生抑郁、易怒、乳房胀痛、痛经、眼部干涩等症。角调式乐曲亲切爽朗,代表曲如《胡笳十八拍》,欣赏该曲,有利于平调旺盛的肝气,起到疏理肝气的作用。

脾:宫调式乐曲　脾胃为后天之本,气血生化之源。饮食不节、思虑过度等常损

tack it, as shown in bloated stomach, semi-liquid excrement, ulcerous mouth, obesity, sallow face, small amount of pale menstruation blood, exhaustion and prolapse of viscera. Music of note 1, such as *Ambush in all Directions* (Shi Mian Mai Fu), is melodious and tranquil. Enjoying the music during meal or within an hour afterward regulates the function of the spleen.

害脾胃之气,产生腹胀、便溏、口唇溃疡、肥胖、面黄、月经量少色淡、疲乏、内脏下垂等。宫调式乐曲悠扬沉静,代表曲如《十面埋伏》。在进餐期间,或餐后一小时内欣赏这类乐曲,有助于调节脾胃功能。

Lungs: music of note 2. The lungs, governing breath exchange with the outside, are prone to the effect of polluted air, shown in cough (phlegm), blocked nose and breathlessness. Music of note 2, such as *Snow in Sunny Spring* (Yang Chun Bai Xue), is high-pitched and tragically soul-stirring, sonorous and grand. It can help adjust breath and so replenishes the qi of lungs and promotes its functions of diffusion, purification and descending.

肺:商调式乐曲　肺主气,司呼吸,主管人体气体交换,与环境直接相通。环境污染,空气质量下降,各种病邪容易袭肺,引起咳嗽、咯痰、鼻塞、气喘等症状。商调式乐曲高亢悲壮,铿锵雄伟,代表曲如《阳春白雪》。在这类音乐旋律中,不断调理呼吸,能起到调补肺气,促进肺的宣发肃降作用。

The kidney: music of note 6. The spleen stores the primordial yin and yang. A long sapping of the qi in the storehouse of the spleen gives rise to dark complexion, cold limbs, water-like and long urination, aching waist and knees and frigidity. Music of note 6 is fresh and clear, like flowing cloud and brook, demonstrated by *Three Echoes of the Plum Blossom* (Mei Hua San Long), which furnishes the essential qi of the spleen.

肾:羽调式乐曲　肾藏元阴元阳,是人体精气的储藏之所。当人体精气较长时间耗损,会产生面色晦暗、形寒肢冷、小便清长,腰酸膝软、性欲低等现象。羽调式乐曲清纯,如行云流水,可调理肾气。代表曲如《梅花三弄》,欣赏此类乐曲,可以促长肾中精气。

3 Keys

A good environment is a priority for a better effect of the music nourishment, so please choose a quiet and elegant place with fresh air, plus a cup of

3 注意事项

要达到比较好的养生效果,首先应当营造一个良好的环境。最好能选择静谧、

tea, rid of nervousness and irritation, and play music with hi-fi. The walkman or the headphone is only good for lesser conditions.

优雅、空气清新的地方，泡上一杯茶，排除心理上的紧张烦乱情绪，使用高保真音响播放音乐。只是在不得已情况下，可利用随身听，用封闭式耳机来欣赏音乐。

Enjoy the music as background when getting up and going to bed or at siesta. Close your eyes, collect your spirit, calm down and savour the music. It had better be fixed time so that the music can play on the body regularly. Note that perseverance is a key for the long-term project.

应选择适当的时间段，如在起床、午休或就寝时，可用作背景音乐，闭目养神，静心体味。最好能有比较固定的时间段，使音乐能有规律地对身体机能产生作用。需要的是坚持不懈的恒心，才能收到效果。

The volume makes little difference in the curing effect of the music. But a large one brings discomfort as noise.

欣赏音乐时，音量的大小，对人体的良性作用只有很小的区别，但太大的音量却具有不良作用，甚至变成一种噪声，给身体带来不适。

People of different constitution feel music differently and choose what they like. Generally, the choice is a good one when they feel the music pleasant and adjust their mood quickly.

不同体质、不同身体状态的人对音乐的感受不同，除五音选择外，音乐种类的选择主要根据自己的体验。当聆听不同音乐的时候，某种音乐能让欣赏者感到身心舒畅，能很快地调整心情的时候，一般来说，那就是比较适合身心需要的音乐。

It should be noted that music with a strong rhythm, like the march, enhances starvation when enjoyed with an empty stomach; during meal percussion music is a taboo, as it is rhythmic and mighty, which diverts the attention from the food and spoils appetite and digestion; crazy and stimula-

还需注意空腹时忌听进行曲及节奏强烈的音乐，会加剧饥饿感；进餐时忌听打击乐，打击乐节奏明快，铿锵有力，会分散对食物的注意力，影响食欲，有碍食物消

ting rock-n-roll adds fuel to fury; and sleep is a worse time for the music above, as is known to all, especially for the insomnia patients.

化;生气忌听摇滚乐,怒气未消又听到疯狂而富有刺激性的摇滚乐,会火上加油,助长怒气;睡眠时上面几种音乐也不宜,会使人情绪激动,难以入眠,特别是失眠人群,更不宜听这类音乐。

Section 2 Chess Playing

第2节 弈棋养生

In chess playing, players calm down and concentrate on the fun of chess, hence improving their organ functions and inner environment of yin and yang, qi and blood. More than an intelligence competition, chess-playing is a wholesome entertainment that prolongs life.

弈棋养生是指人们在对弈的过程中,享受弈棋的乐趣,使人的精神情绪专一宁静,从而使脏腑机能、阴阳气血等内环境得到改善,达到调养身心、保持健康的养生方法。弈棋不仅是智力竞赛,更是有利身心、延年益寿的娱乐活动,是一种良好的养生之道。

There is a variety of chess in China, such as the Go, Chinese chess, military chess, skipping chess and gobang, the first two of which are complex that take a long practice or serious study, while the latter three are simple for folk entertainment.

中国棋类有很多,如围棋、象棋、军棋、跳棋、五子棋等,民间还有很多简约的棋法,如打三棋等。有些棋法很繁复,需要较长时间的学习磨练,或研究前人的相关著述,才能登堂入室,如围棋、象棋。而军棋、跳棋、五子棋类则比较简单易学,适宜于普通大众娱乐。

1 Mechanism

In chess playing, one collects mind, calms down, concentrates on the board, rid of wild thoughts, moves in a set frame and finishes the game in laughter, which serves the function of adjusting the breath as in Qigong, thus good for disposition and health. Changes on the board train the players' reaction by making the spirit tense and relaxed in fine rhythm. So chess playing is an entertainment that cultivates intelligence and disposition. Apart from that, chess playing is especially important for the elders, in that it keeps their brain nerves working, thus preventing Alzheimer's disease, and that it gives them a good mood in the atmosphere of friendliness.

1 养生机理

弈棋需要精神专一，凝神静气，意守棋局，全神贯注，消除杂念，谋定而动，谈笑之间决胜负，可起到气功练习中的调息、吐纳作用，从而有益于健康，培养良好的性情。棋局变化使人精神有弛有张，神凝则心气平静，专注则杂念全消。棋局的变化，又可以锻炼人的应变能力，既是一种休息、消遣，也是一种益智养性的活动。下棋是一种积极的脑力活动，棋盘上瞬息万变的形势，要求对弈者全力以赴，开动脑筋，以适应不同的棋局变幻。两军对垒，这是智力的角逐，行兵布阵，是思维的较量。经常下棋，能锻炼思维，保持智力聪慧不衰。特别是中老年人，经常弈棋可以保持活跃的脑神经活动，防止老年性痴呆。与棋友会棋，切磋技艺，能增进朋友之间的往来，特别是中老年人，下棋作为一种活动，还可使人精神愉快，有所寄托，使身心舒畅。

2 Essentials

A good environment is prerequisite for chess playing in that one run takes a long time, and so a good mood is necessary. Generally the best places

2 养生要领

首先要选择良好的下棋环境。一盘棋的胜负，往往难以在短时间内决出，对弈

are the chess room and home, where tea and snacks are easily available, which add to comfort. Outdoor playing can occur under the shade in summer or spring or autumn, but be wary of the wind.

双方会较长时间处在单一环境中，因而要选择良好的环境，以使身心舒适。一般来说，可选择在棋室或家中对弈，这样能方便地获取茶水、点心等，增加对弈舒适度。若在户外对弈，夏天可在树阴之下，凉爽而不受暴晒；春秋季节宜选择风小之时，避风、避寒而弈；冬天应避免在户外对弈。

Playing with a chess pal of a similar level can be mutually beneficial in terms of challenge and growth, which sustains passion for the game.

其次要选择水平相当的棋友。下棋既是一种雅趣，也是一个学习提高的过程，因此与水平相当或稍高的棋友下棋，才能更好地提高自身的棋艺。若总是与水平低的棋友下棋，胜利得来太易，对棋的热情反而会很快消退。

Be sure to stretch oneself in the intervals. Being static physically for a long game is bad for blood circulation, especially in the case of those who crouch or sit on a low stool, where paralyzed and hurting legs would ensue, and a sudden standing-up would cause low blood pressure temporarily by body position, which is fatal to the elders. So one should take advantages of the time for the other's move to exercise a little, such as standing up slowly, stretching oneself, moving the neck, shoulders, waist and hips, to ensure smooth circulation of qi and blood.

再者，利用棋局间隙活动身体。在对弈过程中，双方往往都会长时间处在一种姿势，直至棋局结束，这样不利于周身气血的流通，尤其对于深蹲或坐低凳弈棋的人，骤然站起会引起体位性低血压，老年人甚至会因此而危及生命。所以弈棋期间，可在等待对方落子的间隙起身稍作活动，以流通气血。

3 Keys

3 注意事项

Chess playing is a beneficial activity. But it

下棋固然是有益的活

should be moderate, otherwise it will do harms to health. Therefore, we should be cautious about the following taboos.

Do not play chess right after meals. Rest a while for better digestion and absorption, otherwise the brain grows tense, taking more blood supply from the digestive system, thus indigestion and related disease.

Do not sit for a long time. Have some movements like standing, stretching legs and twisting head, shoulders, waist and arms to maintain proper qi and blood circulation. Sitting for a long time will lead to obstructed backflow of venous blood in lower limbs, causing numbness and pains.

Do not take victory hard. Do not work oneself up in aggressiveness, but have the broad mind to laugh failure off. Calm down with skill practice as the aim. Over excitement in the elders triggers stroke and breast-pang.

Do not burn midnight oil. Declining in physiological functions, the elders are prone to fatigue that is hard for recovery. Lack of rest at night undermines the immune system and diseases slip in.

动，但不掌握适度，以致废寝忘食，反而有损于健康，故而应注意以下几点：

饭后不宜立即弈棋 饭后应稍事休息，以利于对食物的消化吸收。若饭后立即面对棋局，必然会使大脑紧张，减少消化道的供血，导致消化不良和肠胃病。

棋局间要适度活动 下棋时间要适度，要注意活动肢体，适当地站立、伸腿、活动颈、肩、腰、臂，保持良好的气血循环。坐的时间过长会使下肢静脉血液回流不畅，出现下肢麻木、疼痛等症。

不要得失心过重 两军对垒，总会有输有赢，不要因为棋局的输赢而过分激动或争强好胜，要有一笑对输赢的宽阔胸怀，不计较得失，以探讨技艺为出发点和目的，才能心平气和。过度激动对老年人十分有害，往往可诱发中风、心绞痛。

不要挑灯夜战 老年人生理功能减退，容易疲劳，且难以快速恢复，若夜间休息减少，身体抵抗力下降，容易发生疾病。

Section 3 Calligraphy and Painting

第3节 书画养生

As a traditional means of regimen, calligraphy and painting create an atmosphere where one collects spirit and calms down, which cultivates the mind, invigorates intelligence and pleases the heart.

书指书法，画指绘画。书画养生是通过凝神静气、心神专注于书法绘画中，用以陶冶性情、活跃心智、愉悦心理的一种养生方法，是传统的养生方法之一。

Chinese calligraphy and painting, especially the former, is an art with a strong national characteristic. More than a way to express ideas, calligraphy boasts various artistic ways of writing the Chinese character, which are so intoxicating that both copying in study and dancing the brush casually put one in a merry mood. Calligraphy and painting, with study, health-building and artistic enjoyment all in one, is a great way of cultivating health.

中国书画，特别是书法，是汉字独有的艺术，是具有浓郁民族特色的艺术表现形式。汉字的书写不仅仅是一种表意的方法，而且通过对字的不同书写手法，形成了一种独特的艺术形式。几千年传承的书法，无论楷书、行书，还是草书，其神韵、美妙都足以令人神往。无论是临摹习学，还是信手挥毫，都能让人有一种心旷神怡的良好心境。在生活中经常练字或作画，融学习、健身及艺术欣赏于一体，是养生的良好途径。

1 Mechanism

1 养生机理

Calligraphy and painting regulate qi and blood, and smooth meridians and collaterals. It requires concentration of the mind, harmony of heart and qi, and a flexible coordination of moving the hand, wrist, elbow and hip, so as to involve qi and strength of the whole body. Hence a smooth flow of

书画可调血气，通经脉。写字作画必须集中精力，心正气和，灵活而协调地运用手、腕、肘、臂等部位，从而调动全身的气和力。这样，身体内气血畅达，五脏和谐，百

qi and blood, harmony among the five solid organs, dredged collaterals, regulated visceral functions, balanced excitement and restriction in the brain nerves and naturally vigorous spirit.

脉疏通，机体各部分功能得到调整，大脑神经兴奋和抑制得到平衡，精力自然旺盛。

The painter's enchantment with the creation and strokes during painting form a unified and harmonic relation among his spirit, movement and breath, thus regulating the nervous system and function of heart and lungs. One practicing calligraphy and painting can remove strain and show composure in a crisis in that he must control the brush with his concentrated will, that is, to master "movement " with "quiescence ".

书画活动可以静心宁神，使心理达到平衡。书画作者在创作过程中往往注意力高度集中在构思上，运笔时呼吸与笔画的运行自然地协调配合，形成了精神、动作、呼吸三者的和谐统一关系，对人的身心健康、神经系统和心肺等脏腑均能起到调节作用。作画习书必须用意念控制手中之笔，绝虑凝神，志趣高雅，便能以"静"制"动"，消除紧张而变得遇事沉着。

Calligraphy and painting cultivate noble sentiments, termed "book aroma" by the ancients. The book aroma adds wisdom to the atmosphere of calligraphy and painting, and also dispels gloom.

书画创作又是一个培养高尚情操的理想行为。在书画创作中体现出来的高尚情操古人称"书卷气"。这种书卷气又使书画娱乐的境界提高，从而增强了书画养生中的智慧含量和解郁力量。

So calligraphy and painting can help cure disease. In terms of psychology, regular script drives irritation away, official scrip calms one down, running and cursive scripts inject passion, so calligraphy is acclaimed as qigong and Taiji Quan on paper. Collect your spirit, concentrate your mind, calm down, set the core of breath down the abdomen and push your flexible movement with the breath, and the qi and blood of the whole body can be worked

书画也是一种防病、治病的手段。在心理方面，楷书能除烦，隶书使人恬静，行草给人激情，所以，有人称书法是纸上进行的气功和太极拳。写字要求凝神静虑，集中精力，心平气和，意沉丹田，气运形体，灵活自如地运动手、腕、臂以至全身，这就

up and organ functions regulated, hence promoting circulation and metabolism.

会自然地通融全身的气血，使体内各部机能得到调整，促进血液循环和新陈代谢。

2 Essentials

2 养生要领

It is important to get into a good habit of keeping the head erect, setting the shoulders level, spreading the chest and straightening the back, and standing with the feet parallel, which balances strain and relaxation of the gesture, thus free exertion.

习书作画要头部端正，两肩平齐，胸张背直，两脚平放，这样才能使全身松紧有度，才能在书画时养成良好的习惯，也不至于太疲倦。

It is advised to keep practicing calligraphy and painting regularly, preferably by a schedule. The regularity alone can furnish progress in art and health.

作为一种养生方法来习字绘画，要有规律地进行，最好制定并遵照一个时间表，按规划从事这一艺术，坚持下来，才能取得书画技艺方面的提高，又有养生延年方面的收获。

A calm state of mind is a must for calligraphy and painting and health therein. Chinese calligraphy and painting lay emphasis on the atmosphere, momentum and romantic charm, to achieve which, one must collect spirit and be engrossed in the brush, getting rid of worldly thoughts.

作书绘画必须要保持平静的心态，烦躁激动都难以入静，起不到养生的效果。中国书画都特别注重追求意、气、神，意指意境，气指气势，神指神韵。既要求书画时要静息凝神，精神专注，也要求全神贯注于笔端，令作品体现出自身的气势和神韵。习书时心要完全静下来，排除一切杂念，思想高度集中。

3 Keys

3 注意事项

Do not force energy in exhaustion or recovery from disease, since calligraphy and painting consume the qi and burden the frail condition.

劳累之后或病后体虚，不必强打精神，勉力而为，本已气虚，再耗气伤身，会加重身体负担，不易恢复。

Do not take up the brush in fury, astonishment, terror or bad mood, since the violent feelings block the transportation of qi movement, and so hinder fine fruit of the art, thus worsening the mood and attacking health.

大怒、惊恐或心情不舒，不宜立刻写字作画。此时气机不畅，心情难静，很难写出好字、绘出好画，会使情绪更糟，影响身体。

Do not paint or write shortly after meals, for fear of indigestion, as is mentioned above.

饭后不宜马上写字作画。饭后伏案，会使食物壅滞胃肠，不利于食物的消化吸收。

Section 4 Reading and Reciting

第4节 品读养生

Reading and reciting include reciting and savouring poetry and prose, appreciating calligraphy and painting and singing.

品读养生是指以读唱为主要方式的养生方法，包括品读诗文、吟诵歌赋、品鉴书画、学唱戏曲等。

The myriad cultural gems in the thousands of years' human history offer glorious objects for appreciation, which add to wisdom, cultivate morals and sentiments and refine life. Traditional literary works are gorgeous fountains for such nourishment.

人类在几千年的历史中积淀了无数的文化精品，是用来行养生品鉴的优秀资源。品鉴它们能增长智慧，涵养德行，陶冶情操，优化生活，归根到底就是养心。在养心这一基点上，传统诗书词画就和养生有共同的源泉。

The ancient book, scrolls of painting included, is the prime means of culture appreciation. Book fragrance is a term for the refined air of a book lover, and there are book-loving families also termed "clan of book fragrance".

传统文化都是以书为载体（包括画卷）的，书是人们品鉴文化的主要方式。古人说"书香"，把读书人脱尘出俗的气质称为"书香气"，把喜爱读书的人家称为"书香门第”,把喜爱读书的国家称为“书香国度”。要培养自身高尚的气质,多读书、读好书是非常有效的方法。

1 Mechanism

Reading nurtures the heart and pleases the spirit. Spirit nourishment is a vital notion of TCM, held to count more than physical nourishment. The great works of poetry, prose, novels and paintings with their profound literary mood, elegant sentiments and interests, inspiring spirit and insightful philosophy intoxicate and elevate the reader.

1 养生机理

读书具有养心怡神的作用。中华民族养生理念中最重要的一点是“养神”,很多养生家都认为养神重于养形。古今各种优秀的文化成果,无论是诗词、书画,还是散文、小说,那些深远的意境,优雅的情趣,激扬的精神,精深的哲理,都能使人沉醉,在心理上获得不同感受,不断提高自身的心理素养。

Reading inspires the mind. A healthy state of mind and a refined personal quality greatly furnish health. People who read a lot can always cultivate an elegant bearing and a fine realm of thought.

读书能激励心智。健康的身体需要有健康的心态,良好的素质,很重要的途径就是品读欣赏古今的文化成果。平常欣赏阅读大量的书画诗词的人,多会保有优雅的精神气质和良好的精神境界,就是得益于此。

Reading adjusts the mood. A book in hand preserves one from sadness in sorrow, frustration in setback, and rapture in favour, and he can always be philosophical, poised and elegant, unrestrained and optimistic, like the flowing cloud and a leisurely crane.

读书能调整情绪。一书在手,受苦而不悲,受挫而不馁,受宠而不惊,如闲云野鹤,能保持着一种雍容恬雅,潇洒达观的境界。

Reading postpones aging. The ancient Chinese doctors held books as a prime approach to health preservation. Aging starts with the brain, which de-

读书可延缓衰老。中国古代养生家认为,书卷乃养生第一妙物。人的衰老,首

velops with use. Reading exercises the brain and thus helps eschew Alzheimer's Disease and promotes longevity.

先是脑的衰老。大脑用则进,不用则退。读书可使脑功能得到锻炼,延缓大脑衰老,有助于预防老年性痴呆,进而延年益寿。

2 Essentials

Reading and appreciating books and paintings should keep one company throughout life, but to do it for health, we should give heed to some knacks.

2 养生要领

对于每一个人来说,品读欣赏书画都是一个需要终身矢志不渝的工程。但从养生的角度来品读欣赏文化,则需要掌握一些要领。

Have a rich variety of positive tastes. Calligraphy, painting and classic literature should all be embraced by one's appreciation. Different objects contribute more to health.

有益身心书常读 品读内容需要选择,应当有计划地购置积累积极健康高雅的书籍和画作,培养自己读书赏画的兴趣爱好。有益身心的书画应当包容广泛,不仅仅局限于一种一类,要有书法的鉴赏,名画的品鉴,名著的咀嚼,诗词的韵味,从不同的艺术角度去品味,才能有益于养生。

Develop interest to make the most out of reading. One needs a careful chew rather than skim to savour and grasp the flowing calligraphy, grand and subtle poetry, and unrestrained prose. An excellent work is worthy of repetitious recital and learning by heart. Only in this way can one draw real nutrition from reading and promote health.

要读出兴趣、读出营养 书法的秀美飘逸、雄浑豪迈,需要细细欣赏;诗词的激扬豪壮、凄婉缠绵,需要慢慢咀嚼;文章的潇洒激越,需要反复领会。养生的读书品画,不能如过眼云烟,蜻蜓点水,一部好的作品,需要仔细品味,反复吟咏,甚至熟读成诵,铭记于心,真正领会到作品的精彩,这样才能读出兴趣，吸取到营养，达到养生的目的。

Develop the appreciation into a habit. Literary appreciation is an elegant pursuit above many people. One should cultivate a constant taste for it in order to earn health. Especially the elders, who are retired without regular work to do and have an abundance of leisure, are advised to fill it with reading and try to be a connoisseur of art. It is a great way to prevent functional retrogradation, such as Alzheimer's Disease.

养成读书品画的习惯

书画欣赏是一种高雅的情趣，并不是所有人都有这样的爱好，大多需要自我培养，持之以恒，才能养成品读欣赏的能力，成为养生的有益方法。特别是老年人，离开了工作岗位，没有规律性的工作做，又多半在生活上静多动少，可以用读书来填补这一空缺，从而养成一种勤读书、善品鉴、会欣赏的习惯，这对于预防很多老年性的生理退化，如老年性痴呆，都是很好的途径。

3 Keys

Several keys in reading should be observed before it can promote health.

3 注意事项

品读具有良好的养生效果，但也要注意正确的品读习惯，否则达不到养生的目的。

Establish confidence. Do not feel awe-stricken by mistakenly taking literary appreciation for the privilege of the literati. But be confident to chew and savour excellent works and enjoy their flavour, turning it into a habit, and the level of appreciation can be lifted, which benefits health more.

建立品读养生的信心

首先，对诗词书画、妙文博论的爱好和欣赏并不仅仅是读书人的专利，要意识到欣赏品读具有养生的良好效果，并不仅仅只是闲来无事的浏览，要选择一些优秀文化成果，细细咀嚼，反复品味，品出了其中的真味，发现了其中的情趣，养成品鉴阅读的习惯，才能登堂入室，取得理

Read widely. Do not limit the reading material to popular novels, but hug all cultural treasure of poetry, calligraphy and painting, prose, philosophy, at home and abroad. Besides the materials above, philosophy and popular novels can also be embraced into reading, which provides overall nutrition.

Develop reading into a habit. Make a reading schedule and observe it; do not read shortly after meals for better digestion and blood circulation; do not sit reading for a long time, but season it with a little exercises such as stretching oneself, changing reading gesture and looking into the distance, or intersperse it with other health-building practice. Be sure not to read for a long time lying in bed or sitting on the toilet, which hinders blood circulation.

想的养生效果。

要选择广泛的品读内容

不要仅仅局限于通俗流行的小说故事，应该根据养生的要求，唐诗宋词、书法画卷、散文哲学、古今中外各种优秀文化，都应根据自身的条件纳入养生品读的范围，才能广泛获取营养。

养成良好的品读习惯

如制定一个适合自身的品读时间表，持之以恒；饭后不宜立即读书，以防影响消化机能，应先活动一会儿再开始品读，使气血流通；不宜长时间坐着不动，要注意调节肢体活动；不宜单一进行某一种活动，品读期间要适当地改换姿势，如极目远眺、伸腰蹬腿、听听音乐等，或者穿插施行其他养生方法；注意良好的体位，躺在床上、蹲在马桶上均不宜长时间阅读，容易阻滞气血流行。

Section 5 Fishing

第5节 垂钓养生

Fishing, which calms, concentrates, relaxes and refreshes the mind, is a positive way to nurture the temperament and intelligence, especially to the old and the frail and those in recovery.

垂钓养生是指通过钓鱼为主的野外活动，以得到恬淡凝注、悠闲清爽心境的养生方法。自古以来，垂钓就是人们所喜爱的活动。尤其对久病康复，年老体弱者，是一种积极的修身养性，益智养神的好方法。

1 Mechanism

Health strengthening. The beautiful nature is an ideal place for health preservation. Fishing by the sparkling lake or lush field with fresh air and sunshine, free from pollution and noise, benefits health immensely. Fresh air furnishes fine physiological reaction; ultraviolet in the sunshine enhances blood circulation in the skin and organs, thus promoting metabolism, which shows in healthy skin and ruddy complexion. In addition, fishing by serene waterside diminishes strain of the ears caused by noise pollution in the city, thus preserving hearing.

Spirit setting. A settled heart is crucial to the smooth transportation of yin and yang and qi and blood. Fishing in the green sets the heart down in leisure and worldly thoughts are naturally gone. So fishing elevates the mind and invigorates physiological functions, hence a fine way to preserve a healthy psychology, shutting the door on melancholia, depression, agitation and hot temper. After fishing, people go home in a relaxed spirit and tired body,

1 养生机理

强身健体 环境优美的大自然，本身就是养生保健的良好场所。垂钓于江河湖畔，空气清新，阳光充足，避开污染，没有噪声，有碧波粼粼的湖光，有苍青翠绿的田园，有利于身体健康。经常呼吸新鲜空气，可引起人体各种相应的良好生理反应；经日光中紫外线照射后，可以增强皮肤和内脏器官的血液循环，促进体内的新陈代谢，可使人获得健美的皮肤、红润健康的面容，有助于保持良好的身体功能。另外，城市噪声已构成环境的严重污染，经常到空旷宁静的水域垂钓，幽静的环境能消除两耳的疲劳，有助于保持良好的听觉功能。

宁神静心 心神的静谧对人体阴阳气血的运行调理非常重要。垂钓在青山绿水，薄雾蒙蒙之中，投竿于湖塘江河，眼神贯注着浮漂的动静，心神宁静闲逸，会自然而然地排除杂念，达到静心怡神的功效。因此，垂钓有助于提高生活情趣，活跃各

fall into a sound sleep and wake up more energetic, as is shown in the fact that many who suffer from insomnia find it easier to sleep after fishing.

种生理功能，是保持心理健康，防止抑郁症、精神沮丧及焦急、暴躁等不良情绪的好方法。而垂钓归来，精神松弛，心舒体倦，又可获得香甜一梦，醒来一身轻松。许多失眠患通过钓鱼而能安眠就是最好的说明。

Temperament transforming. The tranquil fishing environment, concentration and joy in fish on hook can turn impetuosity and fury into peacefulness and leisure, so one feels purged and merges into nature.

移情易性 垂钓环境的清幽，垂钓所需要的专注，守候浮漂的雅致，钓来鱼儿的愉悦，都可以移浮躁于平静，转愤激于悠闲，使人融入自然，净化身心，达到移情易性的效果。

2 Essentials

2 养生要领

One had better fish in warm and mild weather rather than hot summer with the hazard of heat stroke and injury to people of cardio cerebral vascular disease triggered by heavy perspiration.

气候适宜 最好在天气暖和，气候宜人的时候从事垂钓。太热的天气容易中暑，出汗太多对心脑血管患者均不适宜。

Select fishing pals of a pleasant temperament, with whom chatting and mutual care are available.

钓友合宜 选择性情脾气相宜的钓友，既可相互照应，又可闲谈交流，于悠闲中获得一份感情的深化。

3 Keys

3 注意事项

Do not take the result seriously. Fish for fun and pleasure, and take the leisurely state of mind as the best fruit.

得失心不要太重 垂钓以悠闲娱乐、愉悦身心为主，收获大固然可喜，空手而回也无需失落，把垂钓的良好心境作为最大的成果，才是养生的要领。

Do not fish beyond one's physical condition.

把握自身的健康状态

Fishing takes a long time, plus violent elements in nature, so it is advised to measure oneself and be sure of one's physical endurance in case of emergency.

垂钓活动常常需要较长的时间,需要正确估计自身的健康水平,天有不测风云,风雨无常,烈日暴虐,身体需要有一定承受能力,以防意外发生。

Try not to fish alone. The middle-aged and the old need mutual care in the event of physical emergency and sudden changes in the elements.

尽可能不独钓。孤身独处并不利于垂钓养生,特别是中老年人,无论身体的意外,还是气候环境的突变,都需要相互关照。

Section 6 Gardening and Petting

第6节 花鸟养生

Growing flowers and keeping pets can contribute to health physically and mentally, apart from beauty and amusement. Luxuriant plants render the home calm and pleasant, while lovely pets bring vitality into the family.

花鸟养生指通过培植花卉、驯养鸟兽宠物、养鱼等,达到愉悦身心的养生方法。尽管现代人们居住环境拥挤,很少能拥有供栽花种树的庭院,但在有限的空间里,只要兴趣所在,养花种草、养鸟训宠物,赏心悦目,可锻炼身体,可修身养性。即便在阳台少量养些花草,也可以给生活带来美的享受,绿的生机,花的芬芳,带来好的心情和体魄,别有一番情趣。繁茂的花草还能在家庭中创造一种恬静和快乐的气氛,使人获得精神上的愉悦和享受,消除生活中的单调和烦闷。至于宠物的活泼可爱,亲昵怡人,更能增加生活的气息。

1 Mechanism

Regulating the mood. The stressful modern life with pollution in air, food and noise is apt to be annoying and injure psychological health. But plants, birds, fishes, cats and dogs can calm one down quickly and regulate the state of mind, especially for the elders, who can take a walk with the bird cage, or the dog in the park or under the shade, enjoying the twitter of birds or admiring colourful flowers and breathing fresh air, much pleased in spirit.

1 养生机理

调节情绪 现代人的生活环境、工作环境充满压力、竞争,也充斥着空气、食物、噪声的污染,很容易使人烦躁,情绪不稳定,影响正常的心理健康。若能时常在家中侍弄花草,或逗弄鸟儿,或观赏金鱼,或与驯养的宠物嬉戏,很快可使情绪平静下来,起到调节心境的养生作用。特别是老年人,手提鸟笼,或溜宠物,在花园,在树阴,在路边花坛,倾听鸟儿的鸣叫,欣赏美丽的鲜花,呼吸清新的空气,能愉悦情志,是非常好的养生方法。

Keeping qi and blood smooth. TCM maintains that a fixed gesture blocks the circulation of qi and blood, causing functional deficiency which, however, is not what we can say about gardening and petting. In so doing limbs are in frequent movement, eyesight is nourished and mind is pleasantly distracted, hence conducive to smooth blood flow, relaxed spirit and boomed metabolism that restores and enhances the function of the heart and lungs.

疏通气血 中医认为,一种相对固定的姿势都会影响气血流通,导致人体机能的障碍。看电视,读书作画,写作,以及其他工作,都需要保持某一姿势,而观花赏鱼,逗弄笼鸟等,既可活动肢体,也可休养视力,转移脑力,使气血流畅,精神松弛。

2 Essentials

Make full use of unoccupied space and time. Enliven the room with the use of every possible inch of space and occupy one's intervals between work tending the plants and pets. With the pets, birds or plants on the balcony, roof or in the living room,

2 养生要领

充分利用闲散空间与时间 有私家庭院者应当合理规划,选择种植一些花草树木蔬菜,精心培植,利于欣赏。城市居民在高楼林立

life will be brighten up and health will be improved.

中,可在阳台、客厅、露台、屋顶等处,根据兴趣所在,或驯宠物,或养鸟,或种花卉,不要让室内了无生气。有了这些,就必须经常去侍弄它们,无形中增加了生活情趣,增加了活动身体的机会,丰富了增进健康的途径。

Develop interest. Love the plants and pets and you will find their intelligence. Although not everyone is interested in plants and pets, a long-term accompany and appreciation will raise the interest in and establish emotional bond with them.

培养观赏逗弄兴趣 对于花卉虫鱼,或者猫狗宠物,不是任何人都具备兴趣。人们应该把这些作为养生的方法,渐渐培养自己的兴趣,经常细心观赏,耐心侍弄,建立和它们的感情,发现它们的灵性。

Carry it along. Only constancy and persistence in the two practices can enhance the interest in life and further health!

持之以恒 半途而废的任何养生方法,都起不到养生作用,只有坚持下来,品到个中妙趣,才能深刻地体会到那种途径的养生乐趣和良好的养生效果。

3 Keys

Take family members into considerations. If someone is allergic to the odor or feathers of a certain pet, do not keep it. If there are kids, it is proper not to keep large pets or birds in case kids are injured.

3 注意事项

顾及家庭成员的适应性

并不是所有人都适应猫狗鸟类,如有人对某种宠物的气味、毛羽过敏,则这类宠物显然不宜在家庭中驯养。如家庭中有小孩子则最好不要养大型宠物或鸟类,以防危害到幼儿。

Be hygiene in gardening and petting. Train the cats and dogs in toilet habit, be sure to vaccinate

要有良好的卫生习惯

一方面要训导好宠物的卫生

them, clean their hair or feather and sterilize the place in case of disease. And remember to weed the garden, drive worms and spray leaves to keep them glistening.

习惯，另一方面需注意预防宠物病，及时清理打扫粪便羽毛，经常进行消毒，以预防豢养宠物可能带来的疾病。养花草时，要注意定期清除花盆内的杂草和植株上的害虫，定期用水喷冲叶片上的灰尘，以保持清洁。

Section 7 Travel

第7节 旅游养生

As is known to all, travel relaxes the mind, eliminates strain, restores energy and pleases the spirit.

旅游养生是通过长距离旅游、远足郊游，以观赏风景、游乐嬉戏的方式，来舒缓心情、缓解压力、恢复精力、愉悦心境的养生方法。

Its comprehensive benefits lie in enjoying nature and cultural sites, exercising the physique and tempering the will, broadening the horizon, and venting sentiments. The ancient Chinese drew inspiration from hiking a lot and composed many famous poems. Most temples are situated in marvelous landscape where people can draw the essence of nature, thus a better place for cultivating health and character.

旅游是一种综合性的养生方法，不仅可以欣赏自然美景、人文景观，又可锻炼身体、锤炼意志，更可以开阔眼界，拓展知识，舒畅情怀，锻炼身体，增长见识，是一种有益于身心调养的活动。古人非常推崇远足郊游活动，特别是文人墨客，常悠游于山水之间，激发创作灵感，很多佳句诗作由此而成。尤其是道家、佛家的庵、观、寺、庙，大多建立在环山抱水，风景优美之处，得山水之清气，修身养性。

1 Mechanism

Enjoying nature and breathing fresh air. People are refreshed by air in mountains, forests, rivers and seas. Fresh air means the air with a large proportion of oxygen anion and a small one of sulphur dioxide and dust. Researches indicate that a concentration of oxygen anion smaller than 25/m^3 would cause headache, sickness, dizziness and fatigue, while that larger than 10 000/m^3 vitalizes metabolism, cheers one up and makes one energetic and improves his appetite, and that larger than 100 000/m^3 can cure diseases. So fresh air is essential to health. The oxygen anion likes the sea and waterfall best, though air in the countryside and mountain is sufficiently fresh. So, one should travel more to inhale fresh air in health pursuit and disease treatment.

Cultivating character and broadening horizon. Negative feelings simply melt away when one climbs to the top of mountains for a grand view or enjoys the music of waves or roams in the woods. Poets, musicians and painters never fail to be inspired by the vast expanse of grassland and rushing rivers and surging seas.

1 养生机理

领略自然风光，呼吸新鲜空气 当人们投身于大自然，欣赏领略深山密林、江河湖海、溪泉潭瀑、田园花草风光，能使人耳目为之一新；呼吸大自然的新鲜空气，神情为之一爽。新鲜空气主要指含污染物，如 SO_2、粉尘等极少，负氧离子含量高，清新、洁净的空气。研究表明，负氧离子含量若小于 25 个/m^3，人就会头痛、恶心、晕眩、疲劳；含量大于 1 万个/m^3，人就会因代谢活跃，心情舒畅，精力充沛，食欲增加；大于 10 万个/m^3，就可用来治疗某些疾病。可见，空气是否清新对人的健康很重要。乡村、山地负离子则较多，海边、瀑布等地含量最多。经常能够去空气新鲜的地方游玩，对人的身体会有好处，既可预防疾病，保持身体健康，又能对某些疾病起到良好的康复治疗作用。

陶冶性情，增长知识 登高望远、临水听涛、濒海观潮、花丛漫步、山谷跋涉、林中暇游之时，广阔无垠的原野，苍翠幽深的崇山峻岭、变幻莫测的云雾，奔腾不息的江河大海，可以使人神清意爽，消除不良情绪。诗人、音乐家、书画家更可以从中找到艺术创造的灵感。所以旅游不但可以陶冶性情，还能增长知识，开阔眼界，既有修身养性的作用，又能提高文化和鉴赏水平。

Building the physique. It is natural that hiking exercises limbs, conducive to smooth blood circulation, flexible joints and strong tendon and bones. The elder do not have to aim higher than a leisurely stroll. And the weighty can travel a lot to lose weight.

锻炼体魄　在远足跋山涉水之中，可以活动身体筋骨关节，锻炼体魄，使人气血流通，关节灵活，筋骨强健。年老体弱者不必求快求远，可于漫步闲游中获得锻炼。对体胖者，旅行是减轻体重的好方法。

2 Essentials

2 养生要领

Targeting at suburbs. Hiking in the suburb for a short time benefits health enormously. Go to a nearby countryside with your family or friends, and the joy and fresh air immediately alleviate fatigue and stress.

郊游为主，适当远游　他乡异国的远游固然很好，但不可能经常进行，最具养生价值的是短距离、短时间的郊外远足。宜选取较近的田园旷野、江河湖海、林谷幽泉，或一家游乐，或呼朋聚会，以欢愉畅快的情绪，呼吸新鲜空气，缓解疲劳，消除压力。

Joining in group activities. Group activities promote communication and emotion in a cheerful atmosphere. While traveling alone gives rise to loneliness, a negative feeling injuring health.

适当的群体活动　群体活动既能沟通情感，相互交流，又可制造出更多的欢乐气氛。适宜的游伴有利于身心愉快感的形成，独自一人的旅游容易产生孤独感，不利于身心健康。

3 Keys

3 注意事项

Be moderate in labour and mind safety. Inordinate activities do harm to the viscera. And be wary

劳逸适度，注意安全　过度活动反倒容易影响健

of external dangers as well as one's own health problems, such as heart disease, hypertension and neurotic disease in participating in certain sorts of activities and note the degree.

康，甚或导致组织器官的损伤。旅游时应注意防范野外环境的不安全因素，另外还得考虑自身的健康因素，如患有心脏病、高血压、神经精神类疾病时，必须注意活动的种类和强度，避免发生意外。

Do not be pretentious. Do not pretend to be man enough in climbing, swimming, hiking and adventure, especially in the case of the elders and the frail.

不要做超过自身能力和承受力的攀爬游泳、登高涉险，必须量力而为，不可硬充好汉，争强好胜，特别是年老体弱，或身体状态不好时，更要倍加小心。

Take the season into account. Spring is ideal for hiking, and summer for the sea and forest, while the crisp autumn provides a golden time for all activities. Take care to escape the scorching sun at noon, and one can choose to paddle on the lake of lotuses in the evening when and where coolness reigns.

注意季节因素 一般来说，逢春季应顺应自然之生机，踏青便是一项有益活动。夏季天气炎热，若去海滨或森林，则可避暑养气。若旅游外出，也应择时而往，避免太阳直射，尤避免长时间在阳光下暴晒。傍晚时分，泛舟湖上，观赏荷花，能使人顿感凉爽。秋高气爽的季节，是旅游的最佳时候。无论登山临水，还是游览古迹，均不失为最使人惬意的黄金季节。

Section 8 Tea Drinking

第8节 品茗养生

In tea drinking, one savours the subtle fragrance and rejoices in communication with tea pals,

品茗养生是指在品赏茶饮的过程中，享受茶茗的韵

hence attaining health.

味、茶友交流的乐趣、饮茶趣谈的氛围，从而获得养生保健的效果。

Among three natural drinks in the world, the other two being coffee and coco, tea is spread most widely. WHO dictated that tea is the best drink for the middle-aged and the old. China claims credit for her long history of tea culture. The ancient Chinese endowed the tea with ten virtues: dispersing melancholy, sobering the sleepy, enlivening the energy, curing disease, serving ceremony, showing reverence, amusing the palate, nourishing the viscera, furnishing the Tao and refining the spirit.

茶与咖啡、可可被公认为世界三大天然饮料，而以茶叶的饮用流传最广。世界卫生组织认为，茶为中老年人的最佳饮料。源远流长的中国茶文化堪称世界之最、中华“国粹”。中国古人就认为茶有十德：以茶散郁气，以茶驱睡气，以茶养生气，以茶除病气，以茶利礼仁，以茶表敬意，以茶尝滋味，以茶养身体，以茶可行道，以茶可雅志。

The ancients held up as the essence of tea aesthetics “flavour savouring”, a taste of subtle sweetness after bitterness. It is for the enjoyment of solitude, but admiring it at a tea party can be a more enlightening experience and the cheerful atmosphere better promotes health.

古人认为真正的喝茶不为解渴，只在辨味，在“品”，体味那苦涩中一点回甘。品茗固然可以独享，但更多的则是茶友的共同品赏，才能品出个中的真味，达到养生的境界。

1 Mechanism

1 养生机理

Refreshing the sleepy. The tea is always a saviour to people who are fatigued, sleepy and drunk.

提神醒脑 茶具有提神醒脑的功效。对于健康长寿者来说，饮茶更是功不可没。没有茶，人就难得清醒脱困。所以疲倦、劳累、酒困之后，人们都寄望于饮茶解困、消倦、醒酒。

Medium for chatting. Drink tea not only for elegance, but also for the chatting atmosphere that

趣谈养性 品茗养生之“品”，不仅要求细细体会茶

pleases the spirit, as is described in the play *Tea House* (Cha Guan) by Lao She, an illustrious Chinese writer. And people drink in the modern tea house savouring life and regulating mood.

中滋味，还包括对因茶而来的各种有益身心健康因素的体味。品茗养生之乐并不全在于品饮，更在于茶友之间天南海北地聊侃，交流趣谈，从而愉悦身心。作家老舍的《茶馆》，以及现实生活中的茶厅茶馆，起意只在提供休闲趣谈的场所，让人们在一杯茶中体味生活，消除烦恼，平静心绪，调整情绪。

Curing disease. The tea promotes digestion, lowers the fat in the blood, helps lose weight and urinate, alleviates the swelling and inflammation, resists germ and radiation, prevents coronary heart disease, atherosclerosis and cancer, cushions exhaustion, promotes body fluid, relieves internal heat and protects teeth.

却病延年 茶的本身具有养生保健作用，茶有助消化、降血脂、减肥、利尿、消肿、抗菌消炎、抗辐射、防治冠心病、抗疲劳、防癌、抗癌、生津解渴、抗病毒、解毒、抗动脉硬化、保护牙齿等作用，经常品茶，不仅能预防疾病，还能延年益寿。

2 Essentials

Develop a habit of tea drinking. Many people worry that the dark colour of tea would affect the skin. But the fact is that the medical function of tea can eliminate accumulated pigment in the skin and thus preserve its original colour. As for the bitterness, it is actually a prelude to the subtle sweetness in its wake, where the elegant pleasure of tea drinking abides.

2 养生要领

养成饮茶的习惯 很多人不喜饮茶，认为茶水的颜色深暗而会影响皮肤颜色。其实，茶叶的保健作用本身就可以清除皮肤的色素沉着，保持皮肤的正常颜色，有美肤效果。至于茶饮的苦涩，也只是未解其中味，坚持品饮一段时间，习惯之后，就能体会到苦涩之后的甘甜回味，从而得到饮茶之乐。

Eschew artificial drinks. The rich variety of

用茶饮代替其他饮料

tea—green tea, white tea, yellow tea, brown tea and black tea, each with its own nutrition and fragrance—offers a wide choice for people with different physical needs.

茶水含有天然的营养成分，是上佳的饮料。茶叶种类繁多，香味清雅，且绿茶、白茶、黄茶、青茶、红茶等，寒温各具，各类人群均可找到适合自己的茶叶品种，这种特点是其他饮料所不具备的。

Savour tea in communication. Entertaining the guest with tea at home or meeting friends in the tea house, one can enjoy tea while savouring life and the mood is well regulated.

邀朋结友共品茗 品茗，最好的方式是与茶友共同品味。无论何种茶，在茶友的共同品赏中，其价值都不尽在饮茶中，而在品茶的乐趣，品茶中的交流。客人来家以茶相待，或邀约于茶馆，一杯茶在手，一边品味茶饮，一边品味人生，吐出腹中牢骚，抒发心胸浩气，可达到舒展情绪的良好效果。

A quality tea cup is indispensable. If you cannot be fully equipped as those in the coastal regions south of the Yangtze River, who are particular about the elegant tea set for the tea art, you should at least prepare a pottery or porcelain cup, and cup of stainless steel or enamel will not do.

茶具不可或缺 品茗需要特定器具和茶叶。茶叶可根据喜好，无论绿茶花茶，红茶黑茶，均有益于养生。而饮茶还应当配备相应的茶具。江南沿海地区功夫茶的器具非常讲究，品茶也很讲究。内地和北方相对较少使用专门的茶具，但至少要有专用的茶具，最好是陶、瓷杯具，不锈钢和搪瓷杯并不是饮茶的好器具。

3 Keys

Avoid making the tea too strong. Extremely strong tea harms the stomach. So be mild in your

3 注意事项

浓淡适宜 茶的浓淡可根据个人喜好和茶的种类而

freedom to make tea. A serious warning to the vantage drinkers who, with the palate increasingly insensitive to bitterness, would make their tea stronger and stronger unconsciously. Generally 3 - 4 grams of leaves is appropriate. In the case of green tea, pour in 300 ml of boiled water at the temperature of 80-90 degrees Celsius, let it brew for 1-3 minutes and drink it, and it can be refilled 3 times; brown tea and black tea like boiling water, but the best result can only be attained by special cup and method; note each kind of tea requires a method suited to its character. The curing function of the tea can only be brought about by habitual drinking, so people are not recommended to drink only for sobering or the subtle sweetness.

Avoid drinking at the wrong time. Do not drink tea after a meal or before sleep, as tea stimulates the brain, which affects digestion and sleep.

Try not to drink tea left over from the previous day. Such tea would go rotten in summer, yet even in winter it is not good to keep tea soaked for too long. So newly made tea is preferable.

调整，但不宜过浓，过浓则伤胃。一般来说，干茶一次用3～4克为宜。其中，绿茶用300毫升80～90℃热水冲泡1～3分钟后品饮，可反复加水三次；青茶、红茶用沸水冲泡，为达到最佳的品饮效果，最好使用专门的器具和手法；其他茶类则根据茶叶的各自特性进行冲泡。品茗养生的目的是利用茶叶防病保健，因此重在养成习惯和爱好，日日品饮，渐渐积累养生效果，决不能追求浓茶极苦回甘的口感和快速醒神的作用。

掌握品茶时间 大部分人在饱餐后、睡觉前均不宜喝茶，更忌浓茶，茶对大脑的刺激作用会影响食物的消化，也会影响睡眠。

隔夜茶最好不饮 有人认为茶叶浸泡时间太久，会有过多的单宁酸溶解于茶叶中，对健康不利，也有研究认为并不构成对健康的影响。但不管结论如何，浸泡时间太长，特别是炎夏时节，茶水容易变质，故饮茶以新鲜泡制的为好，特别是隔夜茶，放置时间若过久，则不要饮用。

Chapter 5 Breathing (Qigong) Exercise Approach to Health Preservation

第5章 功法养生

Qigong exercise means exercising the body led by the mind and regulating breath to go with it, hence dredging meridians and collaterals and blood flow and toning function of viscera. It dates back to the remote antiquity. As is recorded in *Chronicles by Lü Buwei* (Lü Shi Chun Qiu), the tribe of Yao, famous king in the primeval tribal period, lived in a damp and cold place, and so suffered from blocked and slow-flowing circulation of qi and blood, shrunken tendon and bone, and swollen legs and feet and had difficulty in walk. So the people danced to promote blood flow and lubricate joints. It is based on the spontaneous health-preserving exercise of the primitive people that the ancient breathing exercises were born and developed by exploration and practice of doctors of later generations into the various breathing exercises with characteristics in the major forms of physical exercise, breath regulating exercise and spirit calming exercise.

功法养生，是以意识为主导，通过形体的导引运动，配合呼吸吐纳，来畅通经络气血、调节脏腑机能，而达到强身健体、延年益寿、促进身心健康目的的养生方法。养生功法源远流长，《吕氏春秋》记载，原始氏族部落时期的陶唐氏部落，由于天常阴雨，而水道淤塞不畅，居地阴凉潮湿，而容易导致人体内气血抑郁瘀滞，筋骨萎缩，腿脚肿胀，活动困难。于是人们就编创舞蹈来宣导气血，通利关节，以形体运动的方式来养生保健。古代的养生功法正是起源于原始人类的这种自我运动保健行为，我国历代医家和养生家在不断的探索和实践中，创造出了许多具有鲜明特色的，以形体运动、调节气息、宁静心神为主要形式的养生功法。

Section 1 Health Preservation Functions of Qigong

第1节 功法的养生作用

Through movement, daoyin, breathing, mind concentrating and resting, traditional Chinese exercises can promote the circulation of qi, blood and meridians, regulate the organ functions and minds, cultivate origin qi and strengthen the body, bones and sinews.

中国传统养生功法，通过运动导引、呼吸调息、意守静养各种手段和方法，来达到畅通气血经络、调节脏腑机能、和畅精神情志、培育元真之气、强健躯体筋骨的养生保健功效。

1 Clearing Channels and Circulation of Qi and Blood

1 通畅经络气血

The body channels make up a special web that transports qi and blood, connects organs and limbs, top and feet, and interior and exterior, receives sensory messages and regulates body functions. By regular circulation and communication, the system of meridians and collaterals incorporates all the organs, senses, limbs, bones, skin and flesh into an organic whole, thus guaranteeing normal life activities.

经络是运行全身气血，联络脏腑肢节，沟通上下内外，感应传导信息和调节人体功能的特殊网络系统。经络相贯，遍布全身，通过有规律的循行和联络交会，组成了经络系统，把人体五脏六腑、肢体官窍及筋骨皮肉等紧密地联结成统一的有机整体，从而保证了人体生命活动的正常进行。

The TCM qigong regulates the channel system by various means, major ones being three: stretching the limbs with muscles and tendon to the fullest, like yoga, thus dredging the channels and blood flow, as in sinew-transforming exercise (Yi Jin Jing); stretching the end of limbs so as to invigorate qi movement in the channels, the end being taken as root of the channels in TCM, while the head and organs their end, as in the exercise body-

中医养生功法通过各种手段和方法对人体的经络系统进行调节，从而达到疏通经络、畅通气血的功效。具体而言有以下三种形式：其一，通过肢体的抻拉，牵拉肌肉经筋，进而疏通经络，畅通气血，如“易筋经”功法中大部分动作都是通过抻筋拔

mind exercise (Xing Shen Zhuang), which moves the head and the end of limb to trigger all the channels and push blood flow; keeping the mind reigning, or tapping and massaging certain channels or acupuncture points on them, so as to fuel the qi movement in the channels.

骨、牵拉肢体来引动经络、调畅气机；其二，通过牵动经络之根结调动经络气机，经络学说把四肢末端视为经络的根本，而头与躯干的内脏部位为它结束的标位，如“形神庄”功法依据此理论，安排头部和四肢末端的动作，来引动全身经络、畅通周身气血；其三，通过意守或拍打按摩某经络或其上的穴位，来激发经络气机。

2 Regulating Visceral Functions

A harmony of visceral functions guarantees normal life. The qigong of TCM aims to regulate organ functions and attain their stability, to which there are three ways: dredging channels of the body, which are closely related to organs, such as 8-brocade exercise (Ba Duan Jing), a traditional exercise combing body movement with breathing, which falls into 8 sets of movement in stretching of the body, bending forward and backward, and stretching and bending of limbs, matched with breathing, so as to exercise the organs; regulating organs by different pronunciation, which leads the entry and exit of qi movement of organs, such as six-character chant exercise (Liu Zi Jue), in which the pronunciations of “si, he, hu, xü, chui, and xi”, accompanied with leading movement, serve to regulate organ functions; breathing by the abdomen that raises and lowers qi movement of organs.

2 调节脏腑机能

脏腑功能活动的稳定协调是人体生命活动得以正常的重要保证。中医养生功法就是通过多种形式的手段和方法来协调脏腑的功能活动，以维护其系统的稳定，从而避免和纠正脏腑功能太过或不及的病理状态。具体而言，其调节脏腑机能方式有以下三种：其一，通过经络系统，调整脏腑机能，脏腑和经络密切相关，养生功法，通过畅通经络，进而调节脏腑，如八段锦，它是形体活动与呼吸运动相结合的传统运动，其八个动作分别以躯体的伸展、俯仰，肢体的屈伸运动，伴随呼吸来加强对五脏六腑的功能性锻炼；其二，通过发音调整脏腑机能，引导脏腑气机的开合出入，如“六字诀”通过呬、呵、呼、嘘、吹、嘻六个字的不同发音，配合一定的动作导引，以调节不同的脏腑机能；其三，通过呼吸吐纳，尤其是腹式呼吸，来导引脏腑气机的升降。

3 Harmonizing Spirit and Temperament

The qigong of TCM improves spirit of the exercisers, calming them down and cheering them up, from the following aspects: It emphasizes the reign of will throughout the process, which is shown in relaxing the mind, matching movement with spirit, concentrating on the postures and moving qi with them. The key is to merge movement and will in one, conducive to calming down; the qigong improve spirit by such physical means as leading body movement, stretching tendon and bones and channels, dredging qi and blood circulation and tuning qi movement of organs, as is evident in the saying "A well-tuned breath ensures fine spirit"; certain moves can regulate the mind directly. Holding palms in the Buddhist way at the chest, for instance, can collect mind and settle breath. And the posture of "dragon stretching the claw" in sinew-transforming exercise (Yi Jin Jing), can disperse the knotted liver qi and so cheers one up, by turning the body, stretching hands left and right and bending, thus the two sides get tense and relaxed alternately.

3 和畅精神情志

中医养生功法能有效地改善人体的精神心理状态，许多练功者都在习练养生功法后，感到心情舒畅，心态平和。中医养生功法产生心理效应的机理可概括为以下三点：其一，养生功法的锻炼十分强调将意识的运用贯穿始终，即做到精神放松、形意相合、神注庄中、气随庄动。在练功过程中，注重形体导引与调神相配合，做到形神合一，从而有利于心神的宁静。其二，养生功法通过动作导引，抻筋拔骨、牵引经筋、经络，畅通气血，调畅脏腑经络气机，从而改善精神情志，所谓“气和则志达”。其三，养生功法中有些特定动作对神有直接调节作用。如：养生功法中常有两掌合于胸前的动作，就可以起到敛神定气的作用；如“易筋经”功法中的青龙探爪式，通过转身、左右探爪及身体前屈，使两胁交替松紧开合，以达到舒肝理气、调畅情志的功效。

4 Cultivating Primordial Qi

TCM holds jin, qi and shen as the fundamental elements of life activities. Cultivating health means preserving and strengthening the three. The exercise with its will-governing, breath regulating and postures aim at tuning body message, energy and mutual transformation, hence invigorating jin, qi and shen and attaining longevity.

4 培育元真之气

中医养生学把精气神看成是人体生命活动的基本要素，健身修炼、养生延年的根本都是保养和强壮人体内的精气神，中医养生正是以保养精气神为要务。这正是古人对人体生命过程的认识。中医养生功法通过运用意识、调节呼吸及动作来调控机体信息、能量、物质相互转化，从而使精充气足神旺，达到却病延年的目的。

5 Strengthening Sinew and Bones

Most of the qigong cultivate jing, qi and shen and build tendon, bone and skin, by physical movement, such as sinew-transforming exercise (Yi Jin Jing), Taiji Quan, and body-mind exercise (Xing Shen Zhuang), which, by physical movement and limb pulling, can stretch muscles, tendon and membrane, promote smooth flow of qi and blood, and improve pliability and flexibility of muscles and ligament, and movability of bones and joints.

5 强健躯体筋骨

传统养生功法，有很大一部分从形入手，内炼精气神，外练筋骨皮。诸如易筋经、太极拳、形神庄等，就是注重对形体锻炼和调控，通过肢体运动，抻筋拔骨，从而牵拉人体各部位大小肌群和筋膜，促进活动部位的气血畅通，提高肌肉、肌腱、韧带等组织的柔韧性、灵活性和骨骼、关节、肌肉等组织的活动功能，以达到强筋壮骨的目的。

Section 2 Common Qigong Exercises

The rich varieties of breathing exercises are sparkling gems in TCM. Here is an introduction of some traditional exercises and some that have been popular and effective in China in recent years.

1 8 Brocade Exercise (Ba Duan Jing)

As a traditional exercise, the Ba Duan Jing was practiced widely in the North Song Dynasty, and was still recorded in many health works in the Ming Dynasty. The name refers to 8 sets of moves, and it is compared to resplendent brocade, on account of its rarity arising from classic arrangement of postures and marvelous health-building effect. There are many schools of this exercise, categorized in "8 sets of sitting postures" and "8 sets of standing postures", in which the latter is more popular for its friendliness to common folks. The exercise falls into units of organs, so it goes without saying that it is most effective in modulating organ functions. As the chant in the book on the in the Qing Dynasty goes, "stretch hands upward, and stretch them on both sides like drawing the bow, and the triple energizer is dredged; stretch one arm upward and the spleen and stomach are soothed; look backward to cure strain and injury; shake the head and bottom to assuage heat in the heart, hold feet with both hands

第2节 常用养生功法

中医养生功法种类繁多,其流派纷呈、特色各异,是中医养生学的璀璨明珠。现择其精要,简单介绍几种传统流派代表性功法,及近年来在社会上流传较广、影响较大,健身效果较好的养生功法。

1 八段锦

八段锦是我国传统的养生功法,据文献记载,北宋期间八段锦就广泛流传于世,明代以后,在许多养生著作中都可见到关于该功法的记述,八段锦的名称是将该功法的八组动作及其效应比喻为精美华贵的丝帛、绚丽多彩的锦绣,以显其珍贵,称颂其精炼完美的编排和良好的祛病健身作用。八段锦流派较多,有"文八段"(坐式)和"武八段"(立式)之分,由于立式八段锦便于群众习练,流传更广。八段锦功法以脏腑分纲,具有较好调整脏腑机能的功效,清末有关书籍将八段锦的功法特点及其功效以歌诀形式总结为:"两手托天理三焦,左右开弓似射

to fortify the kidney and waist; clench fists and glare to add strength".

雕;调理脾胃须单举,五劳七伤往后瞧;摇头摆尾去心火,两手攀足固肾腰;攥拳怒目增气力,背后七颠百病消。"

1.1 Characteristics

1.1.1 Units of Organs and Coordinated Channels

The 8-set brocade exercise arranges the leading movements by physiological and pathological features based on the TCM theory of visceral manifestation and the theory of meridians and collaterals. Each unit, with its own obvious emphasis, can also echo and coordinates with other units in function, hence accomplishing a physical panoramic modulation of organs and physical condition as a whole.

1.1.2 Reign of Will and Movements Matched with Breathing and Spirit

The exercise lays emphasis on the will's control over movements, so the spirit is injected into the physique. The reign of spirit combined with leading movements pushes the genuine qi flowing in the body, thus attaining a state of breath clinging to movements.

1.1.3 Symmetry and Harmony; Being Mobile and Static

Symmetry and harmony link every two moves. Guided by the will, the body moves breezily and vivaciously, each posture relevant to the next, exuding an air of full spirit inside with leisure outside, fullness with void and firmness with litheness.

1.1 功法特点

1.1.1 脏腑分纲　经络协调

八段锦依据中医藏象理论及经络理论,以脏腑经络的生理、病理特征来安排导引动作。在八组动作中,每一组既有其明确的侧重点,又注重每组间功能效应呼应协调,从而全面调整脏腑机能及人体的整体生命活动状态。

1.1.2 神为主宰　形气神合

八段锦通过动作导引,注重以意识对形体的调控,将意识贯注到形体动作之中,使神与形相合;由于意识的调控和形体的导引,促使真气在体内的运行,达到神注形中,气随形动的境界。

1.1.3 对称和谐　动静相兼

本功法每式动作及动作之间,表现出对称和谐的特点,形体动作在意识的导引下,轻灵活泼,节节贯穿,舒适自然,体现出内实精神,外示安逸,虚实相生、刚柔相济的神韵。

1.2 Essentials

1.2.1 Relax and Calm Down; Match Movement with Breathing

Relax the body and mind first, which ensures harmonious flow of breath. And the movement, breathing and will must work in natural harmony. Natural movement should live up to standard effortlessly, natural breathing not be forced, and natural will be there unconsciously.

1.2 练功要领

1.2.1 松静自然 形息相随

八段锦的锻炼，一方面要求精神形体放松，心平方能气和，形松意充则气畅达。另一方面，要求形体、呼吸、意念要自然协调。形体自然，动作和于法度；呼吸自然，要勿忘勿助，不强吸硬呼，形息相随；意念自然，要似守非守，绵绵若存，形气神和谐一体。

1.2.2 Right Moves and Smooth Relevance

One should carefully learn the postures with their void and fullness, relaxation and firmness, so as to move up to standard, and after practicing for some time, aim at cohesion between void and fullness of postures, smooth like flowing cloud and brook in a harmonious continuity, and finally attain the consummation of movement, breathing and spirit all in one.

1.2.2 动作准确 圆活连贯

八段锦动作安排和谐有序，在锻炼过程中首先要对动作的线路、姿势、虚实、松紧等分辨清楚，做到姿势工整，方法准确。经过一段时间的习练力求动作准确熟练、连贯，动作的虚实变化和姿势的转换衔接，无停顿断续，如行云流水，连绵不断。逐步达到动作、呼吸、意念的有机结合，使意息相随，而达到形气神三位一体的境界和状态。

2 The Five-animal Exercises (Wu Qin Xi)

The Wu Qin Xi is one of the representatives of traditional exercises with a long history. It was created by imitating 5 animals: the tiger, the deer, the bear, the monkey and the bird. It had been passed down orally until the North and South Dynasties

2 五禽戏

五禽戏是古代传统导引养生功法的代表之一，具有悠久的历史。它是通过模仿五种禽兽——虎、鹿、熊、猿、鸟的动作而编创成的导引功

around 500 A. D., when it was recorded in *Character and Longevity* (Yang Xing Yan Ming Lu) of TAO Hongjing. Now it has developed into several schools. The exercise, by imitating gestures and bearing of different animals combined with the reigning will, can dredge channels, strengthen organs and lubricate limbs and joints.

法。五禽戏开始时并没有文字流传，到了南北朝时期，陶弘景的《养性延命录》用文字将其记录了下来。随着时间的推移，该功法辗转传授，逐渐形成了各流派的五禽戏，流传至今。该功法通过模仿动物们不同的形态动作及气势结合各自的意念活动，能起到舒经通络，强健脏腑，灵活肢体关节的功用。

2.1 Characteristics

2.1.1 Emulating animals in gesture and bearing

The Wu Qin Xi is mostly on the move, which leads qi movement up and down, open and closed. The moves emulate the awesomeness of the tiger, comfort of the deer, stability of the bear, litheness of the bird and agility of the monkey with their matched bearing.

2.1 功法特点

2.1.1 模仿五禽 形神兼备

五禽戏模仿动物的形态动作，以动为主，通过形体动作的导引，引动气机的升降开合。外在动作既要模仿虎之威猛、鹿之安适、熊之沉稳、鸟之轻捷、猿之灵巧，还要求内在的神意兼具“五禽”之神韵，意气相随，内外合一。

2.1.2 Overall movements with details

The Wu Qin Xi involves the whole body, with the moves of bending forward and backward and sideways, twisting around, spreading & closing and coiling & straightening, etc, which exercises the cervical vertebra, the sternal vertebra and the lumbar vertebra; stretches the governor meridian on the back and the urinary bladder meridian, and stimulates acupoints on the back. Meanwhile, it also exercises such small joints as fingers and toes, which, by moving the extremities of the 12 channels, serves to smooth channels and qi and blood circulation.

2.1.2 活动全面 大小兼顾

五禽戏动作体现了身体躯干的全方位运动，包括前俯、后仰、侧屈、拧转、开合、缩放等不同的姿势，对颈椎、胸椎、腰椎等部位进行了有效的锻炼，并且也牵拉了背部督脉及膀胱经，刺激了背部腧穴。同时功法还特别注重手指、脚趾等小关节的运动，通过活动十二经络的末端，以畅通经络气血。

2.1.3 Combination of Being Mobile and Static, and Preservation and Exercise

The exercise consists mostly in mobile exercising, which stretches the body, moves tendon and bones, and dredges channels, yet it also emphasizes the opening and closing of the movements, plus a short pose at the end of each game, which induces one into a comparatively static condition and the mood of the 5 animals, so as to regulate breath and calm the mind.

2.2 Essentials

2.2.1 Standard Movements and Matched Breathing

One should try to move up to standard in accordance with the name of each posture, that is, "to move like a tiger in the exercise of tigers, and a bear in that of bears". Special heed should be paid to the rise and fall, slowness and forcefulness of the moves, striving for its agility and softness, continuity and smoothness. And make sure to match the moves with breathing on the principle of rising with inhaling and falling with exhaling, stretching with inhaling and withdrawing with exhaling, inhaling ahead of exhaling, and storing breath in for breath out.

2.2.2 Envisioning for Bearing

It is important to study the habit and bearing of the 5 animals. Envision their bearing and enter into their mood in practicing the game. Take the tiger set, for example, imagine oneself as a tiger in mountain stretching and pouncing on the prey in an awesome manner, and in the deer set, envisage oneself to be a deer playing on the prairie stretching limbs in a relaxed stroll; and in a bear set, as a bear in the forest, turning and walking with a steady and

2.1.3 动静结合　练养相兼

五禽戏虽以动功为主，舒展形体、活动筋骨、畅通经络，但同时在功法的起势和收势，以及每一戏结束后，配以短暂的静功站桩，以诱导练功者进入相对平稳的状态和"五禽"的意境当中，以此来调整气息、宁静心神。

2.2 练功要领

2.2.1 动作到位　气息相随

练习五禽戏要根据动作的名称含义，作出与之相适应的动作造型，并尽量使动作到位，合乎规范，努力做到"演虎像虎""学熊像熊"。尤其要注意动作的起落、高低、轻重、缓急，做到动作灵活柔和、连贯流畅。并且注意呼吸和动作的协调配合，遵循起吸落呼，开吸合呼，先吸后呼，蓄吸发呼的原则。

2.2.2 以理作意　展现神韵

练习五禽戏时，要注意揣摩虎、鹿、熊、猿、鸟的习性和神态。通过以理作意，即意想"五禽"之神态，进入"五禽"的意境之中。如练习虎戏时，意想自己是深山中的猛虎，伸展肢体，抓捕食物，有威猛之气势；练鹿戏时，要意想自己是原野上的梅花

lovable gait; in the monkey set, a monkey in the wild playing with agility; and in the bird set, a crane by the lake spreading wings and sailing lithely and elegantly.

鹿，众鹿抵戏，伸足迈步，轻捷舒展；练熊戏时，要意想自己是山林中的黑熊，转腰运腹，步履沉稳，憨态可掬；练猿戏时，要意想自己置身于山野灵猴之中，轻松活泼、机灵敏捷；练鸟戏时，要意想自己是湖边仙鹤，轻盈潇洒，展翅翱翔。

3 Sinew-transformation exercise (Yi Jin Jing)

As a traditional exercise, the tendon-changing exercise was created by Damo, an Indian monk, and practiced on by monks of Shaolin Temple before the Song and Yuan Dynasties (1000s—1300s A. D.), not popular until the Ming and Qing Dynasties (1300s—1900s A. D.), when several schools were developed. The exercise lays emphasis on postures, breathing and will, with moves focusing on the flow of 12 channels and the two channels of Ren channel and the governor meridian, in the course of which one feels breath and channels flow smoothly and peacefully. The exercise builds tendon, bones and muscles, dredges channels, strengthens constitution, energizes and prolongs life.

3 易筋经

易筋经是我国传统的养生保健功法之一，相传为印度达摩和尚所创，宋元以前仅流传于少林寺僧众之中，自明清以来才日益流行于民间，且演变为数个流派。“易”者，变易、改变也；“筋”指筋肉、经筋；“经”指规范、方法。该功法重视姿势、呼吸与意念的锻炼，按人体十二经与任督二脉之运行进行练习，锻炼起来，气脉流注合度，流畅无滞，有强筋健骨、壮实肌肉、和畅经脉、增强体质、充沛精力、延年益寿的良好效果。

3.1 Characteristics

3.1.1 Stretching Tendon with Will Matching

Governed by the will, the tendon-changing exercise stretches the body with the emphasis on the tendon and membrane, so as to dredge the 12 channels and the eight extra channels with their qi movement, hence regulating organ functions.

3.1 功法特点

3.1.1 抻筋拔骨 形气并练

易筋经功法从练形入手，以神为主宰，形气并练，通过形体动作的牵引伸展、抻筋拔骨来锻炼筋骨、筋膜，以畅通十二经络与奇经八脉之气机，进而调节脏腑机能。

3.1.2 Dredging Jia Ji and Stimulating Acupoints on the Back

Focusing on the governor meridian and acupoints on the back closely related to organs, the exercise conducts a lot of bending forward and backward and sideways and twisting, so as to stimulate acupoints on the back, dredge Jia Ji, harmonize the two channels of Ren channel and the governor meridian, thus regulating organ functions.

3.1.2 疏通夹脊 刺激背俞

背部分布有督脉，脊柱两侧膀胱经上分布有与脏腑密切相关的“背俞穴”，本功法安排有较多的身体俯仰、侧弯及旋转动作，通过脊柱的旋转屈伸运动以刺激背部的腧穴、疏通夹脊，和畅任督二脉，调节脏腑机能，达到健身防病、益寿延年目的。

3.1.3 Body Naturally Spread in Harmony

One should strive to spread the body naturally, especially in bending inward and outward and twisting, and attain a symmetric harmony between limbs and the body, left and right, upper and lower parts of the body, so as to exhibit a relevant and harmonious flow of the generous air. This set of exercises moves evenly and slowly, combining softness with strength, a strength that is lithe and supple. So the exercise can regulate organ function and dredge qi and blood circulation by stretching muscles and channels.

3.1.3 舒展大方 协调美观

本功法的动作，不论是上肢、下肢还是躯干，其动作的屈伸、外旋内收、扭转身体等都要求舒展大方，上下肢与躯体之间，肢体与肢体之间的左右上下，以及肢体左右的对称协调，彼此相随，密切配合，呈现出动作舒展连贯、柔畅协调的神韵。而且整套动作速度均匀和缓。动作刚柔相济，用力轻盈圆柔，不使蛮力，不僵硬。其目的就是通过“抻筋拔骨”，牵动经筋、经络，进而调节脏腑机能，畅通气血，达到强身健体的目的。

3.2 Essentials

3.2.1 Will Zeroing in on the Moves

One must relax and calm down to practice the exercise, so as to follow the moves with the will, which, mind you, should be done naturally and un-

3.2 练功要领

3.2.1 神注庄中 形神合一

本功法的习练，要求精神放松，意识平和。通过动作变化引导气的运行，做到

consciously without being forced.

神注庄中，意气相随。运用意念时，不刻意意守某一部位，而是要求将意识贯注到动作之中，并注意用意要轻，似有似无，切忌刻意、执著。

3.2.2 Breathing Maturally Matching Moves

Do not force the breathing to be long, but keep it going with the moves naturally and harmoniously. A smooth breathing furnishes a relaxed and peaceful mind.

3.2.2 自然呼吸　动息相随

习练本功法时，要注意把握动作和呼吸始终保持柔和协调，不要刻意执著于呼吸的深绵细长。练功呼吸时，要求自然流畅，不喘不滞，这样更有利于身心放松、心气平和。

3.2.3 Alternating Void with Fullness and Softness with Force

Void and fullness, softness and force must work in alternation, in that too much force bring about rigidity, which blocks smooth flow of qi and blood, while too much softness makes the moves slack and empty, which cannot perform the function of triggering qi movement and stretching muscles and joints.

3.2.3 虚实相间　刚柔相济

习练本功法时，要注意动作刚与柔、虚与实相协调配合。因为，用力过“刚”，会出现拙力、僵力，以至于影响气血的流通和运行；动作过“柔”，则会出现松懈、空乏，不能起到引动气机，抻筋拔骨的作用。

4 Tai Ji Quan

Tai Ji Quan boasts a long history as a traditional exercise. The name “taiji” probably derives from the pair conceptions of yin and yang, fullness and void, mobile and static, minus and plus in *the Book of Changes* (Yi Jing), the former two of which run through the whole process of the exercise. The postures keep to circles or curves, with change between yin and yang, opposites in unity and round harmony in every move. By the leading physical movements,

4 太极拳

太极拳是我国传统养生功法之一，其历史源远流长。太极拳名为太极者，盖取法于《易经》阴阳动静之理，盈虚消长之机。太极拳在整个运动过程中自始至终都贯穿着“阴阳”和“虚实”，其运动作势，圆活如环之无端，循环往复，每个拳式都蕴含阴阳

Taiji Quan merges will, breath and moves in one and accomplishes the effects of harmonizing spirit, dredging channels and qi and blood circulation and energizing organ functions, hence the balance of yin and yang and harmony of qi and blood.

变化之道,及对立统一、圆活一致的太极之理。太极拳通过形体导引,将意、气、形结合成一体,使人体精神和悦、经络气血畅通、脏腑机能旺盛,以调整机体的阴阳、气血达到平和的健康状态。

4.1 Characteristics

4.1 功法特点

4.1.1 Movements in Circles and Balance of Yin and Yang

4.1.1 势正招圆　阴阳相济

Circles and curves make up the foundation of Taiji Quan, which resemble the taiji diagram. The postures must be standard, rid of sluggishness, recoil or tilt. In a word, Taiji Quan moves in generous circles and curves with perfect relevance and continuity attained in the absence of punctuation.

太极拳的形体动作以圆为本,一招一式均由各种圆弧动作组成。拳路的一招一式又构成了太极图形。并且其势端正,不散漫,不蜷缩,不歪斜。故从其外形上看,太极拳动作圆满,舒展不拘不僵,招招贯串,连绵不断,整套动作要一气呵成。

4.1.2 Will Zeroing in on the Moves

4.1.2 神注庄中　意随庄动

Taiji Quan exercise requires coordination of hands, eyes, body and steps, governed by the will. The exercise moves in the shape of taiji diagram, with the spirit also governed by taiji. Taiji Quan produces yang with mobility and yin while being static, in which way the yin and yang, qi and blood of the player are agitated. The will leads the breath in an overall endless circulation.

太极拳的锻炼要求手、眼、身、法、步动作协调。注重心静意导,形神兼备。其拳形为"太极",拳意亦在"太极",以太极之动而生阳,静而生阴,激发人体自身的阴阳气血,以意领气,运于周身,如环无端,周而复始。

4.1.3 Even Breathing and Generous Gentleness

4.1.3 呼吸均匀　舒展柔和

Taiji Quan demands breathing to be even, long, slim and slow and match movements, so as to lead the exit and entrance of qi movement. Generally, inhale in withdrawing moves and exhale,

太极拳要求呼吸匀、细、长、缓,并以呼吸配合动作,导引气机的开合出入。一般而言,吸气时动作为合,呼气

spreading. Note that the moves should be steady, supple and generous.

4.2 Essentials

4.2.1 Calm Down and Match Movements with Will

Like other exercises, Taiji Quan requires firstly the removal of worldly thoughts. Calm down with the will zeroing in on the movements. The will governs and follows the moves in the company of the eye, by hands moving outside and qi moving inside, hence attaining a sublime life state of tri-movements of limbs, qi and will all in one.

4.2.2 Serene and natural with even breathing

A priority of doing Taiji Quan is to relax, lowering shoulders and elbows naturally, and removing the strain in hips and waist, for a smooth flow of channels and qi and blood. Breathe deeply and evenly and keep it long enough to go with the gentle curve of movements. Breathe in as deep as the abdomen in withdrawing moves and breathe out from the abdomen in spreading ones.

4.2.3 Move in Harmony with the Waist as the Axis

The waist, as the axis of all moves, initiates the changes between void and fullness. The key of doing Taiji Quan is to stand upright, with perfect harmony between upper and lower body, front and back, left and right, all of which depend on the waist as the axis.

4.2.4 Agile Footsteps with Void Distinguishable from Fullness

To do Taiji Quan, take note to move in curves,

时动作为开。而动作宜平稳舒展，柔和不僵。

4.2 练功要领

4.2.1 心静神宁　神形相合

太极拳的练习，首先要排除各种思想杂念，保持心神的宁静，将意识贯注到练功活动当中。神为主帅，身为神使，意识始终照顾到动作，配合眼神，手动于外，气动于内，达到形到、意到、气到的境界，也就是形气神三位一体的生命优化状态。

4.2.2 松静自然　呼吸均匀

太极拳的锻炼要求全身自然放松，上身要沉肩坠肘，下身要松胯宽腰，以使经脉畅达，气血周流。呼吸要求深长均匀，与动作之轻柔圆活相应。吸气时，动作为合，气沉丹田；呼气时，动作为开，气发丹田。

4.2.3 以腰为轴　全身协调

腰是各种动作的中轴，动作的虚实变化皆由腰带动。太极拳要求立身中正、上下协调、前后兼顾、左右呼应，就必须以腰部为轴，方能带动全身，上下前后左右协调一致，浑然一体，这是练好太极拳的关键所在。

4.2.4 步伐灵活　虚实分明

练习太极拳要注意动作

exert strength as if drawing silk and take footsteps with the agility of the cat. Be sure to put the weight of the body on a certain foot and change it accordingly, which, in distinguishing full step from void one, ensures the balance of the body.

圆融，步伐要灵活，运劲如抽丝，迈步如猫行。运动时两腿要分清虚实，随着重心的转移，两足要交替支撑重心，以保持全身的平衡。

5 Six-character Chant Exercise (Liu Zi Jue)

5 六字诀

The Liu Zi Jue is an exercise by breathing and pronouncing. The likes of which were recorded in ancient literature such as *Chronicles by Lü Buwei* (Lü Shi Chun Qiu) in the Qin Dynasty 2 000 years ago. And the earliest record of it was found in *Character and Longevity* (Yang Xing Yan Ming Lu) of TAO Hongjing of the North and South Dynasties 1500 years ago, since which time more theories and practices of the chant exercise have been developed and supplemented.

六字诀，又称六字气诀，是以呼吸吐纳发音为主要手段的养生功法。关于呼吸吐纳发音的功法，历代文献均有不少论述，秦汉时期的《吕氏春秋》中就有关于用导引呼吸治病的论述。而最早记录六字诀功法的当属南北朝时期陶弘景的《养性延命录》，嗣后有关六字诀的功理功法及其应用，历代都有不少发展和补充。

According to researches, the moves had not been included in the chant until the Ming Dynasty 600 years ago. Based on the TCM theory of five elements and five solid organs since the Tang and Song Dynasties, the chant has developed a steady system that stipulates the standard breathing and mouth shape and pronunciation, with moves and leading will observing the rules of TCM channel circulation. The six characters correspond with the organs in the way of "si" to lungs and medal, "chui" to the kidney and water, "xu" to the liver and wood, "he" to the heart and fire, "hu" to the spleen and soil, while "xi" to the triple energizer.

根据文献研究，明以前的六字诀不配动作，明以后的六字诀有多种动作配合。六字诀流传至今，在功法上已形成了较为稳定的体系，即功法理论保持了唐宋以来以中医五行五脏学说为理论基础，对呼吸口型及发音有了较明确的规范，肢体的动作导引与意念导引遵循中医经络循行规律。六字与脏腑配属为：呬属肺金，吹属肾水，嘘属肝木，呵属心火，呼属脾土，嘻属三焦。

Based on the TCM theory of visceral manifesta-

该功法是根据中医藏象

tion, the exercise matches pronunciation with breathing, and will with moves, hence regulating and controlling rise and fall, exhale and inhale of the breath, and the balance of qi movement in the viscera.

学说理论，通过呼吸吐纳及意念和肢体的导引，配合特定的发音，来调整与控制体内气息的升降出入和脏腑气机的平衡，以达到养生保健，延缓衰老的目的。

5.1 Characteristics

5.1 功法特点

5.1.1 Pronunciation Leading Breath and Regulating Organs

The pronunciation of the exercise initiates and regulates the rise and fall, exhale and inhale of qi movement of organs, with the 6 pronunciations echoing the 5 solid organs plus the triple energizer. So there are special rules governing the pronunciation and mouth shape to achieve a better effect.

5.1.1 以音引气 调节脏腑

六字诀的锻炼通过特定的发音来引动与调整体内气机的升降出入。以"嘘、呵、呼、呬、吹、嘻"六种不同的特殊发音，分别与人体肝、心、脾、肺、肾、三焦六个脏腑相联系，从而达到调整脏腑气机的作用。在六字的发音和口型方面有其相应特殊规范，目的在于通过发音来引动相应脏腑的气机。

5.1.2 Exhale and Inhale Accompanying Pronunciation

Each move with accompanying breathing echoes the feature of qi transformation of the corresponding organs, such as the rise of liver qi, and concealment of kidney qi. So a perfect harmony of pronunciation, breathing and moves is of vital importance for dredging channels and qi and blood, and regulating organ functions.

5.1.2 吐纳导引 音息相随

六字诀功法中，每一诀的动作安排、气息的调摄都与相应脏腑的气化特征相一致，如肝之升发、肾之蛰藏等。练习过程中十分注重将发音与调息吐纳及动作导引相配合，使发音、呼吸、动作导引协调一致，相辅相成，浑然一体，共同起到畅通经络气血、调整脏腑机能的作用。

5.1.3 Generous Curves Combined with Stillness

The Liu Zi Jue boasts moves that are generous and gentle in curved flexibility and continuity, like

5.1.3 舒展圆活 动静相兼

六字诀功法其动作舒展大方、柔和协调，圆转灵活，

flowing clouds and brook, and attains a fabulous air of the player and qi in a harmonious and tranquil merge. Moreover, the breathing and pronouncing should be even, thin, soft and long, with matching stillness in the move that cultivates qi, thus achieving a combination of mobility and quiescence.

如行云流水,婉转连绵,具有人在气中,气在人中的神韵,表现出安然宁静与和谐之美。并且其吐气发音要求匀细柔长,配合动作中的静立养气,使整套功法表现出动中有静、静中有动、动静结合的韵意。

5.2 Essentials

5.2.1 Standard Pronunciation with Breath

Exhaled pronunciation is unique to the Liu Zi Jue with the objective to lead qi movement. So the right mouth shape with its standard pronunciation is vital to the function. Beginners can adopt the way of pronouncing during exhaling to correct the mouth shape and pronunciation, in case of being out of breath; and after getting a hang of it, they can change it to exhaled whispering pronunciation, gradually making it even, thin, soft and long, while noting the subtle change of breath.

5.2.2 Note Breathing without Forcing It

The Liu Zi Jue adopts reversed abdomen-breathing, that is, swelling the chest and withdrawing the abdomen when inhaling instead of swelling the abdomen as in abdomen breathing, and vice versa. This way of breathing can enlarge the scale of rise and fall of the diaphragm, so as to massage organs in some sense, conducive to the flow of qi movement in the triple energizer. Take note not to be forceful in breathing, keeping it thin and slow naturally and unconsciously. Only in this way can the tri-harmony of moves, will and breathing be attained and life activities sublimated.

5.2 练功要领

5.2.1 发音准确 体会气息

吐气发音是六字诀独特的练功方法,发音的目的在于引导气机。练功时,必须按要求,校准口形,准确发音。初学时,可采用吐气出声发音的方法,校正口型和发音,以免憋气;在练习熟练后,可以逐渐过渡为吐气轻声发音,渐至匀细柔长,并注意细心体会气息的变化。

5.2.2 注意呼吸 用意轻微

六字诀中的呼吸方法主要是采用逆腹式呼吸。其方法与要领是:鼻吸气时,胸腔慢慢扩张,而腹部随之微微内收,口呼气时则与此相反。这种呼吸方法使横膈膜升降幅度增大,对人体脏腑产生类似按摩的作用,有利于三焦气机的运行。练功时要注意呼吸,但用意微微,做到吐惟细细,纳惟绵绵,有意无意,绵绵若存,这样方能将形意气息合为一体,以使生命活动得到优化。

5.2.3 Relaxed Movements in Coordination

The exercise focuses on breathing, which is led by moves. The combination invigorates qi transformation activities of organs. So the moves must be relaxed, gentle, slow and natural, to match qi movement change of the even and long breathing and pronunciation.

5.2.3 动作舒缓 协调配合

六字诀功法以呼吸吐纳为主，同时辅以动作导引。通过动作的导引来协调呼吸吐纳发音引动的气息，以促进脏腑的气化活动。因此，习练时要注意将动作与呼吸吐纳、吐气发音协调配合，动作做到松、柔、舒、缓，以顺应呼吸吐纳和吐气发音的匀细柔长的气机变化。

Chapter 6 Acupuncture, Moxibustion and Tuina Approach to Health Preservation

第6章 针灸推拿养生

Based on the TCM theory of meridians and collaterals, acupuncture, combustion and tuina stimulate acupoints and regulate the passageways and qi and blood circulation, thus invigorating the flow of nutritive and defensive qi and blood, balancing yin and yang, nourishing organs and enhancing constitution. The human body is a unified whole with organs as the centre that radiates in channels, limbs and apertures. So the channel theory plays an indispensable role in health preservation.

针灸推拿养生是以中医经络学说为基础，以刺激腧穴、调整经络气血为基本手段，从而激发营卫气血的运行，和阴阳、养脏腑，以增强体质、防病治病、益寿延年的养生方法。人身是一个以脏腑为中心，由经络外络肢体、官窍的统一整体，就其养生理论而言，经络学说有着不可替代的作用。

Section 1 Acupuncture

第1节 针刺养生

Acupuncture is a way of pricking certain acupoints with a needle, with extra ways of lifting, inserting, twisting, turning and channeling out, etc, to stimulate the function of channels, which can dredge channels, smooth qi and blood circulation, coordinate nutritive and defensive qi and enhance constitution. This ancient way of building health was firstly recorded in *Yellow Emperor's Inner*

针刺养生，是运用针具通过对特定穴位的刺激，施以提、插、捻、转、迎、随、补、泻等不同手法，激发经络本身的功能，以达到疏通经络、调畅气血、和谐营卫、增强体质、延年益寿的目的。针刺用于养生保健，由来已久，早

Canon (Huang Di Nei Jing), with more works on it developed from the Tang through the Qing Dynasties.

在《内经》中就有阐述。发展到唐、宋、明清时期，出现了较多的针灸著作。在这些著作中，记载了大量针刺养生的内容。时至今日，针刺养生成为一种别具特色的防病治病、延年益寿的养生方法。

1 Functions

1 针刺养生的作用

1.1 Dredging Channels and Smoothing the Flow of Qi and Blood

If some part of qi and blood flow is blocked, we can resort to acupuncture to stimulate the qi in the channels and dredge it, the whole process, including urging the arrival of qi and awaiting qi beforehand and obtaining qi afterward, serving this purpose. So "dredge" is the key word in reference to its function. Only a smooth flow of channel and qi and blood circulation can connect each part of the body in a harmonious cooperation for normal life activities.

1.1 疏通经络 和畅气血

针刺的作用主要在于疏通经络，使气血流畅。针刺前的"催气""候气"，刺后的"得气"，都是在调整经络气血。如果机体某一局部的气血运行不利，针刺即可激发经气，促其畅达。所以，针刺的作用首先在于"通"。经络畅通无阻，气血通畅，机体各部分才能密切联系，共同完成生命活动，人才能健康无病。

1.2 Regulating Deficiency and Excess; Balancing the Viscera

In life activities, organ functions and the rise and fall of yin and yang, and qi and blood would shift to void or fullness with the change of outside environment and living habit. While acupuncture can restore it to balance, by filling the void and draining the fullness.

1.2 调理虚实 平衡脏腑

在人体生命过程中，机体的脏腑机能，阴阳气血的盛衰，都会随着外环境以及生活习性的变化而产生虚实盛衰的偏差。针刺养生则可根据具体情况，纠正这种偏差，虚则补之，实则泻之，补泻得宜，可使弱者变强，盛者平和，阴阳平衡，健康延年。

1.3 Harmonizing Yin and Yang and Prolonging Life

The relative equilibrium of yin-yang is the key to health. Acupuncture by dredging channels and regulating qi and blood can furnish communication among parts of the body, circulate the nutritive and defensive qi and harmonize yin and yang, hence a flourishing life.

2 Common Acupoints

Zu Sanli (ST 36): three inches below the knee, on the major tendon by the shin bone in the outward direction. A key acupoint for the overall health, it can fortify the spleen & stomach, promote digestion, furnish breath and strength and improve immunity. Method: prick it vertically to 1-1.5 inches with an acupuncture needle. One can prick it on one leg or both at the same time. The prickling can be short for common people, but should stay for 5-10 minutes for the old and the infirm. It can be conducted every day, or on alternate days.

Guan Yuan (CV 4): three inches below the naval. It is a key acupoint to improve health. Prick it askew to half an inch, and draw the needle out after obtaining qi. Conduct it once or twice a week, and health can be improved.

Qi Hai (CV 6): one and a half inches below the naval. It is also a strengthening acupoint. Prick it askew with an acupuncture needle to half an inch, and draw it out after qi arrival. Do it once or twice a week, preferably with acupuncture in Zu Sanli (ST-36), and immunity can be enhanced.

Qu Chi (LT 11): On the fibula at the elbow. Bend the elbow and the acupoint is at the end of the

1.3 谐和阴阳　延年益寿

“阴平阳秘”是人体健康的关键。针刺可以通经络、调气血，使机体内外交通、营卫周流、阴阳和谐。如此生命力自然会健旺，从而达到养生保健，延年益寿的目的。

2 针刺养生常用穴位

足三里：位于膝下3寸，胫骨外大筋内。为全身性强壮要穴，可健脾胃，助消化，益气增力，提高人体免疫机能和抗病机能。刺法，用毫针直刺1～1.5寸，可单侧取穴，亦可双侧同时取穴。一般人针刺得气后，即可出针。但对年老体弱者，则可适当留针5～10分钟。隔日一次，或每日一次。

关元：位于脐下3寸。本穴为保健要穴，有强壮作用。用毫针斜刺0.5寸，得气后出针。每周针1～2次，可起到强壮身体的作用。

气海：位于脐下1.5寸。常针此穴，有强壮作用。毫针斜刺0.5寸，得气后，即出针。每周1～2次，可与足三里穴配合施针，可增强机体免疫机能和抗病能力。

曲池：位于肘外辅骨，曲肘时肘横纹尽头处。此穴具

horizontal wrinkle. It regulates blood pressure and protects eyesight of the old. Prick it vertically with an acupuncture needle to 0.5-1 inch, and draw it out after obtaining qi, but keep it there for 5-10 minutes in the case of the infirm. Do it once a day or on alternate days.

有调整血压、防止老人视力衰退的功效。可用毫针直刺0.5～1寸，针刺得气后，即出针。体弱者可留针5～10分钟，每日一次，或隔日一次。

Sanyin Jiao (SP 6): three inches above the ankle top on the inside by the shin bone in the inside direction. The acupoint is responsible for enhancing organs in the abdomen, especially the fertility system. Prick it vertically with an acupuncture needle to 1-1.5 inches and draw it out after obtaining qi, but keep it there for 5-10 minutes for the infirm. Do it once a day or on alternate days.

三阴交：位于足内踝高点上3寸，胫骨内侧面后缘。此穴对增强腹腔诸脏器，特别是生殖系统的功能有重要作用。可用毫针直刺1～1.5寸，针刺得气后，即出针，体弱者，可留刺5～10分钟。每日一次，或隔日一次。

3 Keys

3 针刺养生的注意事项

3.1 Less and Accurate Acupoints

Choose one or a couple of acupoints at a time, according to one's condition: just one acupoint for a particular function to make it stand out, or a set of acupoints to make it stronger for overall improvement.

3.1 选穴要精当

一般而言，针刺养生一次不宜选穴太多，应少而精。要根据不同的养生需要选择不同的腧穴，可选用单腧穴，也可选用几个腧穴配伍而成。欲增强某一方面机能者，可用单腧穴，以突出其效应；欲调理整体机能者，可选用配伍腧穴，以增强其效果。

3.2 Be Moderate in Pricking

Do not be too forceful in pricking. Generally the needle should be withdrawn after obtaining qi. And the depth varies with different people, greater depth for the fat than for the elders and children.

3.2 施针要和缓

针刺操作手法宜和缓，刺激强度适中，不宜过大。一般说来，留针不宜过久，得气后即可出针，针刺深度也应因人而异。年老体弱或小儿，进针不宜过深，形盛体胖之人，则可酌情适当深刺。

3.3 Taboos in Pricking

Some acupoints as taboos must be remembered. Do not apply acupuncture to the hungry, the overfull after meal, the drunk and those susceptible to pain, and do not apply it to the waist and hips of the pregnant in case of miscarriage.

3.3 把握针刺宜禁

针刺方法有一定的禁忌症，特别是禁针穴位，必须牢记。空腹、过饱、醉酒、惧怕针刺者，不宜针刺；妇女妊娠期间，腰骶部一般不宜针刺，以免堕胎。

3.4 Handle Emergencies in Time

There can be such emergencies as comatose, blocked needle, bent needle and broken needle, for which immediate treatments are imperative. Comatose means the patient faints in the course of acupuncture. Withdraw the needle and make him lie for a while if it is not so serious, and in a more severe case, prick Shui Gou (GV 26), Nei Guan(PC 6), Su Liao (DU 25), Zu Sanli (ST 36), and apply acupuncture to Bai Hui (GV 20), Guan Yuan (CV 4), Qi Hai (CV 6). If it does not work, more emergency measures are necessary.

Blocked needle means the needle is stuck in the body without easy movement, which is often caused by muscle tension or wrong operation. So the patient should adopt a comfortable gesture and relax the muscle and spirit. But when it happens the doctor can press the muscle around the needle or give another prick nearby so as to eliminate tension.

Bent needle means the needle handle deviates from the original angle when pricking in, which renders it difficult to lift and insert, twist and turn and withdraw the needle. When it happens, the

3.4 及时处理针刺意外

针灸过程中，由于各种原因，可能出现晕针、滞针、弯针、折针等特殊情况，应当针对不同情况，及时处理。晕针是针刺过程中发生晕厥的现象，轻者将针全部拔出，静卧休息一会儿即可恢复，重者可刺水沟、内关、素髎、足三里等穴，灸百会、关元、气海等穴，促其恢复；若情况更重，则进一步采取急救措施。

滞针是针在体内捻转不动，行针困难的现象，多由局部肌肉紧张或行针手法不正确而导致。因此，针刺前要保持较为舒服的姿势，并解除精神紧张，放松局部肌肉，以预防滞针。发生滞针时，可在针刺部位周围巡按，或在附近再刺一针，慢慢解除肌肉紧张。

弯针是针柄改变了进针或刺入留针时的方向和角度，提插、捻转及出针均感困难的现象。如针柄轻微弯

needle should be withdrawn slowly. If it bends too much, withdraw it from the direction of the bending. Never force it out in case of broken needle left in the body.

曲，应慢慢将针起出。当弯曲角度过大时，应顺着弯曲方向将针起出。切忌强行拔针，以免将针体折断，留在体内。

In the case of the broken needle in the body, just pinch it out with either the fingers or the tweezers if the end is exposed. If not, surgery is inevitable. Acupuncture for health preservation, however, requires gentle operation on only a couple of acupoints, so the broken needle is quite a scarce occurrence.

断针是行针时或出针后发现针身折断，其断端部分尚露于皮肤外，或断端全部没入皮肤之下的现象。若部分针身显露于体外时，可用手指或镊子将针起出。若完全没于皮肤之下，则需要手术取出。针刺养生要求手法轻柔，行针较少，因此一般不会出现断针的情况。

Section 2　Moxibustion

第 2 节　艾灸养生

Moxibustion means combusting certain acupoints with the moxa roll or the moxa cone, which serves to harmonize qi and blood, adjust channels, nourish viscera and so prolongs life. It is applicable to normal people who try to preserve health as well as the infirm who have been sick for a long time.

艾灸养生又称保健灸，是用艾条或艾炷在身体某些特定穴位上施灸，以达到和气血、调经络、养脏腑、益寿延年的目的。艾灸养生不仅用于强身保健，亦可用于久病体虚之人的调养。

1　Functions

1　艾灸养生的作用

1.1　Warming and Dredging Channels; Invigorating Qi and Blood Circulation

1.1　温通经脉　行气活血

The qi and blood circulation is accelerated by warmth and decelerated by coldness. That is why the hot moxibustion can warm up channels and in-

气血运行具有得温则行，遇寒则凝的特点。灸法其性温热，可以温通经络，促

vigorate qi and blood circulation.

进气血运行。

1.2 Cultivating the Primordial Qi and Warding off Disease

1.2 培补元气 预防保健

The primordial qi is the sovereign of the human body, the absence of it meaning death. Moxa, a pungent and warm medicine, furnished with fire, can cultivate yang and the primordial qi. It is termed "the priority for preserving life" in the *Book of Bian Que's Secrets* (Bian Que Xin Shu), a renowned doctor in ancient China.

人体真元之气是一身之主宰，真气壮则人强，真气虚则人病，真气脱则人死。艾为辛温阳热之药，以火助之，灸法具补阳壮阳、培补元气之功。《扁鹊心书》将其称之为"保命第一要法"。

1.3 Fortifying the Spleen and the Stomach

1.3 健脾益胃 培补后天

The moxibustion exerts an obvious effect on the spleen and the stomach, which are responsible for postnatal health. Moxibust Zhong Wan (CV 12) and the spleen yang is warmed and transported and qi furnished. Do it over Zu Sanli (ST 36), and the digestive system can thrive and absorb nutrients better, which helps to nourish the whole body.

灸法对脾胃有着明显的强壮作用。如在中脘穴施灸，可以温运脾阳，补中益气。常灸足三里，不但能使消化系统功能旺盛，增加人体对营养物质的吸收，以濡养全身，亦可收到防病治病、抗衰防老的效果。

1.4 Raising Yang and Fortifying the Skin

1.4 升举阳气 密固肤表

Moxibustion can raise yang and fortify skin, thereby guarding against pathogenic factors and regulate the whole body, so it is often resorted to in the treatment of qi deficiency that sinks and unsteady defensive yang.

灸法有升举阳气、密固肌肤、抵御外邪、调和营卫之功，常用于气虚下陷，卫阳不固之证。

2 Common Acupoints

2 艾灸养生的常用穴位

Shen Que (CV 8): A key acupoint on Ren channel just at the naval, this acupoint cultivates yang and promotes qi, warms the kidney and fortifies the spleen. Moxibust it indirectly with salt filling the naval, and apply the moxa cone 7 to 15 rounds.

神阙：位于当脐正中处。神阙为任脉之要穴，具有补阳益气、温肾健脾的作用。可灸七至十五壮，灸时用间接灸法，如将盐填脐心上，置艾炷灸之，有益寿延年之功。

Zu Sanli (ST 36): Moxibust it often and the

足三里：常灸足三里，可

spleen and the stomach can be fortified and thus digestion and absorption promoted. Stroke can be prevented for the old. Both moxa roll and moxa cone can do. The time limit is 5-10 minutes.

健脾益胃,促进消化吸收,强壮身体,中老年人常灸足三里还可预防中风。用艾条、艾炷灸均可,时间可掌握在5～10分钟。

Zhong Wan (CV 12): Four inches above the naval. It fortifies the spleen and stomach and thus plays a key role in improving postnatal health. Do it 5 to 7 rounds.

中脘:位于脐上4寸处。为强壮要穴,具有健脾益胃、培补后天的作用。一般可灸5～7壮。

Gao Huang (BL 43): Three inches beside the point below the jutting part of the 4th chest vertebra. Moxibust it often and overall health can be improved. Do it with the moxa roll for 15-30 minutes, or with the moxa cone 7-15 rounds.

膏肓:位于第四胸椎棘突下旁开3寸处,常灸膏肓穴,有强壮作用。常用艾条灸,15～30分钟,或艾炷灸7～15壮。

Yong Quan (KI 1): Bend the foot and the acupoint lies in the pit in the centre of the front half of the foot. It replenishes the kidney and thus cultivates yang, nourishes the heart and calms the mind. Moxibust it often and the heart and the whole body can be strengthened. Do it 3-7 rounds.

涌泉:脚趾卷屈,在前脚掌中心凹陷处取穴。此穴有补肾壮阳、养心安神的作用。常灸此穴,可健身强心、有益寿延年之功效。一般可灸3～7壮。

Qi Hai (CV 6) and **Guan Yuan** (CV 4): Qi Hai (CV 6) lies 1.5 inches below the naval, and Guan Yuan (CV 4), 3 inches below. Both are key acupoints for overall health. Do it once a day and immunity can be promoted.

气海、关元:气海位于腹正中线脐下1.5寸处;关元位于腹正中线脐下3寸处。均为人体强壮保健要穴,每天艾灸一次,能调整和提高人体免疫机能,增强人的抗病能力。

3 Keys

3 艾灸养生的注意事项

Taboos: Moxibustion benefits yang and impairs yin. So it is forbidden from those with yin deficiency or evil heat inside, and also from the facial parts with major blood vessels, and the abdomen, the waist, hips and the genital of the pregnant.

把握施灸禁忌:灸法能益阳伤阴,阴虚阳亢的患者及邪热内炽的病人,禁施灸法;颜面五官,有大血管的部位,孕妇的腹部、腰骶部及阴部,不宜施灸。

Sequence: Moxibust from the upper body to the lower and from yang part to yin. Do it first in fewer rounds, and with smaller moxa cones.

注意施灸顺序:艾灸时一般是先灸上部,后灸下部,先灸阳部,后灸阴部。壮数一般是先少后多,艾炷是先小后大。

Dose: Two to three rounds suffices for replenishment. The size and number of moxa cones vary with people and acupoints. Generally, one should apply smaller and fewer cones to the infirm and the head, hands and feet, and bigger and more cones to the strong and the waist and the abdomen.

掌握艾灸剂量:灸疗穴位一般 2～3 壮,即具补益功效,不宜过多。艾炷灸的多少、大小当因人及所灸部位的不同而有所区别。一般体弱者,宜小宜少;体壮者,宜大宜多。就部位而言,头部宜小宜少;腰腹部可增大增多,四肢末端宜少。

Accidents Avoidence: Observe rules when moxibusting in case of burned wound and fire to the house.

防止施灸意外:实施艾灸时要需严格操作,避免烧伤、烫伤及火灾。

Section 3 Tuina

第 3 节 推拿养生

A traditional approach to health preservation, Tuina stimulates channels and acupoints in the surface of the body in diverse ways, thereby dredging channels, smoothing qi and blood circulation, tuning viscera and facilitating recovery.

推拿养生法,是我国传统的保健养生方法之一,是通过各种手法刺激体表经络或腧穴,以疏通经络,调畅气血,调整脏腑,达到防病治病、促进病体康复目的。

1 Functions

1 推拿养生作用

1.1 Dredging Channels and Invigorating Qi and Blood Circulation

1.1 疏通经络 行气活血

Tuina follows channels and stimulates acupoints, which naturally promotes the circulation of

推拿按摩大多是循经取穴,按摩刺激相应穴位,从而

channels and qi and blood.

推动经络气血运行，以达到疏通经络、畅达气血、防病强身的目的。

1.2 Smoothing Qi and Blood Flow; Tuning Nutritive Qi and Defensive Qi

Tuina with its gentle strength follows channels and presses acupoints, hence regulating the whole body by transmission of channels, including tuning nutritive qi and defensive qi and blood, and balancing yin and yang.

1.2 通畅气血 调和营卫

推拿以柔软、轻和之力，循经络、按穴位，施术于人体，通过经络的传导来调节全身，借以调和营卫气血，平衡机体失衡的阴阳而达到增强机体健康，预防疾病的目的。

1.3 Cultivating and Replenishing the Primordial Qi

According to the ancient doctors, tuina normalizes qi movement, tunes spirit and qi, sharpens ears and eyes and prolongs life. To cultivate the primordial qi, tuina Guan Yuan (CV 4), Qi Hai (CV 6), and Yong Quan (KI 1); to fortify the spleen and stomach, tuina Zu Sanli (ST 36).

1.3 培补元气 益寿延年

古代医家认为，推拿按摩使人气机运行正常，神气和畅，耳目聪明，身体强壮，从而延年益寿。如经常揉按关元、气海、涌泉等穴，可以培补元气；经常揉按足三里，能增强脾胃功能，起到却病延年的效果等。

1.4 Tuning Viscera and Enhancing Their Function

Tuina various parts of the body and the corresponding organs with their qi movement can be tuned—fortifying the spleen and stomach, strengthening the major vessels of the heart, enhancing the diffusion, purification and descending functions of lungs, promoting free coursing of the liver and furnishing storage of the kidney.

1.4 调理脏腑 强化功能

推拿相应的经络腧穴，可强化内脏功能。通过手法对不同的部位推拿，可调畅脏腑气机，健运脾胃功能，加强心主血脉的功能和肺的宣发肃降功能，促进肝的疏泄以及肾脏的潜藏功能。

2 Methods

2 推拿养生的方法

2.1 Medium

2.1 推拿养生的介质

The media of tuina can be selected according to

推拿介质的选择，可以

the season, habit and experience of the tuina practioner and the condition of the patient. In summer, safflower oil liniment and Tong Zhong Ling liniment are preferable for their functions of relieving blockage and invigorating blood flow, eliminating bloat and pain, deterring dampness and evil wind in the body; in spring and autumn, French white is a splendid lubricator, and ginger juice, egg white, tea oil, sesame oil and wine are also good. Besides, there are some media with a particular aim for a particular part on the body, such as tuina cream and jelly prescription for tuina of the face.

根据推拿者的习惯、经验以及季节结合患者的具体情况合理选用。夏季，可以选用一些具有活血化瘀，消肿止痛，散风祛湿等功效的擦剂如红花油擦剂、痛肿灵擦剂等。秋冬和春季一般用滑石粉作为介质，有很好的润滑作用。也有人用姜汁、鸡蛋清、茶油、香油、白酒作为介质。还有一些针对性较强的用于特殊部位的介质，如用于面部的按摩乳、膏摩方等。

2.2 Tuina Gesture

There are six basic gestures of pressing, swinging, wiping, pinching, hammering and moving joints, each with its special function. Choose them according to physical needs.

2.2 推拿手法

常用的基本手法可分为按压类、摆动类、摩擦类、捏拿类、捶振类和活动关节类等六大类，每一类手法其作用各不相同，临床上可根据具体的养生需要，选用不同的养生方法。

2.2.1 The Pressing Type

This type consists of pressing, rubbing, clicking, and pinching. Pressing means putting fingers or the palm on the skin and gradually pressing deeper. The thumb works more than other fingers in the finger press; while in palm press, the joint between the hand and the wrist, the fleshy part behind the thumb, and the whole palm can be used, which can press a larger part than the finger press whose merit is stimulating a particular point with greater strength. Pressing often goes with other types, such as rubbing.

2.2.1 按压类手法

包括按法、揉法、点法、压法、掐法等方法。按法将手指或掌面置于体表，逐渐用力下压，也称为“抑法”；用拇指或食指、中指、环指（无名指）指端或指腹面按压，称为“指按法”，其中又以拇指按法较为常用；用掌根、鱼际或全掌按压，称为“掌按法”，作用面较大，但其局部刺激强度则弱于指按法。按法常可与其他手法结合使用，如与揉法结合，称为“按揉法”。

2.2.2 The Swinging Type

Consisting of thumb pushing, encircling, and rolling, the swinging type means rhythmic sway of the wrist, rendering the pressure strong and light alternately and keep working on the body like pulse. Take the thumb pushing for instance. Put the thumb tip, the fleshy part or the outer side on the body. Swing the wrist, which leads the bending and straightening of the thumb joint, so strong and light pressures keep working alternately on the treated point. Do it at a frequency of 120-160 times per minute. This type applies to all acupoints since it covers a small part and so infiltrates better.

2.2.2 摆动类手法

包括一指禅推法、缠法、滚法等，是通过腕部有节奏的摆动，使压力轻重交替地呈脉冲式持续作用于机体的一类手法。如一指禅推法，是将拇指指端、指腹或桡侧偏峰置于体表，运用腕部的来回摆动带动拇指指间关节的屈伸，使压力轻重交替，持续不断地作用于治疗部位上。每分钟 120～160 次。本法接触面小，渗透力强，可广泛用于全身各部穴位上。

2.2.3 The Rubbing Type

In the rubbing type, some methods rub the skin to produce heat, some push it, and some rub in a revolving fashion. Take the first for instance. Rub the skin with the palm in a moderate force forward and backward, long enough to produce heat. This palm rubbing applies to the chest and sides and abdomen; thumb flesh rubbing, as the name indicates, rubs with the thenar part behind the thumb, which applies to the four limbs; side rubbing, in which one rubs with the small thenar part of the palm, applies to the shoulders, the back, the waist, hips and legs.

2.2.3 摩擦类手法

是以在肌肤表面摩擦的方式进行的一类手法。其中，有些手法是使之摩擦发热，有些手法是推动向前，有些手法是以轮回旋转的形式揉摩。包括摩法、擦法、推法、托法等。其中擦法将手掌紧贴于皮肤表面，稍用力做来回直线摩擦，使其局部发热。用全掌着力摩擦者，称为“掌擦法”，适用于胸胁及腹部；用大鱼际着力摩擦者，称为“鱼际擦法”，适用于四肢部；用小鱼际着力摩擦时，称为“侧擦法”，适用于肩背、腰臀及下肢部。

2.2.4 The Pinching Type

The pinching type consists of pinching, squee-

2.2.4 捏拿类手法

是用挤压提捏肌肤的方

zing, twisting and pulling methods. Take pinching for example. Pinch the sick part with the fleshy parts of the thumb, the forefinger and the middle finger, or of all fingers and pull it upward. It applies to shoulders, the back and limbs.

式作用于机体的一类手法。包括拿法、捏法、挤法、拧法、扭法、扯法等方法。如拿法是用拇指和食指、中指的指腹,或用拇指和其余四指的指腹,对合紧挟患病部位并将其肌肤提起。适用于肩背及四肢部。

2.2.5 The Hammering Type

The hammering type taps or strikes the body and thus gives it a sense of quake. It consists of tapping, striking, hammering, splitting, pecking, chopping and shaking. Tapping means tapping the sick part rhythmically with the "void hand", such as the joint between the hand and the wrist, and back of the fist, and one can also tap with a mulberry stick, called stick tapping; hammering means striking rhythmically with a fist; splitting refers to striking with the side of the palm; pecking, tapping with five finger tips assembled; chopping, with the back of the bent joints of the forefinger and the middle finger. All the gestures apply to shoulders, the back and limbs.

2.2.5 捶振类手法

是以拍击的方式作用于机体,或使机体产生振动感应的一类手法。包括拍、击、捶(叩)、劈、啄、捣、振、抖等手法。其中拍法是用虚掌有节奏地拍打患部。如用掌根或拳背部击打,称为"击法";用桑枝棒进行击打,称为"棒击法";用空拳有节奏地击打,称为"捶法"(叩法);用手掌尺侧部击打,称为"劈法";用合拢的五指指端敲击,称为"啄法";用屈曲的食指或中指的近侧指间关节的背面进行叩击,称为"捣法"。这些手法适用于肩背及四肢部。

2.2.6 The Joint Moving Type

Also termed "passive movement", the joint moving type means bending, stretching, revolving and pulling the joints, the choice of which depends on the structural feature of the joint and treating requirement. The patient should firstly relax and move his joint gently in a moderate margin, avoiding abrupt forceful pulling in case of aggravating

2.2.6 活动关节类手法

是指对患者的肢体关节进行屈伸、内收、外展、旋转、牵拉等的一类手法,也称为被动运动。其形式可根据关节的结构特点和病证治疗的需要选用。操作时,患者肌肉要尽量放松,活动关节的

muscle spasm and injury. This type consists of shaking, pulling and wrenching. Take shaking for instance. Fix one hand on the end of the joint, and put the other hand on the other end, and one can shake the joint in a clockwise direction or otherwise, which applies to joints of the neck, the waist and limbs. Apart from that, there is another shaking method with a larger margin, there is also a finger rubbing method and revolving-pushing one for children.

幅度、力量要恰当。不可突然强力牵拉，以免加重肌痉挛和引起损伤。包括摇法、拉法、扳法等手法。例如摇法用一手固定关节的一端，一手在关节的另一端对可动关节做顺时针或逆时针方向的摇动，也称“运法”，适用于颈、腰及四肢关节部。活动幅度较大的摇法，又称为“盘法”。小儿推拿疗法中所称的“运法”，除了本操作法外，是指“指摩法”及“旋推法”。

3 Common Parts and Respective Methods

3 推拿养生常用部位及方法

Rub Temple: Press the temples with the middle finger tips moving in circles, clockwise first for 10-15 rounds and turning contrary for equal time. It sobers the mind, prevents and cures headache, dizziness and poor eyesight.

揉太阳：用两手中指端，按两侧太阳穴旋转揉动，先顺时针转，后逆时针转，各10～15次。具有清神醒脑的作用，可以防治头痛头晕、眼花视力下降。

Click Jing Ming (BL 1): Click and press Jing Ming (BL 1) with the forefinger tips roughly 20 times, which nourishes the eye and prevents and cures near-sightedness and eye fatigue.

点睛明：用两手食指指端分别点压双睛明穴；共20次左右。具有养睛明目的作用，可以防治近视眼、视疲劳。

Rub Dan Tian (cinnabar field) : Rub the hands hot and do revolving tuina 3 inches below the naval with 3 fingers in the middle of the right hand, for 50-60 times. Dan Tian (cinnabar field) is held by Taoism as housing sperm in men and womb in women, the nourishing of which can furnish the kidney with sperm and replenish marrow, as well as

揉丹田：将双手搓热后，用右手中间三指在脐下3寸处旋转推拿50～60次。丹田，道家认为是男子精室，女子胞宫所在处。养丹田，可助两肾，填精补髓，祛病延寿。常行此法具有健肾固

improve the digestive system.

Rub Zhong Wan (CV 12): Rub hands hot and overlap them on Zhong Wan (CV 12), and rub it clockwise 30 times and vice versa. This hub of the human body lies in the middle of the line artificially drawn between the naval and the xiphoid. Do it often and the digestive system will be improved and the stomach and bowels tuned.

精，改善胃肠功能的作用。

摩中脘：用双手搓热，重叠放在中脘穴处，顺时针方向摩30次，然后再以同样手法逆时针方向摩30次。中脘位于肚脐与剑突下连线中点，居于人体中部，为连接上下的枢纽。常习此法，具有改善消化系统、调整胃肠道的功能的作用。

Rub Da Bao (SP 21): Rub hands hot and apply one hand on Da Bao (SP 21) and rib part across and rub it, alternating the hands 30 times. A major channel of the spleen and crossed by channels of the liver and gut, Da Bao (SP 21) lies at the rib part. Do it every day and the spleen and stomach can be tuned, liver drained of knotting qi and thus cleared, gut furnished, and straying qi and nerve pain at the sides prevented and cured.

搓大包：双手搓热，以一手掌摩搓对侧大包及胁肋部，双手交替各30次。大包是脾之大络，位处胁肋部，为肝胆经脉所行之处。每日操作此法，有调理脾胃、疏肝理气、清肝利胆之功效。可防治肝胆疾病、岔气、肋间神经痛等疾病。

Rub Jian Jing (GB 21): Press and rub shoulders with palms alternately, and pinch Jian Jing (GB 21) with 3 fingers, 20-30 times a day: This acupoint of shoulders lies at the intersection of the three yang meridians of both hands and feet. Rubbing it can prevent and cure periarthritis of should and cervical spondylopathy.

揉肩井：以双手全掌交替揉摩双肩，以拇、食、中指拿捏肩井，每日20～30次。肩井位于肩部，是手足之三阳经脉交会之处。此法具有防治肩周炎、颈椎病的作用。

Rub Lao Gong (PC 8): Put palms together, press and rub Lao Gong (PC 8) clockwise 30 times; hold one thumb and forefinger in a pinching gesture and rub five fingers of the other hand in turns, and then rub one hand with the other palm and do it alternately; until the palms rub hot. Lao Gong (PC 8) is the spring point of pericardium meridian, and the hand is where three yin meridians and three

搓劳宫：以双手掌心相对，顺时针搓压劳宫穴30次；再用一手的拇、食指相对搓另一手的手指，从指根向指尖，五指依次一遍，再用一手掌擦另一手的手背，双手交替进行；最后将两手掌心劳宫穴相互搓热为止。劳宫

yang meridians of the hand meet. Do it often and the heart can be nourished, mind settled, viscera tuned, blood flow invigorated and skin moisturized.

为心包经的荥穴，手是手三阴与手三阳之脉相交处，每日常行此法，可起到养心安神，调和内脏，活血润肤等功效。

Press Shen Shu (BL 23): Rub hands hot and tuina Shen Shu (BL 23) with the palms forward and backward 50-60 times, both at the same time or alternately. Do it before sleep or after getting up, or anytime in rest. This acupoint lies in the waist, which is maintained to be "the house of kidney" by TCM, and the kidney, as a prerequisite of health, governs bones and accommodates essence. Rub the waist until warmth every day, and the kidney and waist can be strengthened, and waist pain caused by a weak kidney or rheumatism can be warded off or cured, in addition to other waist illness such as ankylosing spondylitis and prolapse of lumbar intervertebral disc.

按肾俞：先将双手搓热，再以手掌上下来回推拿肾俞穴 50～60 次，两侧同时或交替进行。此法可于睡前或醒后进行，也可日常休息时操作。肾俞位于腰部，中医认为，"腰者肾之府"，肾为先天之本，主骨藏精。每日用双手摩腰部，使腰部发热，具有强肾壮腰，防治肾虚腰痛、风湿腰痛、强直性脊柱炎、腰椎间盘突出症等腰部疾患的作用。

Rub Yong Quan (KI 1): Rub hands hot and rub the Yong Quan (KI 1) in one foot with the other palm. Do it in both feet 30-50 times until it feels hot; preferably before sleep or after rising. A better effect can be achieved if it is done after a warm foot bath. It can warm the kidney, nourish brain, tune the liver, fortify the spleen, promote sleep, improve blood circulation and strengthen legs; such illness as insomnia, palpitation, dizziness and ringing ears can be warded off or cured.

擦涌泉：先将两手互相搓热，再用左手手掌擦右足涌泉穴，右手手掌擦左足涌泉穴，可反复擦搓 30～50 次，以足心感觉发热为度。此法适宜在临睡前或醒后进行。若能在操作前以温水泡脚，然后再实施，则效果更佳。具有温肾健脑、调肝健脾安眠、改善血液循环、健步的功效，可强身健体，也可防治失眠心悸、头晕耳鸣等症。

4 Keys

When doing tuina, be sure to concentrate the

4 推拿养生的注意事项

推拿时除思想应集中

mind and relax physically and mentally. Master the right locating method for acupoints and operating skills. Tuina mildly first and add strength gradually but also moderately, since if it is done too mildly, the acupoint cannot be stimulated, while the other extreme injures the skin and gives rise to fatigue. Generally the tuina should gradually escalate in times, strength and number of acupoints. An efficient tuina ends in perspiration, so draught should be avoided for fear of catching cold.

外,尤其要心平气和,全身也不要紧张,要求做到身心都放松。掌握常用穴位的取穴方法和操作手法,以求取穴准确,手法正确。注意推拿力度先轻后重,轻重适度。因为过小起不到应有的刺激作用,过大易产生疲劳,且易损伤皮肤。推拿手法的次数要由少到多,推拿力量由轻逐渐加重,推拿穴位可逐渐增加。推拿后有出汗现象时,应注意避风,以免感冒。

Chapter 7 Materia Medica Approach to Health Preservation

第7章 药物养生

Taking materia medica under the guidance of medicinal theories of TCM is an important approach to health preservation. Doctors have not only discovered many health-preserving medicinals, but also created effective fixed prescription with their rich experience in the thousands of years.

药物养生是在中医药理论指导下，运用药物来强身健体的方法，是中医养生保健的重要手段。千百年来，历代医家不仅发现了许多具有养生作用的药物，而且还创造了不少行之有效的保健方剂和剂型，积累了丰富的药物养生的经验。

Section 1 Mechanism

第1节 药物养生的作用机理

Different medicines with different character and serving channels preserve the body in different ways. The medicinal approach to health preservation is based on the concept of strengthening health qi to consolidate constitution, replenishing deficiency and draining excess, and harmonizing yin and yang of the medicines and their set prescriptions, thereby strengthening the kidney and the spleen that govern prenatal and postnatal health respectively, regulating organ functions and balancing yin and yang, hence longevity.

不同的中药由于其偏性和归经的差异，对人体有着不同的治疗或养护作用。药物养生法是通过药物及其配伍后具有的扶正固本、补虚泻实以及调和阴阳的作用，使先后天之本充实，脏腑功能协调，机体阴阳平衡，从而达到治病强身、延年益寿的目的。

1 Strengthening Health Qi to Consolidate Constitution

The positive qi is especially emphasized in TCM, the lack of which fuels disease though it shows in deficiency and excess. So building the positive qi with materia medica can engage all the positive elements of the body in the improvement of immunity, thus warding off disease.

1 扶正固本

中医的药物养生，特别重视中药对人体正气的扶持作用。尽管病理状态有虚实之分，但发病的根本原因在于正气的虚弱，所以运用中药扶助正气，可以调动机体的一切积极因素，增强抗病能力，以防止病邪的侵袭或及早驱邪外出。

2 Tonifying Deficiency and Purging Excess

A broken equilibrium inside the body shows in deficiency or excess. The former refers to deficiency in qi, blood, yin or yang, which should be tonified by medicine, and the latter to the blockage of qi, blood, phlegm or food, wanting purgation by medicine.

2 补虚泻实

机体的偏颇，不外虚实两大类。虚者表现为气血阴阳的不足，应以药物补虚扶正；实者表现为气血痰食的壅滞，应以药物祛邪泻实，如此才能达到增进健康、促进病体康复、益寿延年的目的。

3 Harmonizing Yin and Yang

A general target of medicinal preservation is to harmonize yin and yang and restore them into a dynamic equilibrium. So, take care to reach a moderate degree without overdoing it. Remember that an orderly and harmonious balance of yin and yang is what medicinal preservation consists in.

3 调和阴阳

药物调养的目的在于协调阴阳，使其恢复“阴平阳秘”的动态平衡，因此，治宜恰到好处，不可过偏。药物养生的关键作用就在于调理机体阴阳的平衡，使生命机能有序和谐。

Section 2 Applying Principles

Materia medica must be taken reasonably under

第2节 药物养生的应用原则

方药养生保健要遵循中

the guidance of basic theories of TCM. Disregard of individual difference when taking them would only work the opposite consequence. So heed must be paid to the principles below.

医药的基本理论,合理使用药物才能有助于身体健康,起到预防疾病、延年益寿之效。如果不根据不同的个体差异,盲目滥用则适得其反。因此运用方药养生保健要注意以下原则。

1 Cautious Medication

Many of the medicines for health preservation are of the replenishing character, which generally suit the old and the infirm with poor immunity, but health preservation is not only a matter of replenishment for the deficiency, but purgation of the excess. Great harm can be done if one replenishes the excess blindly. So perception of deficiency or excess is vital in taking medicinals.

1 谨慎用药 切忌滥用

用于养生保健的方药很多,其中有不少是属于补益药物。一般而言,补益药物主要用于生理机能低下、抗病能力降低的年老体弱、久病体虚者的养生保健。然而养生保健方药不只限于补药,要根据具体情况,当补则补,当泻则泻,如果只限于用补法,病邪留恋不去,反招遗患。所以在运用方药进行养生保健时,切忌随便滥用,一定谨慎用药。

2 Taking Medicinals According to Seasons

Health preservation of TCM should be based on the universal concept of men according to nature and the law of warm spring, hot summer, humid heyday of summer, dry autumn and cold winter, and so medicine should be taken accordingly. Further guided by the principle of "cultivating yang in spring and summer and yin in autumn and winter", one should avoid medicines of the pungent and warm character in spring and summer, in case of impairing qi and yin, and medicines of cool and cold character in autumn and winter, in case of harming

2 天人相应 顺时选药

中药养生必须遵循中医学的天人相应的整体观念,根据春温、夏热、长夏湿、秋燥、冬寒的规律,灵活用药。遵循"春夏养阳,秋冬养阴"的原则,在方药施养方面,春夏季节不宜过用辛温发散之品,以免开泄太过,耗气伤阴;秋冬季节要慎用寒凉药物,以防耗伤阳气。

yang.

Be sure to follow the concept of five solid organs corresponding to 5 seasons: liver to spring, heart to summer, spleen July and August, lungs autumn and kidney winter. Things grow afresh in warm spring, so one should take gentle tonics to replenish mildly; things flourish in the steaming yang of summer, so take medicinals of a sweet and cold character rather than replenishing medicine of a hot character in case of heat impairing body fluid and furnishing fire; while in July and August steaming heat mingles with dampness, and medicines should have a clearing effect, aided by other medicines that promote the transportation function of the spleen, in case of heavy nutrition trapping the spleen; while in cool and dry autumn things withdraw from growth and yang atmosphere in nature gives way to yin, when the dryness impairs yin fluid, lungs prosper, the liver shrinks, and the spleen becomes susceptible, so take medicinals that nourish yin and moisturize, aided by other medicines that cultivate qi and blood, avoiding the medicines that consume body fluid; and when winter comes, yang atmosphere in nature withdraws and hides itself together with living things on the earth, when the kidney turns vulnerable, so take tonics of a warm character that furnish yin in the kidney.

同时要顺应主时脏腑的生理特点,五脏分主五季:肝主春,心主夏,脾主长夏,肺主秋,肾主冬。春季气候渐暖,万物生机盎然,故方药养生以清补、柔补、平补为原则;夏季阳气蒸腾,万物生长最为茂盛,方药养生要以甘平、甘凉之品为主,不宜用燥热补药,以防燥热伤津助火;长夏暑热交蒸,湿气较重,方药养生要以清补之品为宜,辅以芳化运脾之药,以防滋腻困脾;秋季气候由热转凉,万物由“长”到“收”,自然界阳气渐收,阴气渐长,气候干燥,易伤人体阴津,肺旺肝弱,脾胃易受其影响,故秋季方药养生保健要以护阴润燥为主,辅以补养气血,忌服耗散伤津之品;冬季阳气潜伏,万物生机闭藏,肾气最易耗损,方药养生要遵循冬令进补的原则,宜用性温益精之品,以补益肾气。

3 Taking Medicinals Depending on Individual Constitution

3 注重体质 因人用药

People differ from each other in constitution, age and gender, and medicinals should be selected accordingly. In addition, living standard, emotions and living areas also have a role to play in the individual

因人用药是根据人的个体体质、年龄、性别等不同特点,有针对性地选择相应的方药进行养生保健。人的禀

physiological and pathological characteristics.

赋强弱、年龄老幼、生活优劣、情志苦乐、地区差异等，决定了不同个体的生理、病理特点，因而在药物养生方面亦应因人而异。

This concept embodies the dialectic treatment of TCM. Cold or hot, deficiency or excess, yin and yang of the viscera must all be taken into account when one takes materia medica.

注重体质，因人选药体现了中医辨证论治的思想，在实际运用中要求医者一定要根据个体情况进行辨证，分清寒热虚实、脏腑阴阳，合理选用具有针对性的药物和方剂，才能取得养生保健，益寿延年之效。

4　Distinguish Between Deficiency and Excess

4　辨别虚实　审因择药

Deficiency consists of deficiency of yin, deficiency of yang, that of qi and that of blood, the four of which may not show singularly, with one possibly allied to another. So an overall perspective must be taken when one prescribes the medicinals, avoiding being partial and overdoing one aspect, which harms health. Therefore, replenishing prescription demands a match of master medicine with servant medicines, yin medicine with yang medicine, cold medicine with hot, and medicine for qi with that for blood.

辨别虚实、审因择药是方药养生的又一重要原则。如前所述，人的禀赋不同，体质有强弱之分，因此运用方药养生要有的放矢。

Replenishment for deficiency mainly applies to the old and the infirm, while there are others suffering from excess, especially in the modern society where people tend to emphasize replenishment rather than drainage, with the result that they become fat with the potential danger of blockage of qi and blood, phlegm and food. So it is vital to purge evil excess by means of perspiration, excrement, clear-

体虚一般表现有阴虚、阳虚、气虚、血虚等，但临床表现并不一定典型，也不一定单独出现。因此在使用补法时，需要全面考虑，注意补勿过偏，不可矫枉过正，对身体造成伤害。因此，以补益为主的养生保健方，组方必

ing and melting, depending on the condition. But take note not to overdo it, which impairs the positive qi and works the opposite effect.

须注意君臣佐使的配伍，阴药与阳药的并举，寒药与热药的调和，气药与血药的同用。

Just bear in mind the principles of perspiring mildly, avoiding violent excrement, clearing yet not too cold, and melting without consuming qi. Do everything moderately, in one word.

药物养生固然是年老体弱者益寿延年的辅助方法，以补虚为主亦无可厚非。然而，体盛而本实者、体盛而邪实者也有之。现代社会，生活优越，人们往往重补而轻泻。由于嗜食膏粱厚味，现代人多脂醇充溢，形体肥胖，气血痰食壅滞已成隐患。因此，泻实之法也是养生保健的重要方法之一。体盛邪实者，更要注意祛邪，祛邪的方法有汗、下、清、消等，应根据不同的情况采用不同的方法。但又不可因体得其盛而过分地攻泻，攻泻太过易伤正气，不但不能起到养生保健的作用，反而适得其反。故方药养生保健中的泻实之法，以不伤其正为原则，力求达到汗毋大泄，清毋过寒，下毋峻猛，消毋耗气。

5 Taking Medicinals Based on Syndrome Differentiation

5 扶正祛邪 辨证遣药

The old and the infirm do not have sufficient positive qi to combat pathogenic qi from outside and are taken over by it. Deficiency and excess often coexist. So replenishment goes together with drainage, the dominant role relying on the condition,

年老体虚之人正气不足，往往无力抵御外邪，因而容易形成正虚邪盛的险候。虚则补之，实则泻之二者截然不同，但又必须兼顾，要仔

that is, more excess than deficiency requires drainage as the major measure, and vice versa. The ancients have long conducted both together, fluctuating in their percentage or mingling them in a whole with, of course, the weight in just one. So be sure to build the positive qi while attacking the pathogenic factors. In so doing one must fortify the spleen and the stomach, which, responsible for postnatal health, are the fountains of qi, blood and body fluid; and the kidney must also be furnished to cultivate the positive qi, as it is the prenatal governor, which takes the harm to all viscera in one.

细衡量,虚实孰轻孰重。虚少实多,应以攻为主;虚重实轻,应以补为主。因此,前人早有攻补兼施之法,或攻多补少,或补多攻少,或寓补于泻,或寓泻于补。祛邪又要兼顾正气,采用扶正祛邪的方法。脾胃为后天之本,是气血津液生化之源,历代医家扶正都重视调补脾胃。肾为先天之本,五脏之伤,穷必及肾,所以扶正又要注重补肾。

6 Taking Medicinals Step by Step

Aging is a gradual process and a complex phenomenon, since people of the same age show different signs of aging due to different constitution and health-preserving practice. Materia medica can play a part in delaying the effects of aging, but they must be taken step by step, unlike the immediate work of food eliminating hunger.

6 不宜骤补 渐进施药

衰老是一个缓慢的渐进过程,然而由于先天禀赋的不同,平素注重保养有别,所以生理年龄相同的人,体表征象却不完全一样,因此,衰老是一个复杂的生命现象。养生方药作为一种辅助方法,对推迟衰老确有一定效果,但又有别于食物能饱腹之立竿见影,需要有一个循序渐进的过程,急于求成反而有害。所以,不宜骤补,渐进施药,也是方药养生保健中应遵循的重要原则。

Section 3 Common Forms of Materia Medica

第3节 常用养生药物剂型

As is mentioned, medicine falls into the types

临床上中药剂型主要有

of soup, processed pills, powder and liquid while health-preserving medicinals consist of medicinal tea, medicinal wine, medicinal dish and medicinal jelly.

汤剂和制成中成药的丸剂、散剂及水剂，由于药物养生的保养特点，其剂型丰富多彩，常用的有：养生药茶、养生药酒、养生药膳、养生膏方等。

1 Medicinal Tea

Some medicines can be simply put into a glass, and then pour in boiling water and the medicinal tea is ready, or boil them directly for a short time for better effect. The simplicity of preparation makes the tea a very common approach to health preservation. But please note that the simple tea should also conform to the dialectic principle of TCM, with the choice catering to different constitution and specific purpose, so that the ailment can be cured and qi movement tuned.

1 养生药茶

养生药茶，是指某些中药用水泡制或煎制，以当茶饮用。这种剂型制作简单、使用方便，是日常生活中十分常用的一种保健剂型。药茶的运用也必须遵循中医学辨证施治的原则，针对不同体质和保养目的，选择不同的组方，以达到补益虚损、调畅气机的养生保健的功效。

2 Medicinal Wine

Medicinal wine means soaking medicines of the right recipe and proportion in the wine and awaiting them to fully dissolve or release the medicinal elements. A common approach to health preservation and clinical treatment, the medicinal wine was recorded in the *Yellow Emperor's Inner Canons* (Huang Di Nei Jing).

2 养生药酒

药酒就是以酒为溶剂，把药物按照配方比例浸泡在酒中，等到药物充分溶解或释放药性后而得到的液剂。药酒用于治病或保健在我国由来已久，在现存最早的中医典籍《黄帝内经》中，就有记载酒的治疗作用的专篇。时至今天，药酒成为人们养生保健和临床治病的常见剂型之一。

Notes should be taken about the choice of medicines and the doses, as the wrong intake would impair health and even life.

药酒虽然具有治病保健的作用，但是在服用药酒时还是要注意一些问题，从选用药酒到服用剂量，都是有规可循的。正确服用药酒能够养生保健，错误地服用反会伤生损命。所以在饮用药酒时，应该注意以下事项：

Firstly, choose medicines dialectically. Choose medicines according to the constitution, disease and adaptation to the medicine and wine. For example, people with a weak spleen and stomach can take Ren Shen wine and Dang Gui (*Radix Angelicae Sinensis*) wine; those with a weak kidney deficiency, Ren Shen and Lu Rong (*Cornu Cervi Pantotrichum*) wine and three-whip wine; those with failing qi and blood, dragon phoenix wine and all-replenishing wine; those suffering from neurosism, wine of fruit of Wu Wei Zi (*Fructus Schisandrae Chinensis*) and He Huan Pi (*Cortex Albiziae*) wine.

其一，辨证选用。药酒的运用要根据自己的体质、患病历史、对药和酒的适应程度辨证选用。例如：脾胃虚弱者可以服用人参酒和当归酒；肾虚者可以饮用参茸酒和三鞭酒；气血不足者应该选用龙凤酒和十全大补酒；神经衰弱者可以选用五味子酒和合欢皮酒。

Secondly, take the right amount. Due to the alcohol and medicines with their particular character, taste and functions, one must take medicinal wine moderately. An overdose of it would spark sickness, vomit, palpitation and even alcoholic toxin, toxicosis medicinalis. Taking too much Ren Shen wine, for instance, fuels excessive heat in the body, failing appetite, heat caused by phlegm, palpitation and indigestion; an overdose of Lu Rong wine triggers palpitation, insomnia and even bleeding nose.

其二，服用适量。药酒中含有酒精和药剂，这些成分都有着自己特定的性味功效，所以服用时要适量，不能过量。过多的饮用不但不会治愈疾病强身健体，还可能诱发恶心呕吐、心悸甚至酒精中毒、药物中毒等不良的后果。如服用人参酒过量会引起上火、食欲不振、痰热心悸、消化不良等症状。过量服用鹿茸酒还会导致心慌失眠甚至流鼻血等不良的反应。

Thirdly, taboo for people with certain diseases. Those with certain diseases, such as liver disease, coronary heart disease, tuberculosis, peptic ulcer,

其三，注意禁忌证。药酒的运用要注意一些不宜饮酒的病，不能采取药酒保健，

and some skin diseases, should be kept away from alcohol, and thus medicinal wine. It is even worse for those alcohol-allergic, the pregnant and children.

例如肝病、冠心病、肺结核、消化系统溃疡和一些皮肤病。而对酒精过敏的人群及孕妇和婴幼儿，饮酒不仅不能够缓解病证，还可能诱发严重后果。

3 Medicinal Food

3 养生药膳

The medicinal food in general, as the name indicates, is more food than medicine, thus more moderate in the effect. And the medicines commonly used for it can also be food embraced by many people, hence "food serving health".

药膳从广义上说，属于食疗的范围，相比用单纯药物类来调养身体，具有相对平和的特点。可用于药膳的药物，多是药食同用之品，其"寓健康于饮食"，深受广大群众的喜爱。

The medicinal food, like medicine, also varies in material, processing and functions, so certain principles must be observed in application, which brings out the best function and guards against negative reaction in the body. In one word, prepare the medicinal food dialectically based on different people, time and place, and more importantly, illness.

药膳由于使用原料、制作原理、防治功效等方面的不同，其在实际应用过程中需要遵循一定的原则。这样既能达到理想的治疗效果，又能避免由于错用药物而导致不良反应的发生。应用时要重辨证论治，不仅应做到因人施膳、因时施膳、因地施膳，更要根据不同的病证做到辨证施膳。

The food, like medicine, also has the four characters of cold, cool, warm and hot, and as we know, the food has the five tastes of being pungent, sweet, sour, bitter and salty. Characters and tastes and taboos must be considered in grouping materials in case of negative reaction or even disease.

药物和食物的属性有寒、热、温、凉四种；味有辛、甘、酸、苦、咸五味之分。药膳的组成原料中，药物和食物都有其独特的性、味，因此在搭配使用时亦应有所注意，应充分了解药物和食物的搭配、使用禁忌，以免由于错误配致不良反应或疾病的发生。

4 Medicinal Paste Formula

The medicinal paste prescription is processed from medicinal soup of many medicines prescribed according to different constitutions and symptoms of the patient, by boiling the soup further to thickness and adding something special to make it as thick as paste. The formila has diverse merits, such as allying replenishment with treatment, catering to cold and hot diseases, nourishing and promoting, curing the root of the disease as well as symptoms, flexible change in amount, and tailored to the constitution or condition, hence a perfect choice for the infirm and those with chronic diseases. With the right prescription and intake, patients of both acute and chronic diseases can recuperate faster, with flourishing primordial qi and stronger constitution. Owing to the advantages of lasting and mild effect, portability and handiness in intake, the paste formula is indeed a treasure for nourishment in winter.

The paste formula should be taken based on the disease, the constitution of the patient, the season, climate and geography. It is generally taken in winter, lasting roughly 150 days from the end of December to the beginning of February. In the case of taking two formulas in a winter, one can take the first earlier. Surely there are also curing paste formulas aiming at curing, conducted by the doctor all year round based on the disease and season, but they are mostly of a cool character. One had better take

4 养生膏方

养生膏方，一般是以大型复方汤剂为基础，根据病人的不同体质、不同临床表现而确立处方，药物经过浓煎后，掺入某些特殊辅料而制成的一种稠厚的膏状物。膏方具有补中寓治、治中寓补、寒温并用、动静结合、补虚扶弱、标本兼治、随证加减、量体裁方的特点，对多种慢性疾病及体质虚弱者有较好的调理和治疗作用。只要处方得当、服用合理，不仅能促进急慢性病人康复，还可使正气旺盛、身体健康，起到增强体质、防病治病、延年益寿的效果。由于膏方药的药性较缓和而持久，便于携带，服用方便，成为冬令滋补、疗养佳品。

膏方的服用，一是根据病人的病情决定，二是考虑病人的体质，应时的季节、气候、地理条件等因素，因人、因时、因地制宜。服用季节一般以冬季为主，带有明显的季节性。一般从冬至即“一九”开始服用，至“六九”结束，大约 50 天，或服至立春前结束。如果一冬服两料

the paste formula with proper diet, repose and physical exercise, which contribute to the best performance of the functions.

膏方，服用时间可以适当提前。当然，由于现代冰箱等储存条件的提高，调治膏方可根据患者的病情需要或不同时令特点随季节处方，一年四季均可，但这种四季膏方一般以清膏为主。服用膏方时最好配合饮食调理，劳逸适宜，运动保健等，这样才能使膏方的作用发挥至最佳。

The paste can be melted in water and drunk or just melted in the mouth, the former being preferred generally. Take a spoonful of paste and put it in the container and pour in boiled water of 90 degrees Celsius or so, then mix and drink it. If there is a big dose of nourishing medicines such as radices rehmanniae or gelatinous medicines that make the jelly too glutinous to handle, steam it or melt it in the microwave oven first. "Pills" of the paste formula have been produced in recent years, which can be chewed conveniently. The jelly prescription can be best digested and absorbed when taken into an empty stomach upon rising and before sleep, free from interference of other food. If the empty stomach does not feel well after taking it, take it one hour after meal.

膏方的服用方法可以分为冲服和含化。一般人喜欢冲服：取一汤匙膏方，用90 ℃左右白开水冲入，和匀后服用。如方中用地黄等滋腻药或配料中胶类药物剂量较大，膏方黏稠难取，可以隔水蒸化或微波炉小火稀化后取用。所谓含化，即是将膏滋含在口中慢慢融化后吞服。此外，近几年出现的"片"状膏剂可以直接嚼食。膏方一般清晨空腹和晚上临睡前服，因此时胃肠消化吸收能力强，且不受食物干扰。如空腹服感肠胃不适，可在饭后一小时左右服用。

The dose depends on the disease, physical condition of the patient and character of the medicine, and especially on the digestive function of the patient. The general practice is to take one spoon (15-20 ml) of it twice a day. One can start with a smaller dose—once a day—and develop to twice a day

服用剂量根据患者病情或身体情况及药物性质而定，尤其与患者消化功能密切相关，一般一次一汤匙(15～20 毫升)，一日 2 次。一般先从小剂量开始，逐渐

for better effect if he does not feel uncomfortable. Paste formula of a mild character can be taken in greater amount, while that of toxin should be taken in smaller amount, which can be developed gradually, in case of being poisoned and the positive qi being impaired. The dose also varies with constitution, gender and age: the old should take less than the young; the infirm, the strong; women, men; and women in period, pregnancy and after delivery less than usual. In one word, the dose should be determined from a comprehensive perspective.

增加，如每日先服一次，如果无不适感，再加至早晚各服一次，以加强其效果。性质平和的膏方，用量可以稍大，有毒、峻烈的药物，用量宜小，并且应从小剂量开始，逐渐增加，以免中毒或耗伤正气。患者的体质强弱、性别、年龄等不同，在剂量上也应有所差别。老年人用量应小于壮年；体质强者可多，体质弱者宜少；妇女的用药量，一般应小于男子，妇女在经期、孕期及产后，应小于平时。但总须从养生需求等各方面综合考虑、全面衡量。

There are taboos to caution against for safety and better effect. Apart from the “18 incompatibicities” and “19 antagonisms” in food grouping principle, some food taboos should be complied with when one takes the paste formula. It is generally deemed that the radish should be guarded against when one takes medicines that furnish qi such as Ren Shen; strong tea against nourishing jelly, and raw, cold, greasy, spicy, indigestible and stimulating food against all paste formulas.

在使用膏方时，为了注意安全，保证效果，必须重视禁忌问题。除了药物配伍中的“十八反”“十九畏”等用药禁忌外，还有补膏忌口等。通常认为，服用含人参等补气的膏方忌食萝卜；服用滋补性膏方不宜饮浓茶；服用膏方期间忌食生冷、油腻、辛辣等不易消化及有特殊刺激性的食物。

Not only is it required when one takes the paste formula, the food taboo is also demanded by TCM generally. For instance, people of yin-deficiency constitution should not eat beef, ginger, garlic and onion due to their hot and pungent character, and they can be convinced by the symptoms of more severe thirstiness, dry throat, constipation, and even

针对患者的不同体质而忌口，不仅是服用膏方的要求，也是中医养生的要求。例如，阴虚体质，忌食狗肉、牛肉，姜、蒜、葱等辛热食品。否则，轻则口干咽燥加重、大便燥结，重则可见出血症状。

bleeding in a worse case, if they do; while people of yang- deficiency constitution should not abuse medicines that warm up and replenish the yang of the kidney, such as the sheep whip, the cattle whip and mutton, by keeping watch on the possible deficiency fire, which would be encouraged by medicine to a bleeding stage, and they should not eat food of a cold character such as the persimmon and the cucumber, nor should they often eat greasy things in case of clogged circulation of qi and blood.

而阳虚体质,忌滥用温补肾阳之品,如服鹿鞭、牛鞭、羊肉等,应注意观察有无虚火,防助火动血,产生变证;忌服用寒性食品,如柿子、黄瓜等;忌用或过用厚味腻滞之品,防气血运行不畅。

Section 4 Some Prescriptions

第4节 养生方药举例

The Chinese medicine mostly takes the form of prescription that mixes several medicines. Here are some common medicines for health preservation: ① to replenish qi: Ren Shen, Xi Yang Shen (*Radix Panacis Quinquefolii*), Shan Yao, Huang Qi (*Radix Astragali seu Hedysari*); ② to replenish blood: Dang Gui, Shu Di Huang (*Radix Rehmanniae Preparata*), Zhi Shou Wu (*Radix Polygoni Multiflori Praeparata*), E Jiao (*Colla Corii Asini*); ③ to nourish yin: Mai Dong (*Radix Ophiopogonis*), Gou Qi Zi (*Fructus Lycii*), Bai He (*Bulbus Lilii*), Bie Jia (*Carapax Trionycis*); ④ to fuel yang: Lu Rong, Zi He Che (*Placenta Hominis*), He Tao Ren, Rou Cong Rong (*Herba Cistanches*); ⑤ to deter pathogenic factors: Sheng Jiang, Ju Hua, Fu Ling (*Poria*), Jue Ming Zi, Shan Zha, San Qi (*Radix Notoginseng*), Tian Ma (*Rhizoma Gastrodiae*). These medicines make up the set prescriptions that follow up.

中医用药,多以方剂形式,将一种或几种药物配合使用。养生常用药物有:①补气类:人参、西洋参、山药、黄芪等;②补血类:当归、熟地、制首乌、阿胶等;③养阴类:麦冬、枸杞子、百合、鳖甲等;④补阳类:鹿茸、紫河车、核桃仁、肉苁蓉等;⑤祛邪类:生姜、菊花、茯苓、决明子、山楂、三七、天麻等。本节包含的各种养生方,多以这些药物为主而组成。

1 Replenishing Chinese Patent Medicines

1.1 To Nourish the Heart

(1) Si Bu Wan (*Four-replenishing Pill*)

Composition: Bai Zi Ren (*Seman Platycladi*), He Shou Wu (*Radix Polygoni Multiflori*), Rou Cong Rong (*Herba Cistanches*), Huai Niu Xi (*Radix Achyranthis Bidentatae*).

Functions: calming the mind, replenishing blood, fortifying the kidney, nourishing the heart.

Illness: Sour waist and fatigued legs caused by uncollected mind, insomnia, forgetfulness.

Dose: 20-30 pills each time.

(2) Yang Xin Dan (*Heart Nourishing Pill*)

Composition: Zhu Sha (*cinnabar*), Ru Xiang (*Olibanum*), Suan Zao Ren (*Semen Ziziphi Spinosae*), Fu Ling.

Functions: nourishing qi and blood, calming the mind.

Illness: unsettled spirit, insomnia with start from sleep.

Dose: 10 pills each time, washed down with warm water.

1.2 To Nourish the Liver

(1) Qi Ju Di Huang Wan (*Wolfberry, Chrysanthemum and Rehmannia Root Pill*)

Composition: Gou Qi Zi, Ju Hua, Shu Di Huang, Shan Zhu Yu (*Fructus Corni*), Shan Yao.

Functions: furnishing the liver and the kidney, clearing eyes.

Illness: impaired liver and kidney, blurred vision.

Dose: 10 g each time, washed down with warm water.

1 补养类中成药

1.1 养心类

（1）四补丸

组成：柏子仁、何首乌、肉苁蓉、怀牛膝。

功效：安神补血，益肾养心。

适应证：用于心神不摄之腰酸腿软，失眠健忘者。

服法：每服20～30丸。

（2）养心丹

组成：朱砂、乳香、酸枣仁、茯苓。

功效：养气血，安神志。

适应证：用于心神不定，惊悸失眠者。

服法：每服10丸，温开水送下。

1.2 养肝类

（1）杞菊地黄丸

组成：枸杞子、菊花、熟地黄、山茱萸、山药等。

功效：补肝肾，明目。

适应证：用于肝肾亏虚，眼花目昏者。

服法：每服10克，开水送服。

(2) Jue Ming Zi Wan (*Semen Cassiae Torae Pill*)

Composition: Jue Ming Zi, Fu Ling, Huang Qin (*Radix Scutellariae*), Mai Dong (*Radix Ophiopogonis*), Ze Xie (*Alismatis Rhizoma*).

Functions: furnishing the liver, nourishing blood, clearing eyes.

Illness: impaired blood in the liver, illusion of black spots in the vision.

Dose: 20 pills each time, washed down with warm water, twice a day.

(2) 决明子丸

组成: 决明子、茯苓、黄芩、麦门冬、泽泻等。

功效: 补肝养血明目。

适应证: 适用于肝血亏虚,视野中黑蚊乱舞之证。

服法: 每服 20 丸,温汤水下,每日 2 次。

1.3 To Nourish the Spleen

1.3 养脾类

(1) Shou Zhong Wan (*Stomach-guarding pill*)

Composition: Shu Di Huang, Ren Shen, Bai Zhu, Ju Hua, Shan Yao.

Functions: replenishing qi and blood, fortifying the spleen and the stomach.

Illness: infirm kidney and spleen, emaciation, sour and hurting waist and legs, fatigue and sleepiness.

Dose: 50 pills before a meal per day, washed down with light rice wine.

(1) 守中丸

组成: 熟地、人参、白术、菊花、山药等。

功效: 补气益血,健脾养胃。

适应证: 用于先后天不足,伴形体消瘦,腰腿酸痛,体倦乏力者。

服法: 每日饭前服 50 丸,清酒送下。

(2) Da Huang Qi Wan (*Big Root-of-membranous-milk-vetch Pill*)

Composition: Huang Qi, Bai Zi Ren (*Seman Platycladi*), Tian Dong (*Radix Asparagi*), Bai Zhu, Yuan Zhi (*Radix Polygalae*).

Functions: replenishing the spleen and qi.

Illness: the infirm and exhausted, weak spleen.

Dose: 10 pills per day.

(2) 大黄芪丸

组成: 黄芪、柏子仁、天冬、白术、远志等。

功效: 补脾益气。

适应证: 主要用于治疗虚劳脾弱之证。

服法: 每日 10 丸。

1.4 To Nourish Lungs

1.4 养肺类

(1) Qiong Yu Gao (*Jade Paste*)

Composition: Ren Shen, Fu Ling, honey, Feng

(1) 琼玉膏

组成: 人参、茯苓、蜜、生

Mi, Sheng Di Huang.

Functions: replenishing lungs and qi.

Illness: the infirm and exhausted with cough.

Dose: one spoon each time, melted with boiled water.

(2) Bu Fei Wan (*Lung Replenishing Pill*)

Composition: Mai Dong, Kuan Dong Hua (*Flos Farfarae*), Sang Bai Pi Gen (*Radix Cortex Mori*), Gui Xin (*Cortex Cinnamomi*), Wu Wei Zi (*Fructus Schisandrae Chinensis*).

Functions: replenishing lungs, conducive to inhaling.

Illness: inadequate qi in lungs, pain in the chest, asthma.

Dose: 15 pills each time, three times a day.

1.5 To Nourish the Kidney

(1) Zhu Yang Wan (*Yang Fueling Pill*)

Composition: Lu Rong, Tu Si Zi (*Semen Cuscutae*), Fu Zi (*Radix Aconiti Lateralis Preparata*), Rou Cong Rong (*Herba Cistanches*), Huang Qi.

Functions: replenishing the kidney with essence, qi and yang.

Illness: fatigue and sleepiness caused by impaired yang in the kidney, sallow face, sour and weak waist and legs.

Dose: 20 pills, washed down with warm wine.

(2) Er Zhi Wan (*Double-herb Pill*)

Composition: Nü Zhen Zi (*Fructus Ligustri Lucidi*), Han Lian Cao (*Ecliptae Herba*).

Functions: nourishing yin and blood, replenishing the kidney.

地。

功效：补肺益气。

适应证：用于虚劳喘嗽之证。

服法：每服1匙，开水调下。

（2）补肺丸

组成：麦门冬、款冬花、桑白皮根、桂心、五味子。

功效：补肺纳气。

适应证：适用于肺气不足，胸痛哮喘。

服法：每服15丸，每日3次。

1.5 养肾类

（1）助阳丸

组成：鹿茸、菟丝子、附子、肉苁蓉、黄芪等。

功效：补肾益气，填精壮阳。

适应证：用于肾阳亏虚之体倦乏力，面色少华，腰膝酸软。

服法：每服20丸，饭前温酒送服。

（2）二至丸

组成：女贞子、旱莲草。

功效：滋阴养血补肾。

Illness: Symptoms caused by yin deficiency in the liver and the kidney.

Dose: 30 – 50 pills, washed down with warm wine before sleep.

2 Medicinal Dishes

(1) Bai He Yu Zhu Shen Ji Si (*Medicinal Shredded Chicken*)

Ingredients: Bai He (*Bulbus Lilii*) 20 g, Yu Zhu (*Radix Polygonati Officinalis*) 15 g, Dang Shen (*Radix Codonopsis*) 20 g, a loaf of Shan Yao shredded chicken 250 g, rice 80 g, alittle scallion, ginger and salt.

Procedures: Remove the beard of Yu Zhu and wash it, shred it, boil it for thick juice, remove dregs; stir-fry the chicken and put it in the pot with Bai He, Dang Shen , Shan Yao and rice; add the juice of Yu Zhu. and scallion, ginger, salt and more water, boil it over strong fire and simmer it after boiling for 25 minutes.

Functions: nourishing yin and moisturizing lungs, furnishing the stomach and promoting body fluid production; mainly for the illness of qi deficiency, cough without phlegm, consumed frame.

Taboo: forbidden from those who cough due to wind cold, and who suffer from clogged qi and phlegmatic hygrosis.

(2) Yin He Lü Yi Xiao Shu Zhou (*Heat Melting Porridge*)

Ingredients: one loaf of white fungus, one piece of lotus leaf, green bean 30 g, shell of the watermelon 60 g, rice 100 g, a little crystal rock sugar.

Procedures: soak the fungus in water and wait for it to swell; shred the clean leaf; remove the surface of the shell; boil the leaf for thick juice, into

适应证: 适用于肝肾阴虚。

服法: 每服 30～50 丸,临卧温酒服下。

2 养生药膳

(1) 百合玉竹参鸡丝

原料: 百合 20 克,玉竹 15 克,党参 20 克,鲜山药一段,鸡肉丝 250 克,粳米 80 克,葱、姜、盐等少许。

制法: 玉竹洗净,去掉须根,切碎煎取浓汁后去渣,把炒制好的鸡丝与百合、党参、山药、粳米一同放入锅内,加入玉竹的煎液,放入葱、姜、盐,再加水适量,武火烧沸后改为文火煲 25 分钟即可。

功效应用: 养阴润肺,益胃生津。主治气虚咳嗽,身体羸瘦,咳嗽无痰。

使用注意: 风寒咳嗽,痰湿气滞者禁服。

(2) 银荷绿衣消暑粥

原料: 银耳一个,荷叶一张,绿豆 30 克,西瓜翠衣 60 克,粳米 100 克,冰糖少许。

制法: 银耳水发,荷叶洗净切碎,西瓜翠衣去外皮,先煎荷叶取浓汁,加入银耳、西

which add fungus, melon shell, beans, rice and water, simmer it for 25 minutes after boiling over strong fire, add sugar when it turns cooler.

瓜翠衣、绿豆、粳米加适量水，武火烧沸后改为文火煲25分钟即可，待温后加入冰糖即可食用。

Functions: clearing hear, promoting body fluid production, or illness of restlessness and thirstiness caused by summer heat; ulcerous mouth and tongue, heat stranguria, short and reddish urine, hypertension.

功效应用：清热解暑，生津止渴。对于暑热烦渴、口舌生疮、热淋小便短赤、高血压病均有一定的防治作用。

(3) Zhu Yu Zao Tang Zhou (*Bead and Jade Porridge*)

(3) 珠玉枣糖粥

Ingredients: Shan Yao 100 g, fresh Yi Yi Ren 100 g, Long Yan Rou 15 g, 6 small dates, black sugar 10 g, rice 150 g.

原料：生山药100克，生薏苡仁100克，龙眼肉15克，小枣6个，红糖10克，粳米150克。

Procedures: boil Yi Yi Ren and rice to rough readiness; cut peeled Shan Yao into loaves; put them and Long Yan Rou the rice pot, add dates after boiling, simmer them until rice turns extremely soft, add sugar when eating.

制法：先将薏苡仁和粳米煮熟，再将去皮生山药切块和龙眼肉入内同煮为粥，水开后加入小枣，待米煨烂即可，食用时可以兑入适量红糖。

Functions: replenishing qi and blood. Have it during menstruation period and qi and blood can be better restored.

功效应用：气血双补。月经期食用，有助气血恢复。

(4) Fu Ling Qin Cai Zhu Rou Jiao Zi (*Fu Ling Pork Dumpling*)

(4) 茯苓青菜猪肉饺子

Ingredients: wheat powder 1 000 g, lean pork 500 g, Fu Ling powder 50 g, mashed green vegetable 50 g, seasoning with appropriate amount.

原料：精面粉1 000克，精猪肉500克，茯苓粉50克，青菜泥50克，调料适量。

Procedures: chop pork fine enough to be filling, add Fu Ling, vegetable, salt, monosodium glutamate, cooking wine, sesame oil and churn them together; make round wrappings with wheat; put the filling in to make dumplings, and steam them for

制法：将肉剁成馅，加茯苓粉、菜泥、盐、味精、料酒、香油调好。将面发好，压皮，包上肉馅，成提花包，入笼蒸八分钟即可。

8 minutes.

Functions: nourishing the heart, calming the mind, fortifying the spleen and promoting the appetite, melting dampness and phlegm, eliminating dropsy and promoting urination; for the illness of failing transportation of the spleen that leads to liquid swell, failing reception of the stomach. Healthy people can also eat it for a better stomach.

功效应用：养心安神，健脾开胃，除湿化痰，利水消肿。适用于脾失健运，胃纳欠佳，脾虚水肿等。常人食之可益胃健体。

(5) Jiang Zhi Chang Sheng Zhou (*Fat-Melting Porridge*)

（5）降脂长生粥

Ingredients: Ze Xie (*Alismatis Rhizoma*) 200 g sunned and ground into powder, He Shou Wu (*Radix Polygoni Multiflori*) 100 g sunned and ground into powder, Da Zao(*Fructus Jujubae*)6 dates, fresh Shan Zha (*Fructus Crataegi*) 30 g, one piece of fresh lotus leaf, rice 60 g, some crystal rock sugar.

原料：泽泻 200 克晒干研粉，何首乌 100 克洗净晒干，研为细粉，红枣 6 枚，鲜山楂 30 克，鲜荷叶 1 张，粳米 60 克，冰糖适量。

Procedures: shred the leaf and boil it for 200 ml of thick juice, remove seeds of Shan Zha, shred them and boil them with rice; when the porridge is about to be ready, put in 10 g of Ze Xie and 10 g of He Shou Wu, and simmer it to boil, churn and calm it and wait for it to boil again, repeating the process a couple of times and it is ready. Have the warm porridge once a day.

制法：取鲜荷叶 1 张，切细，煎取浓汁约 200 ml。山楂洗净去核切碎，与粳米一起加入锅中加水煲煮。本粥气味清香，善开食欲。先煮米为粥，待米开花后，调入 10 克泽泻粉，放入 10 克何首乌粉，改用文火稍煮数沸即可。每日一次，温热服食。

Functions: furnishing qi in the heart, lowering fat and pressure of blood; for the illness of high fat and pressure of blood, and hardening of the artery. It is especially good for the old with such diseases to take this scented and appetizing porridge in the long run, also good for those with high fat in blood yet without symptoms.

功效应用：益心气，降血脂，降血压。对防治高血脂、高血压、动脉硬化均有效果，宜于老年性高血压、高血脂患者长期食之。本方不仅适用于高脂血症临床症状明显者，也可用于临床症状不明显，但经查血脂水平高者。

Taboo: Do not use iron pot to make it.

使用注意：忌用铁器煮

whole Dang Gui (*Radix Angelicae Sinensis*), Sang Shen(*Fructus Mori*), Ling Zhi (*Ganoderma*), Yin Yang Huo(Folium Epimedii), Zhen Zhu(*Margarita*)powder, Pi Pa Ye.

葚、灵芝、仙灵脾、珍珠粉、枇杷叶。

Illness: impaired qi and blood; for the illness of dizziness, blurred eyesight, palpitation, insomnia, cough caused by deficiency of lungs.

应用: 气血亏虚见头晕眼花、心悸失眠、肺虚咳嗽等。

Dose: one spoon of it about 10 g, washed down with water, in the morning and at night.

服法: 每服1食匙,约10克,早晚各一次,开水冲服。

(6) Shi Zhen Gao (*Ten-Gem Paste*)

(6) 十珍膏

Composition: Dang Shen, Huang Qi, Bai Zhu, Dang Gui, Sheng Di Huang, Shu Di Huang,, Mai Dong, Gou Qi Zi, Tian Dong, Wu Wei Zi (*Fructus Schisandrae Chinensis*), Feng Mi.

组成: 党参、黄芪、白术、当归、生地黄、熟地黄、麦门冬、枸杞、天门冬、五味子、蜂蜜。

Illness: replenishing qi and nourishing blood; for the old and the infirm, and those in recuperation after a severe disease.

应用: 补气养血。用于年迈体弱者及大病后调理。

Dose: 10 g of it washed down with water, in the morning and at night.

服法: 口服,一次10克,早晚各一次,开水冲服。

(7) Jian Shen Chang Chun Gao (*All-Spring Paste*)

(7) 健身长春膏

Composition: Hong Shen (*Radix Ginseng Rubra*), Huang Qi, Bai Zhu, Fu Ling, Gan Cao (*Radix Glycyrrhizae*), Shu Di Huang, whole Dang Gui, Chuan Xiong (*Rhizoma Ligustici Chuanxiong*), Gou Qi Zi, He Shou Wu, Nv Zhen Zi (*Fructus Ligustri Lucidi*), Sang Shen, Chen Pi(*Pericarpium Citri Reticulatae*), processed Ban Xia (*Rhizoma Pinelliae*).

组成: 红参、黄芪、白术、茯苓、甘草、熟地黄、全当归、川芎、枸杞、何首乌、女贞子、桑椹、陈皮、制半夏。

Illness: replenishing qi and blood enormously, nourishing the liver and the kidney; for the illness of inadequate qi and blood, dizziness, fatigue, ringing ears, palpitation, insomnia, forgetfulness caused by impaired yin in the liver and the kidney.

应用: 大补气血,滋养肝肾。用于气血不足,肝肾阴亏所致头晕眼花、神疲乏力、耳鸣心悸、失眠健忘等。

Dose: one spoon of it about 10 g, washed down

服法: 每服1食匙,约10

with water, in the morning and at night.

(8) Gui Lu Er Xian Gao (*Double-Fairy Paste*)

Composition: Lu Jiao (*Cornu Cervi*), Gui Jia (*Carapax et Plastrum Testudinis*), Gou Qi Zi, Ren Shen.

Illness: replenishing qi and blood, furnishing essence and marrow; for the illness of emaciation, breathlessness, semen leakage in dream, weak waist and legs, dizziness and deafness caused by exhausted essence and blood and impaired genuine qi.

Dose: one spoon of it about 10 g, melt it in warm wine and drink it in the morning.

克,早晚各一次,开水冲服。

(8) 龟鹿二仙膏

组成: 鹿角、龟板、枸杞、人参。

应用: 益气养血、填精补髓。用于真元亏损、精血枯竭所致瘦弱少气、梦遗泄精、腰腿无力、目眩耳聋等。

服法: 每服1食匙,约10克,早晨温酒下。

Chapter 8 Health Preservation in Different Areas

第8章 不同地区养生

The geographical environment also has a role to play in human physiological activities and life span. All the four renowned longevity areas of the world boast of mountains, woods, rivers, fresh air and smaller population, and are underdeveloped.

人所生活的周边地理环境，在一定程度上影响着人体的生理活动及寿命。比如，世界四个著名的长寿区，毫无例外地都在山峦起伏、环境优美、林木葱茏、水草丰茂、空气清新、人烟稀少而经济欠发达的地区。

As is pointed out in the ancient medicinal works, the climate and altitude are closely related to life span. The yin atmosphere thrives at a higher altitude, where the climate is beaten by the law of nature; and yang flourishes at the low, where the climate beats the law of nature. The growth and activities of the living correspond to the altitude. People tend to live longer in the higher altitude than in the lower. So one must be informed of the climatic law, geographical difference, wax and wane of yin and yang, different life span and growth rules, in order to grasp the outward condition and inward qi movement, and functions and physical changes of people and take a dialectical approach to health preservation. It shows the coherence of climate and geographical conditions to human life span and health. In general, people live longer in cold areas with

古代医籍有谓：天气的寒热与地势的高下与人的寿夭有密切关系，这与地势高低不同有关。凡地势崇高之处，阴气盛；地势低下之处，阳气盛。阳气为主则阳气盛，阳气盛则气候先天时而至。阴气为主则阴气盛，阴气盛则气候后天时而至。万物之生化亦与之相应，这是地势高低与万物生化的一般规律。地势高峻的地区，人易长寿；地势低下的地区，人的寿命相对短些。不管地区范围大小，都各有差异。所以，必须明了气候规律、地理差别、阴阳盛衰、气之先后、

fresh air than on hot plains with polluted air.

寿夭不同、生化常规等各种情况，然后才能掌握人的外在形态和内在气机、功能变化的情况，辨证而养生。充分说明了气候、地理环境对人的寿夭与发病的关系。一般说来，居住在空气清新的高寒山区，其人多长寿；而居住在空气污浊、气候炎热的平原地区，其人寿命较短。

1 Coastal Regions

Teeming with inexhaustible treasures and creatures, the vast ocean is the cradle of life, closely associated with human survival and health. The sea, with its huge capacity of heat, influences the coastal climate by transmission and convection of temperatures. So the coastal regions enjoy a steadier climate than the landlocked area, with a smaller gap between temperatures by day and by night, in summer and in winter.

Thanks to the steady climate, the coastal regions are perfect for health preservation. Besides, the regular wind from the ocean brings high concentration of anion and blows away dust and chemical gases, thus purifying the air and providing "air bath"; the beautiful environment with lashing waves and gentle breeze also refreshes and bucks one up, serving to regulate his spirit, nerves, cardio vessels and the respiratory system; the full sunshine with ultraviolet blesses one with sunbath; sea bath is a matter of course on the beaches, by which the sea water exerts a physics effect on the body, and its elements also play a chemical part on it; and "sand

1 海滨地区

浩瀚的海洋是生命的发源地，蕴藏着无尽的宝藏和丰富多彩的海洋生物，与人类生存和健康密切相关。海水的热容量特别大，通过传导、对流影响海滨的气候。海滨的气温较为平稳，昼夜、冬夏的温差比内陆地区小得多。

由于海滨海岛特殊的地理环境，海洋性气候比大陆气候的冷暖变化大为缓和，十分有利于养生保健。沿海地带昼夜有规律变化的海陆风，使海滨海岛空气洁净，负离子含量高、尘埃及有害化学气体极少，是进行"空气浴"的极佳地区。置身于海滨，碧空蓝天，海浪涛涛，凉风拂面而来，使人精神振奋，心旷神怡，烦恼与倦意全消，有助于调节人的精神、神经、

therapy" is another choice for health preservation.

心血管及呼吸系统功能。海滨地区日照充足,日光散射的紫外线也较多,又为疗养者进行日光浴提供了优越的条件。海滨海岛沿海海滩是进行海水浴的良好场所,海水浴时,海水对机体既可产生物理作用,也可通过所含成分对人体产生某些化学作用。在海滨平坦的沙滩上,还可进行"沙疗法"。

The coastal regions and islands abound in sea food, which is rich in protein, fat and minerals, and so meets the physical demand for all nutrients; coastal regions are also blessed with fruits, such as peaches of Qinhuangdao Isle, apples of Yantai and coconuts of Hainan Island. The happy residents are well provided for in nutrition with their easy access to sea food, fruit, vegetables and other land produce.

沿海区域及海岛,既是海产品生产的主要基地,也是粮食、经济作物的主产地,物产十分丰富。海洋性食物富含蛋白质、脂肪,并富含矿物质,最有利于满足人体对各种必需元素的需要;沿海地区盛产各种水果,如秦皇岛的水蜜桃、烟台苹果、海南岛的椰子等,沿海及海岛居民,既吃丰富的海鲜产品,又吃陆地产品及大量的水果、蔬菜,营养比较全面。

2 Plains and Basin

Plains refer to the vast flat areas with possible hills at an altitude below 200 metres, such as Northeast Plains, North China Plains and plains at the middle-and-lower reaches of the Yangtze River. The basin terrain, as the name suggests, has higher surroundings around the plain, such as Sichuan Basin. The two share low and flat terrain, at an altitude around 50 metres, except higher Northeast

2 平原盆地

平原,指的是地势平坦、地域宽广、或有轻微波状起伏的地区。我国著名的平原有东北平原、华北平原和长江中下游平原。盆地为四周高,中间低的盆状地形,如四川盆地,它们共同的特点是地势低平,除东北平原海拔

Plains. Plains are mostly formed by the reaches of rivers, hence vast fertile fields and mineral springs. The river system, allied with rich rain that "stays mainly in the plain", blesses the region as well as curses it with floods. And the slow flow of the rivulets provides a hotbed for epidemics.

稍高外,大多都在海拔 50 米左右。平原多为江河冲积而成,沃野千里,一望无际。这里雨量充沛,水网交错;三大平原皆临近海洋,易受海洋气候的影响,夏季,东南风带来大量雨水,雨量非常充沛。平原、盆地因地势平坦,地上水位较高,矿泉蕴藏丰富,加之雨量充沛,水域发达,江河支流及湖泊等水网密布,水源十分充足。给当地的生产及生活带来极大便利的同时也易发生洪涝灾害;这些地方水流缓慢,适合某些传染病的宿主动物孳生,从而成为某些历史上有名的自然疫区。

The three plains are of temperate climate with clear-cut four seasons. The rain brings great humidity, and haze frequents the regions. The basin is hot in summer, yet not very cold in winter, thanks to the screen of mountains around. Most plains have great mud deposit brought over by rivers from plateaus, which contains high concentration of some chemical elements that trigger local diseases, such as local fluorine poisoning.

三大平原及四川盆地都属温带气候,夏热冬冷,四季分明。盆地被山脉所环绕,平原地势低平,造成本地域气流缓慢、风速较小,加之雨量丰富,空气湿度大,极易出现晨雾和逆温层;盆地周围的山脉形成天然屏障,阻挡从北方吹来的冷空气,故夏季气温较高,冬季不太寒冷。多数平原盆地的形成来自高原山区河流泥沙的长期沉积,因此会影响地球化学元素分布,使这里某些化学元素富集,成为某些地方病,如地方性氟中毒的发病温床。

3 Plateaus and Mountainous Regions

The plateau above 500 metres in altitude is less favoured by oxygen, thus low air pressure that sparks plateau sickness.

The low plateau temperature shows a vertical gap between mountain top and foot. The heat in the daytime drops sharply to coldness at night, since the long and strong sunshine breaks the thin and dry air to embrace the land with heat, only to be driven away by the gust at night. Such dramatic change in temperature tends to trap people with cold, especially in the upper respiratory system, frozen wound and sunshine-caused dermatitis.

It is well-known that the sunshine, especially ultraviolet in it, is fierce on plateaus, due to thin air and the altitude. While a proper amount of ultraviolet is beneficial, an overdose of it does great harm to skin, eyes and even the whole body.

3 高原山地

居住在海拔 500 米以上的高原山地，海拔越高，空气越稀薄，作为大气成分之一的氧气含量也随之而递减。故高原地区低气压，可造成人体的氧供不足，引起高山反应，具有重要的养生学意义。

高原地区一般气温都较低，且山上山下气温差异很大而呈典型的垂直落差。由于高原山区空气稀薄、干燥，日照强度增加且光照时间延长，因此接受太阳辐射热能较多，使白天地面气温上升很快；夜间由于高原山区风速较快，地面散热往往超过白天所吸收的热，气温急剧下降。形成白天炎热，夜晚酷寒，昼夜温差极大的特点。这种气温的剧烈变化，稍有疏忽，容易受凉感冒，发生感冒、冻伤、日照性皮炎等疾病。

太阳辐射、特别是紫外线辐射强烈。海拔升高，空气逐渐稀薄，大气层对阳光的吸收及反射减弱，太阳辐射与海拔高度成正比。适量的紫外线对人体有益，一旦照射量过大则对人体有害，可引起皮肤、眼及全身性损害。

Plateaus also suffer from light rainfall and thus dry air, except Yunnan and Guizhou Plateaus that are comparatively closer to the sea. The long time of sunshine and sand stirred up by gust accelerate the evaporation, as on Tibetan Plateau and Inner Mongolian Plateaus.

降雨量少而气候干燥。我国除云贵高原因邻近海洋而降水较多外，余皆地处内陆，降雨量少，气候干燥，尤以青藏高原、内蒙古高原为甚。加之日照时间长，风沙大，更加剧了水分的蒸发。

Some regions on plateaus have too high or too low a concentration of some chemical elements, or are affected by heavy metal and radioactive elements, or lack some mineral elements indispensable to the human body, which fuel local diseases.

高原山地的某些地区，化学元素富集或匮乏，或受重金属、放射性元素的影响，或者缺乏人体必需微量元素，进而影响人体的生理功能，引发某些地方病。

The plateaus also benefit health in spite of the demerits. The low temperature and dry air undermine the propagation of mosquitoes, germs and viruses, which, plus the small population, cuts down the spread of epidemics; people here feed on natural food that contain rough fibre, various vitamins and low fat, so cardio vertebral vascular disease is well prevented; and people here are blessed with a peaceful mind and a simple heart with less desires, which contribute to longevity.

古人养生，一般选择海拔 2 000 米以下的中低高原山区地带，其地理气候环境虽与平原明显不同，但尚在人体生理调节适应范围内。人们可以充分地利用这里的有利因素进行养生保健。中低部高原山区，鸟语花香、风景秀美，令人心旷神怡，促使有益人体的激素分泌，松弛神经，有利于调节紧张情绪；瀑布飞溅的水滴产生大量负氧离子，空气格外清新，极大地改善了肺的换气功能，且能醒脑明目；在诸多因素的综合作用下，有助于全身各系统功能的改善和提高，对许多慢性病的调养和康复效果良好。

The ancient Chinese preferred the lower moun-

高原环境气温低而气候

tainous areas below 2 000 metres in altitude, which differ from the environment in plains, yet not beyond the range of human physiology. The mountainous areas, with its birds, flowers and superb scenery, refresh the spirit, promote the production of beneficial hormone and relax the mind; it also boasts waterfalls which produce, with its splashes, a great amount of negative oxygen ion that freshens the air, hence improved lungs, better eyesight and a sober mind. In a word, many benefits combined can improve all systems and aid the cure of chronic diseases.

干燥，蚊虫、细菌及病毒等病源微生物的繁殖受到抑制，而人烟稀少、人口密度低，不利于传染病的传播，而使各种传染病大大减少；人们以自然饮食为主，摄入粗纤维、维生素多，脂肪少，因此，心脑血管疾病的发病率大大降低。人们心态平和，淳朴自然，较少欲求，精神生活安详宁静，这都非常有利于健康长寿。

Chapter 9 Health Preservation in Different Time

第9章 不同时令养生

According to ancient medicinal works, the human body is in an organic whole with nature; on the one hand, human beings must rely on heaven and earth for survival; on the other hand, they are influenced by the changes in the four seasons and rise and fall of yin and yang atmospheres in nature. People should adjust their physical condition in tune with the fluctuation of yin and yang, which fortifies the body and harmonizes spirit.

人体和自然界是一个有机的整体，一方面，人类必须依赖于自然界的天之气、地之物，才能生存；另一方面，自然界的阴阳消长、四时物候的变化，又无时无刻不在影响着人。人通过适时的自身调摄，保持自身的生命节律与自然界的阴阳消长的规律相协调，就能精神调和，形体坚实，不受外界邪气的侵害。

Human life is closely associated with nature. So people should "cultivate health in accordance with seasons", complying with changes of seasons and yin and yang based on the law of nature in their health pursuit. The concept is guided by the prime theory of "man in tune with nature" of TCM. The time falls into the concepts of day and night, months and seasons.

人类生命活动与自然界有着不可分割的联系。自然界四时气候的变化对人体的生命活动会产生极大的影响，人们必须"顺时养生"，应当掌握自然规律，顺应天地阴阳四时的变化，来防病治病，摄生保健。所谓"顺时养生"，即是在中医学"天人相应"理论指导下，按一年四季气候阴阳变化的规律和特点来调节人体，从而达到健康长寿的一种方法。依照不同时令,养生可分为昼夜养生、旬月养生、四时养生等多种方式。

Section 1 Health Preservation by Day and by Night

第1节 昼夜养生

Human metabolism changes with the wax and wane of yin and yang by day and by night, which influences physiology in spite of the smaller scale of change compared to that of the four seasons. The human yang gathers on the surface of the body in the morning, and turns inside at night, which influences pathological changes of the body.

一天之内,随昼夜阴阳消长进退,人的新陈代谢也发生相应的改变,所以养生应重视一日昼夜晨昏的调养。昼夜的阴阳消长变化会直接对人体的生理病理产生影响,虽然昼夜寒温变化的幅度不像四季变化那样明显,但对人体的影响同样是不可忽视的。人体阳气白天多趋于表,夜晚多趋于里。由于人体阳气有昼夜的周期变化,所以对人体病理变化亦有直接影响。

A day can be divided into four parts corresponding to the four seasons: morning to spring, noon to summer, evening autumn and midnight winter. The yang is fresh in the morning and fends off pathogenic factors, when the patient feels better and refreshed; it flourishes at noon and conquers the evil, so the disease appears steady; it wanes in the evening and gives some way to the evil, so the disease deteriorates; it hides itself in the organs at midnight and the pathogenic factor takes fully over, when the disease is at its worst. People can arrange their work and study, making them most efficient

一天可以参照四季进行划分,早晨相当于春季,中午相当于夏季,傍晚相当于秋季,半夜相当于冬季。早晨阳气生发,能够抵御邪气,邪气衰减,所以早晨病情轻而病人精神清爽;中午阳气旺盛,能够制服邪气,所以中午病情安定;傍晚阳气开始衰减,邪气逐渐亢盛,所以傍晚病情加重;半夜人体的阳气都深藏内脏,邪气亢盛已极,

based on this rhythm of yang.

所以夜半病情最重。根据此理论，人们可以利用阳气的日节律，合理安排工作、学习，发挥人类的智慧和潜能，以求达到最佳的效果。

1 Morning

The morning, as the beginning of a day, is the time when everything thrives, thus crucial to the man's condition of a whole day. The yang is freshly reborn, when one should try to conserve and elevate it by working out, thereby promoting blood circulation. With the sunrise, human viscera also grow in absorption, so nutrition is vital for breakfast, which may include ginger soup or shredded ginger that aids the yang. Besides, a regular breakfast plays a part in preventing gall-stone. According to psychology, human sub consciousness transits into consciousness upon getting up, when one should cheer up and encourage oneself, so that he can be happy the whole day.

1 早晨养生

早晨为一天之始，往往被视为充满朝气的时候，对人体而言是一个非常重要的阶段，关系着一天的身体与精神状况。中医认为早晨是人阳气生发之际，而在阳气初生之际做好保养工作很重要，早晨较宜在户外锻炼身体，通过活动，促进血液循环，使阳气得以升发。早晨太阳初升，人体的脏腑功能也处于升发的状态，营养需求量大、代谢也旺盛，所以早饭宜吃好。早餐还可以喝点姜汤或者吃些姜丝、姜片，能够促进阳气的生发、散布。另外，有规律地进食早餐对预防胆囊结石的发生也有一定作用。早上应尽量保持心情愉快。按照心理学的研究，刚起床时是人从潜意识进入意识的分界线，是从潜意识到意识的过渡时期，这个时候保持快乐的心态，或者鼓励自己，那么这一天就可以变得很快乐。

2 Noon

The noon in TCM, termed Wu hour, refers to the two hours between 11 a. m. and 1 p. m., when the yang reaches its zenith and it is perfect time for siesta. Wu hour goes in pair with Zi hour, that is, 11 p. m. to 1 a. m., when the yang starts growing till it flourishes at Wu hour. And from Wu hour the yang at zenith reverts to the opposite yin, which grows till it thrives at Zi hour. So the pair of Zi and Wu hours breeds yang and yin, which should be conserved when newly born.

The noon nap promotes the wax and wane of yin and yang and change of qi movement, refilling the yang consumed in the morning, and aids blood supply to the digestive organs and absorption. The digestive organs grow stronger with the flourishing yang, so lunch is supposed to be sumptuous enough to supply more nutrition for great consumption in the afternoon.

2 中午养生

中午，又称正午，中国古代将一天分为十二时辰，午时即为现代二十四小时制的11:00 至 13:00。此时阳气达到顶点，适宜午睡。半夜11点到1点，为子时，人的阳气开始生发，并逐渐增强，一直到午时，阳气最旺盛；而午时阴气初生，并逐渐生长，一直到子时达到最盛。所以子时和午时，一个是阳气初生的时候，一个是阴气初生的时候，不论阴气和阳气，在初生的时候都很弱小，需要着意保护。

午后的小憩可促进阴阳消长和气机的转换，不仅可以使上午升发耗散的阳气得以培补，还能保证午餐后消化器官血液供应和营养物质的吸收。中午是一天中阳气最旺盛的时候，消化功能强劲，下午人们处在工作或学习中，消耗较大，需要补充较多的营养物质，因此午餐应该丰盛些。

3 Evening and Night

The evening and night refers to the time between 6 p. m. and 5 a. m, when the sun sets and temperature gradually drops until it reaches the bottom at midnight. The yang in the body gradually ebbs away. People move little and their metabolism

3 夜晚养生

夜晚通常指下午6点到次日的早晨5点这一段时间。晚上太阳落山，自然界阴寒之气渐盛，气温通常会逐渐降低，在半夜达到最低。

slows down and demand for nutrition also drops, so a little supper will do, otherwise, a big dinner produces too many calories that cannot be consumed, hence obesity.

人的阳气渐虚，活动渐少，代谢减退，营养需求相对较少，所以晚餐宜少。晚饭如果摄入太多，由于阳气相对较虚，运化无力，加之活动较少，能量消耗减少，极易引起肥胖。

At the depth of night, the yang drops to the lowest and yin takes over, when night snacks impede digestion and absorption and disturb sleep. The yang retires with the closing of pores, so one should refrain from moving a lot in case of being attacked by haze or dew. Never stay up late! The Zi hour is the very hour of thriving yin, when one should sleep to conserve the new-born yang.

到了深夜，阳气降到最低点，体内阴气较盛，此时不宜进食夜宵，不但妨碍消化吸收，还会影响睡眠。夜间阳气收敛内藏，汗孔也随之闭密，所以到了晚上，不要再扰动筋骨，不要受雾露的侵袭，应早点休息，切忌熬夜。子时是一日时辰中的阴中之阴，在子时处在睡眠状态，阳气刚刚来复，不宜耗散。

Section 2 Health Preservation by Months

第2节 旬月养生

The circulation of qi and blood with their ebb and flow is not only associated with seasons and climatic change, but directly related to the intensity of sunshine and the wax and wane of the moon. As is found out by modern medical science, women's menstruation period, body temperature, hormone, state of sex organs, immunity and psychology change in a cycle of a month. Birth rate is also influenced by the moon, highest at full moon and lowest around crescent. The full moon draws full qi and blood to the head and people are apt to get excited with strong hormone.

人体气血的运行及盛衰，不仅和季节气候的变化有关，而且同日照的强弱和月相的盈亏直接相关。如现代医学发现，妇女的月经周期变化、体温、激素、性器官状态、免疫功能和心理状态等都以一月为周期。婴儿的出生也受月相影响，月圆出生率最高，新月前后最低。满月时，人头部气血最充实，内分泌最旺盛，容易激动。

In addition, the wax and wane of human yin and yang varies in different months, in accordance with the five elements that take turns to dominate the cycle of the year. The year falls into four seasons, which further fall into 24 divisions, going in an endless cycle. The doctor prescribes according to seasons and climates, and no less can be said about health preservation, which can be more efficient when done in tune with nature.

另外，中医认为，人体的阴阳消长变化，在每个月都是不同的。一年四时，各随其五行的配合而分别当旺。木、火、土、金、水五行，随时间变化而递相承袭，各有当旺之时，到一年终结时，再开始从头循环。一年分立四时，四时分布节气，逐步推移，如环无端。节气再分候，也是这样推移下去。不但医者治病需要根据气候的不同来区别用药，对于养生而言，也应该了解每个月养生应该注意的事项，顺应天时的变化而动，才能达到事半功倍的效果。

So health preservation should go with the months of the Chinese lunar calendar as follows:

日常应遵循中国农历月份规律逐月施养，具体而言：

The 1st month of spring (roughly February) is a time when everything and yang grow. Lichun, as the first of the 24 divisions, means spring starts. In tune with the growing yang in nature, one should take care to conserve yang in the body. The first month is the early period of transition from concealment to growth, when the kidney is prone to pathogenic factors and lungs are also weak, so one should have more pungent and spicy food, such as fermented beans, onion, coriander, peanuts, Chinese chives, shrimps and dates, which furnish the kidney and lungs, and nourish the stomach; salty and sour food should be avoided, as sourness collects yang into the liver, and thus impedes the growth of yang and free coursing of the liver qi; keep away from

正月，是春季的第一个月，天地之气开始复苏，万物生发。一月包含“立春”和“雨水”两个节气，“立春”位居二十四节气之首，表明春季从这一天开始。养生也要顺应春天阳气生发、万物始生的特点，注意保护阳气。正月是从藏转向生的早期，邪气容易直中伤肾，而肺气亦微弱，饮食上应该少吃咸、酸，增食辛味，如豆豉、葱、香菜、花生、韭菜、虾仁等，这样可以助肾补肺，安养胃气。因为春季阳气初生，酸味入

the draught and cold, and also from over warmth; go to bed late and get up early, and the body and spirit can be relaxed.

肝,具收敛之性,不利于阳气的生发和肝气的疏泄,可少吃。正月既不要冒风受寒也不要太过温暖,应该晚睡早起,以舒缓自己的形体和精神。

The 2nd lunar month (roughly March) is at the mid-spring. At this time the kidney is still weak and the liver qi flourishes, so one should stick to pungent food to replenish the kidney and the liver. Efforts should be made to remove phlegm at the diaphragm; rub the skin to the point of slight perspiration, which takes away the pathogenic factors accumulated in winter. The Chinese chive is of great benefit to health in this month, apart from other yang-replenishing food, such as dates, shepherd's purse, and chicken.

二月,春天将半,包含"惊蛰"和"春分"两个节气。二月时肾气较弱,肝气旺盛,宜少食酸味而增食辛味,这样可以助肾补肝。宜除去胸膈间痰液,将皮肤擦热,使之出微汗,以驱散冬天蓄积在人体内的邪气。二月多食韭菜,于养生大有裨益。除了韭菜之外,还可以食用温补阳气的食物,如大枣、荠菜、鸡肉等。

The 3rd lunar month (roughly April, following this pattern below) is the last month of spring, when everything in nature grows quickly. At this time the kidney qi calms down and the heart qi grows, together with wood qi, so one should keep away from sweet food and stick to pungent food, which replenishes the essence and qi. It turns warmer now and people should go to bed early and get up early to conserve qi in the viscera. Relax the body in tune with nature and take part in more outdoor activities. This is a time when peach, pear and apricot are in full blossom, and willow and poplar catkins dance about in the north of China, which should be guarded against by people allergic to pollen. It is also a month of epidemics, such as acute virus hepatitis, epidemic cerebrospinal meningitis,

三月,是春季的最后一个月,包含"清明"和"谷雨"两个节气,万物萌发,天地充满生气。三月,肾气平息,心气渐渐生发,木气正旺,适宜少食甜味、多食辛味,补精益气,以顺应时令。这时天气转暖,适宜早睡早起,以养脏气。人的形体应该自由放松,使之安泰,以顺应天时。人们的室外活动增加,北方的桃花、梨花、杏花等开满枝头,杨絮、柳絮四处飞扬,对花粉过敏的人应注意防范。此季节还是传染病高发季节,如急性病毒性肝炎、流

measles and mumps. So one should take care to put on more clothes if necessary, to keep them at bay.

脑、麻疹、腮腺炎等。所以要依据天气变化及时增减衣服,预防传染病。

The 4th lunar month is the first month of summer, when everything blooms. The summer corresponds to the heart, that is, yang of the heart prospers in summer, which needs to be conserved. So one should retire late and get up early to take in fresh air of nature. Refrain from fury and other means of venting such as sex, as an effort to reserve water in the kidney and quench fire in the heart, which goes in tune with nature. Have food that clears heat and aids drainage, such as red beans, Job's tears, green beans, white gourd. Add sour food to the diet gradually, yet little bitterness, to nourish the stomach qi; greasy and pungent food should be avoided, such as animal fat, fishes, raw garlic, chili, Chinese chives, beef and mutton. The old should feed on bland food with low fat and salt, in addition to a large amount of vegetables and fruits, and a little low-alcohol wine will do to smooth circulation of qi and blood.

四月,为孟夏之月,即夏季的第一个月,包含"立夏"和"小满"两个节气,是天地交泰、万物花开的时节。中医理论认为,心对应"夏",也就是说在夏季,心阳最为旺盛。因此,夏季需要更多地保养心气心阳。适宜晚睡早起,以受天地间的清明之气,不要大怒、大泄。应少房事以壮肾水,静养以息心火,以使志安宁,顺应天地造化之机。宜多食具有清热利湿功用的食物如赤小豆、薏苡仁、绿豆、冬瓜等;适宜增食酸味,少食苦味,调养胃气;忌食肥甘厚味、辛辣助热之品,如动物脂肪、海腥鱼类、生蒜、辣椒、韭菜、牛羊狗肉等。老年人在饮食上应以低脂、低盐的清淡食物为主,多食用维生素含量高的蔬菜水果,可饮少量低度酒,以保持气血通畅。

The 5th lunar month is when summer really begins and everything in nature has grown up. One should not strain to the point of heavy perspiration, or sleep in open air in case of the invasion of pathogenic factors. Be sure to sleep early and get up early, and take a little noon nap due to the long daytime, which serves to restore energy. It is advisable

五月,包含"芒种"和"夏至"两个节气,是夏天真正开始的时候,天地化生,万物已成。此时要避免大热、大汗,也不要露宿于星月之下,谨防邪气入体导致疾病。要早睡早起,又因此时天气是昼

to be dressed in cotton material that easily draws sweat and take shower more often; one should take precautions against heat stroke, mumps and chickenpox. Rather than sour food, eat more bitter food that drains waste in the body; have more vegetables, beans and fruits instead of spicy and greasy food, such as mutton, beef, chili and onion.

长夜短，中午可以午休一会儿，对恢复体力、消除疲劳有一定好处。由于天气炎热，汗出较多，衣着应以棉制品为好，利于汗液排泄。要常洗澡，保持皮肤清洁卫生，还要防止中暑、腮腺炎、水痘等。饮食调养宜减酸增苦，以清补为主，宜食用蔬菜、豆类、水果等。忌食辛辣油腻之品，如羊肉、牛肉、辣椒、葱等。

The 6th lunar month is when everything in nature flourishes. The yin conceals itself in the body that is steamed by exterior heat, in which condition one is susceptible to plague in bowels if he braves draught or abandons himself to cold food. So one should keep to bland, soft and warm food, such as green vegetables, bitter gourd, cucumber, and watermelon, and guard against unhygienic food. The yang thrives in this period, which needs to be protected by rest during work. People with cardio vertebral vascular disease should make sure to have full sleep and good ventilation, and resort to physical cooling in steaming climate; manual labourers and those working in open air should make a point of drinking more water, and taking a little rendan mini-pills or green bean soup in case of heat stroke. Sleep late and rise early, which goes with the boom of yang and which smoothes the circulation of qi and blood.

六月，包含"小暑"和"大暑"两个节气，生长之气隆盛，主养四时，万物生长茂盛、繁荣。六月阴气内伏，暑毒外蒸，如随意当风，任性食冷，易致泄泻等肠道传染病，须饮食清淡、温软，蔬菜应多食绿叶菜及苦瓜、黄瓜等，水果则以西瓜为好。忌辛辣油腻之品，注意饮食卫生。此时是人体阳气最旺盛的时候，人们在工作劳动之时，要注意劳逸结合，保护阳气。对有心脑血管疾病的人来说，要保证充足的睡眠，并加强室内通风，尤其在闷热的天气中要注意使用物理降温。体力劳动者、室外工作者此时应多饮水，必要时可服少量仁丹，或喝绿豆汤等以防中暑。起居方面，要晚睡早起，以顺应阳气的充盛，

The 7th lunar month starts the autumn. One should calm down, dress loose-fittingly, move slowly and collects the mind. It is warm and dry at the time, which harms body fluid, shown in dry skin, dry eyes, dry throat, yellow urine and constipation, so one should drink more water to conserve body fluid and combat the heat of late summer, and refrain from heavy perspiration. Take more sour food than spicy, such as tomato, eggplant, potato, grape and pear; rather than greasy food, take more food of alkalinity nature, which alleviates fatigue by balancing the element of acid nature produced by exhausted muscles, based on the theory of autumn fatigue being related to body fluid of a more acid nature; have more apples, kelp and fresh vegetables, and less with onion and ginger.

The 8th lunar month is a time when it is crucial to retain the equilibrium of yin and yang in the body, and of no less importance is spirit adjustment. Instead of being susceptible to the gloomy picture of everything declining, one should maintain an optimistic and calm mood, by taking more outings and enjoying nature on crisp sunny days, which pleases the mind and exercises the body. At this time dry symptoms turn more evident in thirstiness, dry lips, dry nose, dry throat, dry excrement and cracked skin, which can be relieved by food with more vitamins, such as cucumber, radish, pear, white gourd, and some medicinals such as Xi Yang-Shen (*Radix Panacis Quinquefolii*), Bei Sha Shen

利于气血运行。

七月，包含“立秋”和“处暑”两个节气，是夏天结束、秋天来临的时候。宜静性情，衣着宽松，行动舒缓，并收敛神气，使心神安宁。初秋温燥伤津，容易出现皮肤干燥、眼干、咽干、小便黄、大便秘结等症状，要注意多饮水，顾护津液，不要大热大汗，适当防暑降温。饮食应多食酸，少食辛。如多吃西红柿、茄子、马铃薯、葡萄、梨等食物，少吃油腻的肉食。秋乏与体液偏酸有关，多吃碱性食物能中和肌肉疲倦时产生的酸性物质，使人消除疲劳。宜多食用的食物有苹果、海带以及新鲜蔬菜等，还要少吃葱、姜等辛味之品。

八月，是秋季的第二个月，包含有“白露”和“秋分”两个节气。八月养生应本着阴阳平衡的原则，使机体保持“阴平阳秘”的状态。精神调养在秋天非常重要，因为秋天万木凋谢，人们容易产生“悲秋”之感，所以要培养乐观情绪，保持神志安宁，以适应秋天容平之气。天气晴好之日，秋高气爽，多外出走走，登高望远，享受大自然的美景，心旷神怡，同时还锻炼了身体，使身心愉悦，排解秋

(*Radix Glehniae*), Bai He (*Bulbus Lilii*), Ku Xing Ren(*Semen Armeniacae Amarum*), Chuan Bei Mu (Bulbus Fritillaria Cirrhosae).

愁。此时养生防秋燥也非常关键，人们往往会出现口干、唇干、鼻干、咽干及大便干结、皮肤干裂等不适，可适当地多吃一些含维生素的食品如黄瓜、萝卜、梨、冬瓜或用中药食疗，如服用西洋参、沙参、百合、杏仁、川贝等。

In the 9th lunar month, the 3rd month of autumn, plants wither and everything tends to conceal itself in the cold climate. One should avoid draught and raw cold food. In the human body the yang withdraws and yin and essence are concealed, which must be conserved in autumn. As in the 8th lunar month, one should retain a positive state of mind and avoid being sentimental about the fallen leaves, and go on to take food that nourishes yin and moisturizes, as dryness still takes charge and threatens yin essence of lungs. Drink more water and eat more Hei Zhi Ma (*Semen Sesami Nigrum*), glutinous rice, rice, Feng Mi (*Mel*), Da Zao (*Fructus Jujubae*) and Shan Yao (*Rhizoma Dioscoreae*) to nourish yin and lungs, less with onion, ginger, garlic, or other pungent and spicy food.

九月，包含“寒露”和“霜降”两个节气，为秋季的第三个月，草木凋零，万物准备进入蛰伏，气候寒冷，须注意避风，少食生冷。当气候变冷时，正是人体阳气收敛，阴精潜藏于内之时，故秋季必须保养体内阴精阴气。精神调养在此时也应受到重视，这是因为气候渐冷，日照减少，风起叶落，特别是北方，万木凋零，草枯叶无，易使人产生悲观情绪。尤其生活、工作中遇到不如意之时，更使抑郁多发。所以，此时人们要注意控制情绪，避免伤感，多做开心喜好之事，保持良好的心态，平安度过秋季。又因金秋之时，燥气当令，所以此时要防燥邪之气侵犯人体而耗伤肺之阴精，饮食上以滋阴润燥为宜。还要多饮水，宜适当多食芝麻、糯米、粳米、蜂蜜、大枣、山药等以滋阴润肺、增强体质，少吃葱、姜、蒜、辛辣等品。

The 10th lunar month starts the winter, when everything is concealed and rivers frozen. Human mood is also susceptible to the effect of the grim nature, so one should take cheer and brighten up. Be sure to retire early and rise late for full sleep, and give heed to the warmth of the back, which serves the concealment of yang and stock of yin essence. Eat more high-calorie food and fresh vegetables for vitamins, such as beef, mutton, black chicken, soy bean milk, milk, radish, green vegetables, fungus and beans, less with sea food due to its cold character, or spicy and bitter food, to cultivate the kidney qi.

十月，包含有“立冬”和“小雪”两个节气，为孟冬之月，即冬季的第一个月，天地都处于闭藏的状态，水冻地裂。人们情绪容易低落，郁郁寡欢，精神养生应做到精神安静，保护阳气，不过度消耗阴精，要保持良好的心态，遇到不愉快的事情要及时排解。生活中做到早卧晚起，保证充足的睡眠，注意背部保暖，这样，有利于阳气潜藏，阴精蓄积，穿着也应注意保暖。饮食宜多吃热量较高的膳食，还要多食新鲜蔬菜，以避免维生素缺乏，如牛肉、羊肉、乌鸡、豆浆、牛奶、萝卜、青菜、木耳、豆类等。少食寒性之品，如海鲜等。宜减食辛味、苦味以养肾气。

In the 11th lunar month, temperature drops sharply and turns freezing. It consists of the vital division of winter solstice, on which day the daytime turns shortest in a year and night longest, and yin in nature reaches its pinnacle and turns down, while yang starts to recuperate. It is a perfect time for nourishment, so people can choose different paste prescription according to their individual constitution. Those infirm with weak digestion should take care to be nourished slowly, with more vegetables. While those of a better constitution should be nourished moderately, avoiding greasy food in case of inner heat triggering disease.

十一月，包含有“大雪”和“冬至”两个节气，为冬季的第二个月，即仲冬，天寒地冻，寒气正盛，气温下降明显。“冬至”是个非常重要的节气，这一天白昼最短，夜晚最长，阴气盛极而衰，阳气开始回升，此时是进补的最佳时令，可根据每个人体质不同选择不同的膏方。体质弱、消化功能差的人，可选择“慢补”，还要多吃蔬菜，切忌过补、急补。体质较好的人选择“平补”，不要过食油腻之品，以防生内热而诱发疾病。

The 12th lunar month, the last month of winter, is the coldest in a year. Be sure to keep warm in case of catching cold; do not strain and impair tendon and bones, or perspire heavily. Eat more mutton, chicken, turtle, He Tao Ren (*Semen Juglandis*), Da Zao, Long Yan Rou (*Arillus Longan*), Shan Yao, Lian Zi (*Semen Nelumbinis*), Bai He Lily and chestnut, which fortify the spleen and the stomach, warm up yang of the kidney, melt phlegm, furnish lungs and stop coughing. But those with more of a hot constitution had better eat less of them and be nourished more slowly. Remember to keep away from cold food in this month.

十二月，包含"小寒"和"大寒"两个节气，是冬季的最后一个月，天地闭藏，阳潜阴施，万物伏藏，是一年中最冷的季节。此时，应去寒就暖，避免感受风邪，不要劳伤筋骨，不要出大汗。可多吃羊肉、狗肉、鸡肉、甲鱼、核桃仁、大枣、龙眼肉、山药、莲子、百合、栗子等，有补脾胃、温肾阳、健脾化痰、止咳补肺的功效。体质偏热、偏实易生痰火的人应注意缓补、少食为好。忌一切寒凉之物，如冰激凌、生冷食品。

Section 3 Health Preservation by Four Seasons

第3节 四季养生

The seasons change in the rule of warm spring, hot summer, cool autumn and cold winter, each in a set degree, to which change the human body should be adapted and thus health can be guaranteed, and vice versa. If seasons change abnormally, or the human body cannot be adapted, disease happens.

自然界四时气候的变化对人的生活产生多方面的影响，尤其是健康受气候的影响更为突出。一年四时的更替，六气的变化，通常是按照一定的次序向前发展和相互转变的，如春温、夏热、秋凉、冬寒都有一定的限度，既不能太过，亦不能不及，人体顺应这种变化，则健康无病。但当气候出现反常变化，或人体不能随季节更替作相应

Seasonal changes influence human physiological functions and pathological changes. In spring and summer yang thrives, and qi and blood flow toward the surface, so one is apt to perspire, while in autumn and winter yang withdraws, so do qi and blood, so one perspires little and water is locked in. Each season with its features gives rise to seasonal diseases. Some chronic diseases such as coronary heart disease and trachitis usually become more severe in the transition between seasons. Therefore, to preserve health, not only should one learn his physiological characteristics in the four seasons, but he should learn and master the pathological rule in the four seasons, thereby taking active precautions with a certain target. Going with the seasonal rule does not mean passive adaptation, but taking the initiative to adjust oneself in tune with seasonal characteristics, hence being fortified against pathogenic factors from outside and achieving health.

Human emotions also shift with seasons, as is shown in the concept of "regulating spirit in the four seasons" in the ancient medicinal works, the four seasons referring to the fundamental seasonal features of warm spring, hot summer, and dry autumn and cold winter. The concept means people should adopt various ways to regulate their mind in

的调整时，则会产生不适，甚至导致疾病的发生。

四时气候的变化对人体的生理功能和病理变化均存在着一定的影响。春夏阳气开泄，气血趋向于表，故腠理疏松多汗；秋冬阳气收敛，气血趋向于里，表现为皮肤腠理致密，少汗多溺。四时的季节气候各有不同的特点，故除一般疾病外，还有些季节多发病。某些慢性的疾病，如冠心病、气管炎等常常在季节变换和节气交替时发作或加剧。所以养生不仅要了解人体在四时的生理特点，更应了解和掌握四时的发病规律，从而采取积极主动的有针对性的预防保健措施，达到防病养生的目的。顺应四季规律并非被动的适应，而是采取积极主动的态度，与天地协调一致、和谐共存，掌握自然变化的规律，按照不同季节特点进行适时的调整，以期防御外邪的侵袭，保证身心健康。

人的情志变化亦是与四时变化密切相关的，所以《素问》有"四气调神"之论。所谓"四气"就是指的春温、夏热、秋燥、冬寒，一年四季气候更迭的基本特征；所谓"四气调神"，是指人们为了顺应

keeping with seasonal changes, thereby preserving health.

时令更迭的自然变化,主动采取各种调神的方法,从而维护身心健康的养生方法。

1 Spring

Spring is a thriving time when everything awakes to warmth and the yang in nature sprouts, in tune with which people should centre their residence, emotions, diet and exercise on the word "growth". The liver takes the dominant position in the five solid organs.

1 春季养生

春三月,从立春到立夏前,包括立春、雨水、惊蛰、春分、清明、谷雨六个节气。春为一年四季之首,乃万象更新之始,天气由寒转暖,春回大地,自然界阳气生发,各种生物萌发生育,一派欣欣向荣的景象。春季是阳气生发之时,五脏应于肝脏,也是肝脏条达之时。所以,春季养生在起居、情志、饮食、运动锻炼诸方面,都必须着眼于一个"生"字,以顺应春天阳气生发、万物萌发的特点。

1.1 Spirit Adjustment

After the long stock in winter, emotions find a chance to be vented in the prosperous spring, so people are prone to irritation, anger and unpredictable moods, and mental diseases occur frequently. To counteract it, they should make conscious efforts to keep a positive attitude, being generous, calm and kind. As is held in *Plain Questions* (Su Wen), one should "grow instead of killing, give in stead of taking, award instead of punishing". In a word, keep emotions open in tune with the growing spring.

1.1 精神调摄

春天的三个月是自然界万物推陈出新的季节,此时自然界阳气生发舒张,万物生机勃勃、欣欣向荣。人们经过漫长冬季的郁积,在春天生发之时,情志也处于一种开放宣达、生发疏泄的状态,情绪易变,易被激惹,精神性疾患较多。根据春时阳气生发舒张的特点,春季养生应使人的精神情绪保持在一种积极乐观、豁达大度、恬静舒畅、与人为善的状态。不要烦恼、躁急、忿怒。要像

《素问》所说，要促进生而不扼杀，要付出而不索取，要多奖赏而少惩罚，以促使志意生发，即是应春气的情志养生之道。

Cultivating qi of the liver helps adjust emotions. As the general in the viscera, the liver is strong in character and governs the lesser yang qi of human body, so it prefers growing and being unrestrained to being knotted in. With the functions of venting emotions, smoothing qi movement, keeping the soul and blood, the liver is at the core of emotion adjustment. To cultivate qi of the liver, firstly, one should cheer up so that the qi movement can be smoothed, qi and blood circulate with leisure, and the liver qi enjoy free coursing; be generous about fame and fortune to avoid extreme emotions, especially melancholy that impairs the liver; secondly, one should calm down, rid of the quick temper. The liver with its general's quick temper would be provoked by irritation or anger, and the liver qi rushes in chaos, which sparks disorder in qi and blood circulation, and in a worse case, the fire character is sparked in the liver, which consumes qi and impairs blood, and thereby the liver itself is injured as a residence of blood, besides causing other damage. Thus the saying "anger impairs the liver"; thirdly, one should take certain medicines or food to regulate the liver and ensure its normal activities. To conclude, one should be generous, kind-hearted and optimistic, or develop positive emotions in travel, which fosters the inner environment of unrestrained growth, the fountain of the activities of the lesser yang qi.

养肝气以调畅情志：肝胆主司人体少阳之气，在四时与春气相应。肝为将军之官，其性刚强，司少阳之气，主生发，喜条达而恶抑郁，功能主疏泄情志，疏畅气机，藏魂，藏血。因此，在五脏中，肝气与情志的关系最为密切，情志调养应重在养肝气。养肝气一是要保持心情舒畅豁达，心情舒畅，则人体气机畅通，气血运行和缓，能协调肝气的条达；心胸豁达，则不孜孜汲汲于名利得失，心情不至于过喜过悲，以防情志抑郁而损伤肝气。二是要忍急戒怒。肝性刚而易躁急，躁急或忿怒之时，情志偏激，肝气因而横逆上冲，使气血逆乱，甚而郁极生火，耗气伤血，肝失其藏血之职，既使肝的本脏受伤，又容易引起其他脏气的失常，所以说"怒伤肝"。三是适时运用药物或食物调养肝脏，从脏腑机能的角度保持肝脏的活动正常。情绪的过度变动最容易损伤肝脏，而格逆少阳春生之气，因而要有容忍之心，开朗之性，助人之德，或踏青郊游，寄情山水，在清新自然中培植良好情绪。情绪的稳定和乐观向上，可造成条达生发的内在环境，是人体少阳之气活动的基础。

1.2 Daily Life

According to Su Wen, on the premise of ensuring basic amount of sleep, people should try to sleep and rise early, dress loose, wear hair naturally, relax and take a stroll, which promote the growth of yang.

There goes a Chinese folklore phrase, "reduce clothes slowly in spring and add them slowly in autumn". The yang is newly born inspring, and climate changes drastically, and in addition, human skin tissue loosens in spring due to growing yang within, so the body is less fortified against pathogenic factors from outside. That is why one should be prudent in taking off the cotton-padded jacket, especially the old and the infirm. So is it with quilts.

1.2 起居调养

《素问》指出人们春季养生在保证基本睡眠的情况下，尽可能晚睡早起，衣着宽松，披散头发，舒缓身体，在庭间漫步，使春季初生的阳气得以升发。

我国民间历来有"春捂秋冻"之说，春季阳气始生，气候变化较大，极易出现乍寒乍暖的情况，加之人体肌表腠理开始变得疏松，对于外邪的抵抗能力有所减弱，所以，此时不宜过早脱去棉衣，特别是年老体弱者，减脱冬装尤应审慎，不可骤减。被褥也不要立刻换薄，以适应春季的气候特点。

1.3 Diet

Governing in spring, the liver is inclined to vent and drain, which goes in tune with the growing yang. The wood quality of the liver overcomes the soil quality of the spleen when it goes too strong, thereby affecting the digestive function. The taste of sourness is taken in by the liver, which collects and contracts and so impedes the growth of yang and free coursing of the liver qi. While sweetness replenishes the spleen and pungent food helps vent

1.3 饮食调养

肝旺于春，与春阳升发之气相应，喜条达疏泄；肝木太过则易克伐脾土，影响脾胃的消化功能。酸味入肝，具有收敛之性，不利于阳气的升发和肝气的疏泄，而甘味补脾培中，故春季宜食辛甘发散之品，不宜食酸收之味，以防肝木太过而克伐脾

and spread, so the two tastes are best choices in spring rather than sourness. Take pungent food of a warm character or sweet food that helps spread, such as wheat, dates, onion, peanuts and coriander, but do not overdo it by taking extra pungent food with a hot character, such as Ren Shen (*Radix Ginseng*), Fu Zi (*Radix Aconiti Lateralis Praeparata*), monkshood and strong wine, which add to heat and spark fire. Besides, metabolism accelerates with the warming up of climate, and viscera are burdened with more work, so the digestive function should be enhanced in spring, by food or medicine rich in protein, thus ensuring full absorption that meets the demand of growing metabolism.

土。如适当食用麦、枣、葱、花生、香菜等辛温升散或辛甘发散类食物,借辛甘温之品发散以助春阳,但也不能多进大辛大热之物如人参、附子、高度白酒等,以免助热生火。另外,春归大地,天气渐暖,人体代谢也加强,各器官负荷增加,因此春季饮食应注意改善和促进消化吸收功能,多吃点富含蛋白质的食物,不管是食补还是药补,应有利于健脾和胃,补中益气,以保证营养品能被顺利充分地吸收,以满足春季人体代谢增加的需求。

In addition, people come out of sort of hibernation with cumulative heat in the body, which undermines immunity, and some chronic diseases, such as hypertension, asthma and allergy may recur in spring, so such patients should refrain from food that awakens illness, such as shrimp, goose and sea food.

此外,春季气候开始由寒转暖,而这时人们经过一冬的蛰居斗室,体内多有积热,人体抵抗力减弱,高血压、哮喘及皮肤过敏等宿疾易在春季复发,有这些疾病的人群应注意饮食上不要食用虾、鹅、海鲜等发物。

1.4 Exercise

Spring is a perfect time for people to exchange old breath with fresh air that melts into essence and blood, and nourishes the viscera. As organs function less in winter, proper exercise in spring aids the growth of yang, improves metabolism, tunes qi and blood, and pushes circulation of qi and blood. People can select exercise based on their individual condition, such as playing balls, jogging, practicing Taiji Quan, and outing in nature, preferably in

1.4 运动锻炼

春天最有利于人体吐故纳新,采纳精气,以化精血,充养脏腑。经过寒冷的冬季,因室外活动减少使各脏腑功能有不同程度下降。春季适量的运动有助于人体阳气的生发,改善新陈代谢,调和气血,增强血液循环。运动锻炼可结合自己的身体条

places with fresh air. And heed should be given to the time and hygiene in exercise, such as breathing with the mouth shut, which warms up and moisturizes the air inhaled, thereby avoiding a dry and sore throat; take off and put on clothes in and after exercise in case of catching cold; never brave draught in wet clothes after exercise; never sit alone in seclusion in spring, which knots in qi and thus impedes the spread of yang. Most people feel sleepy in spring, which is a physiological phenomenon in the seasonal change. It is because the blood vessels and pores in the skin contract in winter and spread in spring, which takes more blood supply that should have gone to the brain. To alleviate the sleepiness, one should ensure full sleep and exercise more outdoors to promote blood circulation.

件,选择合适的运动方式,如打球、慢跑、太极拳、踏青等,形式不拘,与大自然相融,修养身心。运动锻炼最好到空气清新的地方,如公园、广场、树林、河边、山坡等处进行。同时注意锻炼时间与锻炼卫生,如用鼻呼吸,有加温与湿润空气作用,避免咽干咽痛等不良症状;及时增减衣服,预防感冒,运动之后忌穿湿衣让冷风吹。春季切忌独居、默坐,而生郁结之气,妨碍春季阳气的舒发。春季气候温暖,多数人在春天伊始常常觉得昏昏欲睡,精神不振,出现“春困”的现象,这是由于季节性变化而容易出现的一种生理现象。这是由于冬季皮肤血管收缩,春季天气变暖,血管、毛孔扩张,供应皮肤的血流相对增加,供应脑的血液相对减少,从而造成春困。要改善这种情况,一是要保证充足的睡眠,二是要多参加户外锻炼活动,改善血液循环。

2 Summer

The yang flourishes in summer; the sun shines fiercely and rain falls generously. Everything bears fruit and the yin is brewing. In tune with it, the human body also has thriving yang which must be prolonged in conservation.

2 夏季养生

夏三月,从立夏到立秋前,包括立夏、小满、芒种、夏至、小暑、大暑六个节气。夏季自然界阳气旺盛,烈日炎炎,雨水充足,阳极阴生,万物成实。人在气交之中，故亦应之。夏季人体阳气旺盛，心气长旺，所以，夏季养生要注意养护阳气，着眼于一个“长”字。

2.1 Spirit Adjustment

Under the scorching sun the skin tissue loosens and sweat escapes, which consumes the heart as the sweat should have served it, which fuels mental disease. Especially in the heyday of summer when it is humidly hot with no wind and a high temperature with little change from morning to night. Such a climate makes people gloomy and irritated, possibly worsening into mental disease.

As is pointed out in Su Wen works, one should make the spirit as beautiful as buds in summer, without flying into a rage; keep qi movement smooth and show interest in the outside world, that is, to retain a fully positive spirit, which is a premise on which body functions can flourish in harmony, and vice versa.

The heart is at the core of spirit adjustment in summer. As one knows, the heart beats faster with excitement, as it governs blood vessels and spirit, with the former leading up to the latter, that is, a full blood flow ensures a sobre mind, quick wit and

2.1 精神调摄

夏季暑气当令，烈日酷暑，腠理开泄，汗液外泄，而汗为心之液，心气最易耗伤，从而可产生许多精神方面的症状；若是长夏，天气多以湿热为主，表现为气温高，无风，早晚温度变化不明显，这种天气使人感到心胸憋闷，产生焦躁和厌烦情绪，易诱发精神疾病。

《素问》指出，在精神调摄上，夏季要放，要使精神像含苞待放的花一样秀美，切忌发怒，使机体的气机宣畅，通泄自如，情绪外向，呈现出对外界事物的浓厚兴趣。即精神要充沛、情绪要饱满，因为只有神气充足，人体的机能才能旺盛而协调，若神气涣散，就有可能遭到损害。与此相反，举凡懈怠厌倦，恼怒忧郁，则有碍气机，皆非所宜。

夏季调神重在养心。人的精神活动与心的功能密切相关，平静时，心脏跳动平稳，激动时，心脏跳动加快，这是由于心主血脉、主神志

high spirits, while an inadequate blood flow means shortage of blood in the heart, which fuels insomnia, dreaminess, forgetfulness, dizziness and low spirits. So a normal performance of "the heart pushing blood flow" is the premise of high spirits in summer.

的结果。心主神志，是通过它营运血液的作用来实现的。血脉充盈，则神志清醒，思维敏捷，精神旺盛；血脉亏损，心血不足，则常常会导致失眠、多梦、健忘、眩晕以致精神不振等。因此，夏季调神养生的前提，是要保证"心运血脉"的正常进行。

The fierce heat in summer makes people fidgety, which in turn adds to the feeling of heat, so a calm heart is vital in summer. One can take shade in a secluded place, which facilitates harmonious breathing and a clear heart, or better imagine snow and ice to combat the heat. "A calm heart cools one down naturally." There is something in this saying.

夏日炎炎，往往令人心烦，而烦则更热，故宁心静神尤为重要。为了避免暑热，不仅宜在水亭、树阴等洁净而空敞之处纳凉，更宜调息净心，想像一片冰雪在心，就能减少夏季气候给心中带来的炎热感。因此，"心静自然凉"是炎暑季节调养心神的重要法则。

2.2 Daily Life

Go to bed late to draw more yin from nature, and rise early to meet the booming yang. Do more outdoor exercise at dawn to fortify the body in tune with the growing nature of summer.

2.2 起居调养

夏季人们应晚睡以适应阴气的不足，早起以顺应阳气的充盛，清晨多到室外参加一些活动，以增强体质，适应夏长之气。

The summer is characterized by long daytime and short night, high temperature, heavy perspiration that renders yang in the body vulnerable and fatigue ensues. The high temperature not only makes nervus centralis unstable, so one turns dull in nervous reaction, and suffers from poor appetite and low spirits, or even heat stroke and coma in a worse case, but also adds to the excitement of nerves, and one is prone to irritation, headache,

夏季气候的特点是昼长夜短，气温高、汗液排泄较多，阳气易损，使人感觉疲劳。夏季的高温会影响中枢神经系统的稳定，使人的神经反射变得迟钝，胃纳不佳，精神萎靡不振，严重者可出现中暑昏迷。高温还会增加神经的兴奋性，使人烦躁不

faint and insomnia, irritation and fatigue also added to by sweat knocked in owing to the high temperature, severe humidity and low air pressure. And people suffer more from poor sleep resulting from short and hot night. So one should be sure to keep a placid state of mind, which cools one down, and take siesta to make up for the short night, which relaxes the brain and the body, prevents heat stroke and refreshes one for work in the afternoon.

安、头痛、头昏和失眠。温度高，湿度大，气压低，使汗液不易排出和散发，也会让人感到烦躁和疲倦。加上夏天昼长夜短，晚上闷热，睡眠质量不佳，这样，自然影响人的身体。因此，夏季起居要注意防暑降温，保持宁静的心境。由于夏季夜间睡眠时间较短，所以最好保证一定的午睡时间，使大脑和身体放松，有利于下午的工作学习，也是预防中暑的良好措施。

Nowadays there are more electric fans and air conditioners, which should not be abused. Because one sweats heavily and the skin tissue opens and cold wind and evil humidity might slip in, which, in a much cooler environment, would cause disease, such as numb hands and feet, paralysis of the body and face, and other Middle and collateral channels and Collaterals Disease. So one should not abandon himself to coldness by keeping the air conditioner working for a long time or turning it too low, but keep it at about 5 degrees Celsius lower than the outside temperature, in protection of his immunity. A recommended temperature is 26-28 degrees Celsius in extra scorching weather.

现在，人们的防暑降温条件大大改善，有风扇、空调之类，但夏日高温汗出较多，腠理开泄，易致风寒湿邪侵袭。若过分贪凉，使虚邪贼风侵袭，极易引起手足麻木、半身不遂、面瘫等中经络疾病，因此纳凉不能过度，尤其不要长时间吹拂空调，空调温度也不宜调定得太低，以室内外温度相差 5 ℃左右为好，以免降低人体免疫力。若天气特别炎热，则可将空调温度调定在 26～28 ℃。

Taking a warm shower every day in summer can be extremely cooling and also freshen the skin. The water pressure and mechanic massage of the shower can reduce the excitement of the nervous system, expand blood vessels in the skin, accelerate blood circulation, improve the nutrition in skin and tissue, contract muscles, remove fatigue and sleep, and en-

酷暑盛夏，每天洗一次温水澡，是很好的防暑降温措施，还能洗掉汗水、污垢，使皮肤清爽，消暑防病。温水冲洗时水压及机械按摩作用，可使神经系统兴奋性降低，扩张体表血管，加快血液

hance immunity. Wiping the body with a dripping towel can be resorted to in the absence of a shower.

循环,改善肌肤和组织的营养,降低肌肉张力,消除疲劳,改善睡眠,增强抵抗力。没有条件洗温水澡时,可用毛巾蘸温水擦浴全身。

Wear a thin coat in summer and change and wash it often, for a sweated coat on the body for a long time can stimulate skin and trigger many diseases.

在衣着方面,由于夏日天热多汗,衣衫要薄一些,并且勤洗勤换,久穿湿衣、汗衣可刺激皮肤而引起多种疾病。

2.3 Diet

2.3 饮食调养

The heat in summer arouses the fire quality of the heart which, when too fierce, overwhelms the metal quality of lungs. So one can eat food that quenches heart fire and relieve one of heat, such as watermelon, green beans, red beans and bitter gourd. Take a proper amount of cold drinks, which can make up for what is lost in sweat and help disperse the heat in the body, yet not indulge in them and cold melon and fruit, an overdose of which impairs the spleen and the stomach, and leads to disease; especially forbidden are the old and children whose infirm constitution reacts more intensely to stimulation of heat and coldness.

夏季气候炎热,暑热当令,心火易于亢盛,心火过旺则克肺金。所以饮食上宜用清心泻火消暑之物,如西瓜、绿豆、赤小豆、苦瓜之类。暑热天气下,人体出汗较多,可适当用些冷饮,补充水分,帮助体内散发热量,清热解暑。但切忌贪凉而暴食冷饮、生冷瓜果等,否则会使脾胃功能受到影响,甚至酿生疾病。老年人、小儿体质较弱,对于过热过冷刺激反应较大,更不可过贪冷饮之类。

Human qi and blood concentrate in the skin in summer, hence the condition of yang flowing outward and yin withdrawing; moreover, the stomach produces less gastric acid in summer and poor digestion results, which is worsened by humidity in the heat, giving rise to disorder in the transportation of the spleen and the stomach, shown in the sense of suppression in the chest, trance, fatigued limbs, sleepiness and watery excrement. So one had better

夏季气候炎热,人体气血趋于体表,形成阳气在外,阴气内伏的状况,同时夏季胃酸分泌减少,脾胃的消化功能减弱,若暑热挟湿则更易伤及脾胃,致脾胃运化失司,升降失常,出现胸闷、纳呆、肢体困倦乏力、精神萎靡、大便稀溏等症状。因此

take light food in summer that is easily digested, or pungent and spicy food, which is appetizing and which promotes function of the spleen and the stomach.

夏季饮食又以清淡、少油腻、易消化为原则，也可适当选择具有辛辣香气的食物，以开胃助消化，增强脾胃的纳运功能。

Germ propagates readily in summer and so food is vulnerable. As a result, digestive diseases happen most frequently. So one might do well to remember the saying "illness starts from the mouth". Be sure to reheat leftovers before eating and sterilize cookers and dishes and keep them in a clean place.

夏季，致病微生物极易繁殖，食物易被污染而腐败、变质。这个季节是胃肠疾病多发、高发的时期，因此要讲究饮食卫生，谨防"病从口入"。对于剩饭剩菜要回锅加热，经常使用的炊具、饭具、茶具等要及时消毒，妥善保管。

2.4 Exercise

People perspire heavily in summer, which consumes qi and impairs yin, so one should avoid working out under the sun for a long time in case of heat stroke, but exercise at dawn or dusk, and take it moderately, such as walking, jogging, practicing Taiji Quan and qigong. Patients of heart disease, hypertension, hardened arteries, hyperthyreosis and diabetes should take greatest care to avoid hot settings in exercise. Wear clothes that are soft, loose-fitting and of a quiet colour; drink some water when perspiring heavily; never take a cold shower, even only for the head, which fuels cold or rheumatism.

2.4 运动锻炼

暑热使人体汗出较多，易耗气伤阴，若长时间在日光下活动可能引起中暑。所以夏季运动时要避开炽热烈日，并注意加强防护。最好在清晨或傍晚天气较凉爽时进行室外运动锻炼。宜选择运动量适中的运动方式，如散步、慢跑、打太极拳、做广播操、练气功等，不可过度疲劳。患有心脏病、高血压、动脉硬化、甲亢、肥胖病的病人尤其不宜在烈日下或高温环境中进行锻炼。运动时的衣服宜松软、宽大、颜色浅淡、穿脱方便。运动后出汗较多时，可适当饮些凉开水，切勿用冷水冲头洗澡，以免招致感冒，或引起风湿痹痛。

3 Autumn

Autumn is a crucial period when the yang atmosphere in nature gives way to the yin, so do their counterparts in the human body. So health preservation in autumn is characterized by "withdrawal" in every respect.

3 秋季养生

秋季三个月，从立秋开始到立冬前一天止，包括立秋、处暑、白露、秋分、寒露、霜降六个节气。秋令时分，自然界的阳气渐渐收敛，阴气逐渐增长，气候由热转凉，是由阳盛向阴盛转变的关键时期。人体的阴阳双方也随之由"长"到"收"发生变化，阴阳的代谢也开始向阳消阴长过渡。因此，秋季养生，从饮食、起居、情志、运动等诸方面，均要考虑到秋季的特点，以养"收"为原则。

3.1 Spirit Adjustment

As is mentioned above, people, especially the old, are susceptible to sentimentality for the withering scenes in autumn, so the key of spirit adjustment in autumn is to settle one's mind.

3.1 精神调摄

秋天，尤其是深秋，呈现的是秋风扫落叶和万木枯黄的自然景观，使人容易产生风烛残年之情感，这对人的心理及生理都产生负面影响。当人们身临枯草落叶、残花朽木之间，常令人忧愁。尤其是老年人，常引起萧条、凄凉、垂暮之感，勾起忧郁的心绪。所以秋季养生要求人们要尽量地安定其情绪，不要过多地触景生情，应通过精神调摄来克服这种情况，这是秋季调神保健的关键。

According to Su Wen, people should settle the mind and guard the will against irritation, in order to clear qi in lungs and pacify the harsh atmosphere

《素问》认为，在秋天，人们一定要保持精神上的安宁，使意志保持安定，藉以舒

in autumn, and thus cushion its harm to health. In a word, collecting the spirit goes in tune with the feature of autumn. The lungs dominate in autumn, which are prone to sadness and anxiety, so one should "not be overcome by sadness in autumn", but try to conserve the clear qi in the lungs.

缓秋守,不急不躁,使秋天肃杀之气得以和平,不使意志外弛,使得肺气清静。只有这样才能减缓肃杀之气对人体的影响;还要注意不断地收敛神气,以适应秋季的特征;秋应于肺,悲忧最易伤肺,切不可悲伤忧思,正所谓"秋忌悲"。应当保肺之清肃之气,这就是顺应秋季季节特点,在精神上养收的方法。

Emphasis must be laid on the word "harmony" in adjusting emotions in autumn. The middle-aged and the aged are supposed to strive for a harmonious character, that is, not to allow emotions at the mercy of material gain or loss, be optimistic and open-minded, tolerant and generous, adopt a nonchalant and detached attitude toward life, collect the spirit and qi, and retain a peaceful mind, all of which combat the harsh atmosphere of autumn. One can choose exercise according to his individual condition, such as walking, jogging, practicing the five-animal exercise and Taiji Quan and 8-section brocade exercise, doing common exercise and self-massaging for the old, and running, playing balls, mountaineering, taking cold baths and swimming for the middle-aged and youngsters. Better effect can be attained if one combines the "mobile exercise" with "quiescent exercise", with the former building the body and the latter nourishing spirit, hence both achieved.

秋季养生在对精神情志等方面进行调摄时,还应注重一个"和"字,调和情志。对中老年人来说,应养成不以物喜,不以己悲,乐观开朗,宽容豁达,淡泊宁静的性格,收神敛气,保持内心宁静,可减缓秋季肃杀之气对精神的影响,方可适应秋季容平的特征。在此期间可以开展诸多的锻炼项目,应因人而异来选择,如老年人可散步、慢跑,练五禽戏,打太极拳,做健身操、八段锦,自我按摩等;中青年人可跑步、打球、爬山、洗冷水浴、游泳等。在进行"动功"锻炼的同时,可配合"静功",动静结合,动则强身,静则养神,可达到心身康泰之功效。

3.2 Daily Life

People should retire into bed early to collect yin in tune with the "withdrawal" nature of autumn,

3.2 起居调养

秋季,自然界的阳气由疏泄趋向收敛,人的起居作

thereby guarding lungs against the attack of chill, and rise early for the expansion of qi and yang in lungs in case of withdrawing too much.

息也要相应调整。早睡以顺应阴精的收藏，以养“收”气，可以避免秋天晚上凉气伤肺；早起，可以使肺气得以舒展，防止收之太过，以顺应阳气的舒长。

The lungs command in autumn with full qi and blood, but they are prone to the unpredictably cold weather and dry atmosphere, and one tends to catch cold and cough, so lungs are at the core of health preservation in autumn.

肺与秋季相应，与秋气相通，肺旺于秋，秋天肺的气血最充沛，功能最旺盛。秋季天气寒热多变，寒凉之气及秋燥之气极易伤肺，发生感冒、咳嗽等，所以秋季重在养肺。

Do not add thick clothes abruptly even in late autumn. Chill in autumn is an important approach to health preservation. One perspires little in this way, so he can guard his yin body fluid and yang that would otherwise have evaporated with sweat, in tune with the withdrawing nature of autumn and in preparation for concealment in winter. “Keeping chilly in autumn” is a health-preservation concept that covers many aspects of life as follows: people, especially children, should not sleep under a thick quilt, as perspiration impairs yin and consumes body fluid; do not wear too much, and remember to be chilly when exercising, such as playing balls, mountaineering and walking; “taking a cold bath” fits in perfectly with the concept, which had better been kept on throughout the autumn. A proper degree, however, should be noted in “being chilly”; add clothes according to the weather, but do not be bundled up so long as one does not feel cold.

秋季虽然天气逐渐转凉，但衣被要逐渐添加，即使是晚秋，穿衣也要有所控制。秋冻是秋季一种有效的养生方法，有意识地让机体“冻一冻”避免了多穿衣服产生的身热汗出，汗液蒸发，阴津耗伤，阳气外泄，顺应了秋天阴精内蓄、阳气内收的养生需要，也为冬季藏精做好了准备。对于“秋冻”的理解，不应局限于未寒不忙添衣，应从广义上把它引申为秋季的一个养生法则。如睡觉不要盖得太多，尤其是小孩，多盖极易导致出汗伤阴耗液。各种运动锻炼如打球、爬山、冷水浴、散步等，无论何种活动都应注意一个“冻”字。尤其是冷水浴，是符合秋冻的有效方法，可整个秋天坚持，不要间断。但"秋冻"也应掌握好尺度。如衣服的添加与否,应根据天气的变化来决定,只不过不宜添得过多,裹得太紧,以自己感觉不寒为准。

3.3 Diet

The lungs govern in autumn and sourness can help withdraw for their benefit, so one should take more sour food than pungent food, such as onion and ginger, which spreads and drains qi in the lungs.

The dry atmosphere takes over in autumn owing to less rain and high air pressure, and it harms yin body fluid and causes cold. Spicy food can worsen it to the condition of itching throat and bucking; some chronic diseases can recur or deteriorate, such as bronchiectasis and tuberculosis, shown in more evident symptoms of coughing, phlegm-coughing and blood-coughing; those with a hot stomach and inadequate yin body fluid would suffer from constipation, red eyes, sores in the mouth and restlessness, so food should be taken to serve the purpose of moisturizing lungs and nourishing yin.

Naturally, water, vegetable soup, mild tea, juice, soy bean milk, and milk can moisturize and make up for lost fluid; most vegetables and fruits

3.3 饮食调养

秋季肺脏当令,酸味收敛,所以可食用酸味收敛补肺。辛味发散泻肺,秋天宜收不宜散,所以饮食上尽可能少食葱、姜等辛味之品,适当多吃一些酸味果蔬。

每年自秋分到立冬,天气少雨,气压高,空气干燥,为燥气当令之时,燥气容易耗伤人体的阴津,使人出现一派"燥"象。如感受秋燥,易患感冒;如果再多食辛辣之品,很容易出现咽痒、呛咳等咽喉炎的表现;某些疾病在秋燥的影响下,也易复发或加重,如支气管扩张、肺结核等,导致咳嗽、咳痰、咯血等症状加重;平素胃热而阴津不足的人,容易发生大便干结,伴见目赤、口舌生疮、烦躁不安等一系列症状。为防止秋燥对人体带来的不良影响,在饮食上宜以滋阴养肺润燥为法。

具体地说,首先要多喝开水、淡茶、果汁饮料、豆浆、牛奶等流质,以养阴润燥,弥

are succulent, cold or cool in character, thus promoting the production of body fluid, bringing the heat down and smoothing excrement; to clear and nourish lungs one can also take more Feng Mi, Bai He, Lian Zi, Hei Zhi Ma, fungus, white fungus and crystal rock sugar, less with spicy and fried food due to its hot character, such as Chinese chives, garlic, onion, Sheng Jiang (*Rhizoma Zingiberis Recens*), Ba Jiao Hui Xiang (*Fructus Anisi Stellati*) and Xiao Hhui Xiang (*Fructu Foeniculi*).

补损失的阴津;其次宜多吃新鲜蔬菜和水果。秋燥最易伤人的津液,多数蔬菜、水果性质寒凉,有生津润燥、清热通便之功;蔬菜、水果含有大量的水分,能补充人体的津液。另外,还可多吃些蜂蜜、百合、莲子、芝麻、木耳、银耳、冰糖等清补润燥之品,以顺应肺脏的清肃之性。少吃辛辣煎炸热性食物,如韭菜、大蒜、葱、姜、八角、茴香等。

Autumn is abundant in fruits, but most of them are cool or cold in character except longan, grapes and lichee, so one should be moderate in consumption. Especially the old with their weak digestive system would have impaired yang, vomit or have running bowels if they overeat them. In addition, every kind of fruit has its character, so one should select them based on his own constitution. For instance, those with great inner heat, showing in sores in mouth or the tongue and constipation should eat more pear, banana, persimmon, and kiwi fruit for their cool character; while those with running bowels should help themselves to fruit of warm character, such as peach, lychee, longan and cherry.

秋季是大量瓜果上市的季节,但除龙眼、葡萄、荔枝外,大部分水果性偏寒凉,因此在食用时也应有节制。特别是老年人肠胃功能薄弱,多食会损害阳气,影响消化功能,引起腹泻、呕吐等病证,所以更应引起足够的重视。而且每一种水果又都有它自身的特性,要辨清体质加以选择。如平素内火较重,口舌易于生疮,大便秘结者,宜多食梨、香蕉、柿子、猕猴桃等寒凉水果;而素体阳虚,动辄腹泻者则宜食桃子、荔枝、龙眼、樱桃等性温的水果。

Enteritis and malaria are frequent occurrences in autumn, so one should give great heed to food hygiene, avoiding unboiled water and rotten food, and even take precautions by drinking the herbal de-

秋季是肠炎、痢疾多发的时节,所以应特别注意饮食卫生,不要喝生水及食用腐败变质的食物,在肠炎及

coctions of isatis root or herba portulacae in the sweeping period of enteritis and malaria.

痢疾的流行期服用板蓝根、马齿苋等中药汤剂，可起到一定的防治效果。

3.4 Exercise

The golden autumn is a splendid time for exercise, such as mountaineering and playing balls. The old can choose to take a stroll, practice Taiji Quan or the five-animal exercise. The intensity of exercise can be elevated with it growing colder, and health can be evidently improved when winter comes. Be cautious about adding clothes; ensure the supply of water and dissolving vitamins; drink warm water before exercise, and other liquid as is mentioned above, to keep normal secretion of membrane and moistness of the respiratory tube and skin.

3.4 运动锻炼

金秋季节是开展各种锻炼的好时期，可因人而异选择各种运动项目，如爬山、打球等，老年人可选择散步、太极拳、五禽戏等。而随着天气渐冷，可适当增加运动量，到严冬来临时体质会有明显的改善。注意衣物的灵活增减，还要及时补充水分及水溶性维生素。运动前喝些温开水，平时饮用菜汤、牛奶、果汁，可保持黏膜正常分泌，呼吸道湿润，皮肤润泽。

4 Winter

In the freezing winter, the yin atmosphere in nature takes dominance and the yang conceals itself entirely, and human metabolism slows down. So it is vital for people to keep warm, collect their yang and guard yin, based on the principle of concealment.

4 冬季养生

冬三月，从立冬开始，经过小雪、大雪、冬至、小寒、大寒直到立春前一天为止，是一年中气候最寒冷的季节。自然界天寒地冻，阴气盛极，阳气潜伏。人的代谢相对缓慢，故冬季养生，应避寒就暖，敛阳护阴，以闭藏为本。

4.1 Spirit Adjustment

The spirit adjustment focuses on "concealment". According to Su Wen, one should keep serene and try to control his emotions, guarding them in the heart like privacy yet removing grim emotions. The key is to conceal the spirit rather than reveal it, otherwise, the emotions disperse and qi

4.1 精神调摄

冬季精神调摄，要着眼于"藏"。所以，《素问》说冬天要保持精神静谧，尽量控制自己的精神情志活动，最好能做到含而不露，像个人的隐私一样存于胸中秘而不

movement rises and falls in disorder.

宜,又要有如获得期望的结果一样心满意足。其关键是冬季要藏神于内,不要暴露于外。这就是适应冬季在情志方面的养“藏”之道。一旦违反这些要求,就会影响情志的内敛而妨碍气机的升降。

Measures should be taken to prevent seasonal abnormal mentality, such as melancholy, sluggishness, and drowsiness in winter, which recur every year in the young, especially females. To alleviate it, one can resort to sunshine, exercise, fresh vegetables, fruits, beans, dairy products, peanuts and animal intestines.

冬季精神调养还要防止季节性情感失调症,有些人在冬季易发生情绪抑郁、懒散嗜睡、昏昏沉沉等现象,并且年复一年地出现,这种情况多见于青年,尤其是女性。可通过延长光照时间、加强体育锻炼、多吃新鲜蔬菜、水果、豆类、乳类、花生、动物内脏等,进行调养。

4.2 Daily Life

To preserve health in winter, one should retire early and rise late, and preferably move about after sunrise, so as to conserve yang and save yin essence which, naturally, should first be ensured by dressing warmly. So yang is the priority of health preservation in winter. If it is disturbed, also to be upset is the law of “yin coming into form overwhelming yang transforming into qi”.

4.2 起居调养

冬季的起居养生,宜早睡晚起,最好等待日出以后活动,以免扰动阳气;还要注意防寒保暖,护阳固精。在寒冷的冬季里,不应当扰动阳气,破坏阴成形大于阳化气的规律。早睡晚起,日出而作,可保证充足的睡眠时间,以利阳气的潜藏,阴精的积蓄。

With the stimulation of freezing cold air in winter, the respiratory tube turns vulnerable and some chronic diseases tend to recur, such as acute recurrence of chronic arthritis; when the cold spell comes, patients of cardio vascular disease would feel

严冬由于气温下降,冷空气刺激使呼吸道抵抗力下降,易致一些慢性病发作,如慢性支气管炎急性发作;气温骤降或寒潮来临,易使心

stifled in chest, breathless, dizzy, sick and overall discomfort, or even suffer stroke or myocardial infarction; and the freezing air also triggers flu. So one should be sure to put on more clothes and keep himself warm, thereby keeping disease at bay.

血管病患者感到胸闷、气短、头晕、恶心和全身不适,可能诱发心肌梗死和中风;流行性感冒的发生和流行与冷空气的袭击也有密切关系。所以在冬季,一定要适时增添衣物,注意防寒保暖,防止各种疾病的发生。

In tune with the "concealment" nature of winter, one should also be temperate in sexual intercourse to conserve yin essence. Arranging sex discretely and moderately plays a part in preventing hot disease in spring.

在性生活方面,也应注意顺应自然界主收主藏的规律,节制房事,蓄养阴精。性生活应审慎安排,适中为度,对于预防春温病也有一定的作用。

4.3 Diet

4.3 饮食调养

The diet in winter should follow the principle of "cultivating yin in autumn and winter without disturbing yang", high-calorie food that nourishes yin and guards yang being preferable to the raw, cold, dry and hot. The kidney is linked to saltiness, while the heart to bitterness. As the former governs in winter, and saltiness overwhelms bitterness, more bitter food than salty should be taken to guard qi of the heart.

冬季饮食调养,应当遵循"秋冬养阴""无扰乎阳"的原则,既不宜生冷,也不宜燥热,适宜用滋阴潜阳、热量较高的膳食。因冬季是肾主令之时,肾主咸味,心主苦味,咸能胜苦,所以饮食之味宜减咸增苦以顾护心气。

The freezing winter drives yin essence and yang into concealment, and so the spleen and the stomach are boomed in function, which absorb nutrition expectantly, when one should take food rich in protein, such as mutton and chicken, which keeps one warm, especially warming yang and rendering yin inexhaustible. Those with yin-deficiency constitution should take food that nourishes yin, such as E Jiao (*Colla Corii Asini*), tortoise, soft-shelled turtle, and white fungus, to attain the equilibrium of yin and yang, which generates endlessly. Taboo should

冬月天寒地冻,人体的阴精秘藏,阳气内蓄,脾胃的机能每多健旺,是营养物质易于蓄积的最佳时机,饮食应选用蛋白质含量高及可以防寒保暖的食物,如羊肉、鸡肉、狗肉等,以达温阳则阴不穷。而素体阴亏者,宜进食养阴滋补之品,如阿胶、龟肉、鳖肉、银耳等,使阴阳协调平衡,生化无穷。但一些

be taken about some raw, cold and sticky food, such as sticky rice cake, cold drink and melons, which impairs yang in the spleen and the stomach. Hot food makes one cozy in winter, but not in the case of hot and dry food, which fans the concealing yang into flame.

Around the winter solstice yang begins to grow in the body and needs protection, when it is the perfect time to take tonic, as the digestive system turns stronger for more calories to combat the cold climate, and thus nutrition in the tonic can be better absorbed and stocked. The paste prescription is recommended.

生冷黏腻的食物，如年糕、冷饮、瓜果等易损伤人体脾胃的阳气，冬季也要少食或忌食。冬季虽宜热食，但燥热之物不可过食，以免内伏之阳气郁而化热。

冬至前后，人体阳气开始生发，必须保护初生的阳气，此时也是进补的最佳时间。因为气候寒冷，人体对能量的需求较高，消化吸收功能相对较强，而此时进补，补品中的有效成分更易积蓄，一般可选用膏方进补。

4.4 Exercise

Those who persist in exercising in winter are less susceptible to bronchitis, pneumonia, amygdalitis, chilblain and cold, etc. In China, there has been the idea of "keeping exercising even in the harshest winter". Perseverance is vital for exercising in winter. But it should be noted that one is not supposed to brave gust, freezing and heavily snowy, foggy, or frosting days, in case of catching cold or frostbite. Be sure to warm up before exercising; do not take off the coat until one grows warm after exercising for some time, and remember to change the sweated underwear into a dry one afterward; put on the cap and gloves when going outdoors in case of chilblain. Finally, in tune with the "concealment" nature of winter, what is crucial is not to go beyond normal exercise, as it consumes yang in the body.

4.4 运动锻炼

长期坚持冬季锻炼的人，很少患支气管炎、肺炎、扁桃体炎、冻疮、感冒等疾病。我国自古也有"冬练三九"之说，因此，冬季天气虽寒，也要根据自身的情况，持之以恒进行运动锻炼。冬季锻炼要避开大风、大寒、大雪、雾露天气，要注意预防感冒和冻伤。锻炼前应做好准备活动，开始锻炼时衣服要多穿些，待身暖和时再脱去厚衣服，运动后要及时更换衣服，不要穿湿衣。外出活动最好戴帽子和手套，以免发生冻疮。同时应注意运动不宜过量，避免耗损阳气，以符合"闭藏"的养生要求。

Chapter 10 Health Preservation for Different People

第 10 章 不同人群养生

TCM health preservation is individual-oriented. It pays attention to individual difference, emphasizes on choosing proper methods according to individual difference so as to achieve the best results. Everybody is mentally and physiologically unique without doubt. So it is extremely difficult to make a difference of everybody's health preservation. This chapter talks about health preservation application objected on people of different ages, genders, careers and physical situations.

中医养生以"因人制宜"为基本原则，注重养生的个体差异，强调在辨识个体差异的基础上，选择适当的养生方法，以达到最佳的养生效果。当然，每个人从心理到生理都是独一无二的，把每一个体的养生问题都进行区别对待，是极其困难的，本章仅从年龄、性别、职业、体质四个不同角度，以人群为对象，阐述养生应用问题。

Section 1 Health Preservation for Different Ages

第 1 节 辨年龄施养

1 Children

The children here refer to those below 12 years old. It is an important stage of mental and physiological growth. TCM pays attention to the health preservation for children and emphasizes its importance in the lifetime. It needs to follow the principles of cultivating and teaching together according

1 少儿保养

少儿是指从出生到 12 岁这段时期，是人体生理和心理快速成长的阶段。中医十分重视对少儿的保养，强调了"养小"对一生保持健康的重要意义。少儿的养生，

to children's mental and physiological characteristics in order to make them grow healthily.

需根据其特有的生理和心理特点，采用养教并重的原则，促使少儿健康成长。

1.1 Physiological and Psychological Features

1.1.1 Quick Growth and Development

During this stage, the mental and physiological status of children changes very fast. There are three stages for one decade. The first stage refers to the one year after birth. In this stage, a newborn baby gradually grows into a human being who can eat, sit, stand, walk and have emotions. This stage is the period when a child develops fast. Four to six months after birth, the weight will grow from 3 kg at birth to about 6 kg. At the age of one, the child can weigh over 9 kg and the height will be one half times of the weight at birth. The head circumference will grow 10 to 12 centimeters. Mentality also develops fast in the infant period. For example, a child can hold straight the head at 3 months, grab things at 4 months and laugh when seeing relatives, toys and feeders. At the age of 4 to 5 months, he can babble and gradually understand the words of the adults. At 7 months, he can sit; at 9 to 10 months, he can stand; at one year, he can walk.

1.1.2 Tenderness and Fragileness

At the initial stage of the growth and development, a child physiologically enjoys vitality, tenderness and as well as weakness. With weak resistance, he is vulnerable to diseases and the condition develops quickly. In addition, he isn't well devel-

1.1 生理和心理特点

1.1.1 生长发育快速

这一时期少儿的生理和心理变化非常快，十年上3个台阶。如中医认为，从出生到1岁属于变蒸期，即通过变蒸，出生的胎儿逐渐成长为能食谷肉果菜，能坐、能立、能行走，有喜怒情志的人。所谓的变蒸期正是人一生生长发育最快的阶段。出生后4～6月，其体重从出生时约3千克增加至约6千克，到1岁时可增至9千克以上，达到出生时的3倍；1岁时身长为出生时的1.5倍，头围在一年内增长10～12厘米。神经心理发育在婴儿期也很迅速，如3个月会竖头，4个月会抓物，当看到亲人、玩具、奶瓶时，能出声大笑；4～5个月时，可以咿呀作语，逐渐理解大人说话；7个月会坐，9～10个月会站，1岁会走。

1.1.2 脏腑柔弱，形气未充

少儿处于生长发育的初期。在生理上，既有生机蓬勃、蒸蒸日上的一面，又有脏腑娇嫩、形气未充的一面。其抗病力低下，易于发病，病

oped psychologically, timid, easy to be frightened and unstable. Meanwhile, a child can be easily influenced and educated from different aspects. Therefore, targeting at the physiological and psychological features of child, great opportunities can be seized timely to take scientific and preventive measures, which guarantees the healthy growth of a child.

情发展迅速。小儿的心理发育也未臻完善,其精神怯弱,易受惊吓致病,情志不稳,可塑性大,易于接受各方面的影响和教育。针对少儿的生理、心理特点,不失时机地采取科学的保健措施,是促进少儿健康成长的重要保证。

1.2 Essentials for Different Stages

In the rapid growth and development of a child, the mental and physical status will leap several stages, namely, newborn stage, infancy period and childhood. The essentials for health preservation of different stages will be introduced as follows:

1.2 分期养生要点

少儿在快速生长发育的过程中,生理和心理发育会发生几次由量变到质变的飞跃。少儿期可分为新生儿期、婴幼儿期、儿童期三个阶段,兹将各期的养生要点概述如下。

1.2.1 Newborn Stage

The newborn stage refers to the first month after birth. In this stage, keeping warm and proper feeding are the essentials.

(1) Keep moderate temperature: After delivered from womb, the newborn need to get accustomed to the environment outside. Therefore, the temperature needs to be kept moderate. Importance can be attached to warmth keeping, even in summer. Meanwhile, don't overdo it, in case of the internal heat. Used cotton-padded clothes and quilts are advocated. For premature babies, warmth is more important. If possible, nurture them in the special warmer.

(2) Breast feeding: The newborn babies should be fed with breast milk, for it is transformed from

1.2.1 新生儿期

自出生至满月为新生儿期。以保暖、合理喂养为养生保健重点。

(1)寒温适宜,保暖为先:新生儿从母腹出生,对外界环境需有一个适应过程,因此要注意寒温的调适。尤其强调保温的重要性,甚至在夏季也要注意保暖,逐渐减衣。同时,也不可保暖太过,防止产生内热,提倡用旧的棉衣棉被做成襁褓。对于早产儿就更要注意保温,有条件的尽可能在医院的专用保暖箱中进行养护。

(2)母乳喂养,饥饱得当:新生儿应当以母乳喂养,

the blood and qi of the mother and rich in nutrition. Furthermore, the resistance contained in the qi and blood of the mother can pass down to the baby through breast milk. Therefore, breast feeding is of utmost importance to the growth and development of the newborn baby, which means that during the breast feeding, the health condition of the mother can directly influence the baby. If breast feeding is chosen, feed the baby with the breast milk from a healthy mother. During the feeding, the motion, diet and lifestyle need to be cautiously regulated, for it is the best nurturing for the newborn. Meanwhile, don't feed too much, otherwise vomiting and malabsorption will be induced.

因母乳为母亲血气所化生，富含新生儿所需要的所有营养物质，并将母亲血气中抵抗病邪的防御能力传给下一代。因此，母乳喂养对新生儿的健康的发育成长至关重要，这也就意味母乳喂养阶段母亲的健康状况对新生儿有直接的影响。如果请乳母来喂养，一定要选择身体健康的乳母。喂养期间，母亲的情志、饮食、起居均需谨慎调养，这时母亲的养护，就是对新生儿最好的养护。同时，喂养也需饥饱得当，母亲喂养过多的情况比较常见，容易导致小儿吐乳，反而不能很好吸收。

1.2.2 Infancy

Infancy refers to the period from the first month after birth to the first birthday. This is the period when a human being develops fast, a leaping period. In this period, infants need a great demand of nutrition and proteins. However, the digestive system isn't well developed yet. Therefore, digestive and nutritional disorders easily occur. Hence, it is of much importance to feed the infants with breast milk properly. In addition, infants are vulnerable to diseases with weak body resistance. Thus, they need to be vaccinated and develop a healthy lifestyle.

1.2.2 婴幼儿期

从满月到周岁为婴儿期。这是人一生中生长发育最迅速的阶段，是“变蒸”过程，被称作人生中第一个飞跃时期。婴儿期需要摄入的营养素和蛋白质要求特别高，但此时消化功能尚不完善，易发生消化与营养紊乱。所以，提倡母乳喂养和合理的营养指导十分重要。婴儿期抗病能力较弱，要有计划地进行预防接种，完成基础免疫程序，并应注重卫生习惯的培养。

Toddler period refers to the duration between

从1周岁到3周岁为幼

the first year to the third year. Compared to the infant, the toddler develops slowly, especially in physique. However, toddlers can move around, have more access to the surroundings. Although with fast developed mentality and strengthened language and thinking ability, toddlers still lack the ability to sense the risks. Therefore, accidents and poisoning should be prevented. With more access to the surroundings and poor immunity, toddlers are vulnerable to infectious diseases. Therefore, prevention is essential.

儿期。幼儿期生长发育速度较前者慢，尤其在体格发育方面，活动范围渐广，接触事物渐多，智能发育较前突出，语言思维能力增强，但识别危险的能力尚不足，需预防意外事故和中毒。此时接触外界较广，自身免疫力低，传染病发病率较高，防病仍为关键。

Mental care, proper feeding, temperature regulation and timely vaccination are the essentials of health preservation in this period.

精神关爱，合理喂养，寒温调护，按时预防接种等，是婴幼儿期的养生保健要点。

(1) Mental care: Due to underdeveloped shen, infants are easily frightened by external factors and develop diseases like fright epilepsy. Therefore, mental care is much needed. When infants are crying, comfort them immediately. Otherwise, mental needs are not satisfied, and the mental health and the relationship between parents and child will be affected. If infants are comforted every time when they are crying, their communicative ability will develop fast with more facial expressions. Quick response to infants is also conducive to the harmonious relationship between parents and infants. In addition, once needs are met, infants will feel safe and capabilities of every aspect will develop faster.

（1）精神调养，顺其心意：婴幼时期的孩童形神发育未全，容易受外界各种因素的惊吓，而作惊痫等病，所以精神上需要更多的关爱。当父母看到孩子啼哭时，应尽快给孩子以适当的安慰。反之，如果对孩子没有及时的关心，满足其精神需要，可能会影响其身心健康的成长，也影响着父母和孩子之间的关系。每次啼哭都很快得到照顾的孩子的交际能力发育比较快，具体表现在孩子的面部表情比较多。父母对孩子做出敏感快速的反应有助于与孩子形成和谐的关系，同时孩子感到满足，有安全感，各方面能力提高也比较快。

According to psychological researches, attitude towards child is an essential factor behind the physical and psychological development. Infants are rich in emotions and depend on parents in life, psychology and behaviors. Therefore, parents shouldn't be indifferent or indulgent. Instead, proper care is necessary. Parents need to be lenient, kind and strict with both prize and punishment. Support the right behaviors and satisfy their rightful requirement, which will create a favorable environment for their growth.

心理学的研究表明，对孩子持什么样的态度是影响幼童身心发展的重要因素。小儿虽少七情六欲，但仍富有感情，在生活、心理和行为上均有极大的依赖性。父母对孩子不应冷漠无情，也不能溺爱、百般迁就，而应给以足够的爱抚。爱抚是一种宽严相济、恩威并施的意识行为。表现为和蔼的态度、无微不至的关注、怀抱、亲昵与依偎，以及对孩子始终如一的严格要求。支持他们的正确行为，满足他们的正当要求，为他们的成长创造良好的环境与条件。

(2) Proper feeding: Infants grow fast with their body, mentality and organ functions being matured gradually. Diverse nutrition is of great demand. Therefore, diet for infants need to be highly qualified and with full nutrition.

（2）饮食调养，循序渐进：婴幼儿生长发育迅速，体格、智力以及脏腑功能均不断趋向完善成熟，对各种营养物质的需要量较多，婴幼儿膳食构成应做到质量高、营养全，数量由少到多，品种由单一到复杂。

At first, milk is only needed, especially the breast milk. Breast milk is the natural food and especially suitable for infants under six months. If there is no breast milk or the mother cannot feed, substitutes like milk, ewe's milk, milk cake and soybean milk are available. Among them, fresh milk is preferred. If the breast milk is insufficient or the mother cannot feed it with breast milk, mixing milk will be necessary.

母乳是婴儿最理想的天然食品，对 6 个月以下的小儿更适合。若无母乳或其他原因不能哺乳，可采用人工喂养，通常予以牛奶、羊奶、奶糕、豆浆等代乳品，鲜牛奶可作首选。若母乳不足或其他原因不能全部用母乳喂养，可采用混合喂养。

Six months later, auxiliary food like grains, fruits and vegetables are added gradually to supplement nutrition and to promote the development of digestive functions. Spleen and stomach are the acquired root. Infants have weak functions of intestines and stomach and also insufficiency of the spleen. Moreover, they cannot control their intake by themselves. Therefore, improper feeding will impair the spleen and stomach, hinder the digestion and absorption and affect growth and development. Therefore, infantile feeding should focus on preventing the spleen and stomach. Don't feed too much. The auxiliary food should be fluid at first, then semifluid and finally solid. They should be supplemented according to the specific conditions which can be acquired through observing the stools. Milk products are the primary food, and step by step, they will be replaced by grains, vegetables, fish, meat and eggs. If possible, 250 g milk or 40 g milk product, in addition with 50-100 g food of animal origin and bean products, will basically satisfy the needs of protein. Vegetables and fruits are the main sources of dietary vitamins and minerals. Try to keep food diverse so as to guarantee ample supply of nutrition that an infant needs during growth.

6个月以后，要逐渐增加谷物果蔬等辅助食品，既补充营养，又能促进脾胃功能的发育。脾胃为后天之本，小儿肠胃脆弱、脾常不足，饮食又不能自节，喂养稍有不当，就会损伤脾胃，妨碍营养物质的消化吸收，影响生长发育。所以，幼儿的喂养应着眼于保护脾胃，饮食应以易于消化吸收为原则，不可强行填塞。辅食的添加应该由流质到半流质再到固体，由少到多，由细到粗，循序渐进。增加辅食的数量、种类和速度，要视小儿消化吸收的情况而定，宜随时观察孩子的大便以取得了解。食品应以乳类为主，逐渐过渡到粮食、蔬菜、鱼、肉及蛋等综合性食物。条件许可的话可以每日摄入一定量的乳类食品或豆制代乳食品，每日 250 克牛奶或 40 克豆制代乳粉，再加上 50～100 克动物性食品和豆制品，基本上能满足对蛋白质的需要。蔬菜和水果是膳食维生素和矿物质的重要来源，也应尽量做到多样化，以充分保证婴幼期生长发育所需营养物质的供应。

(3) Temperature regulation: According to TCM, outdoor activities are highly recommended

（3）寒温慎护，薄衣为法：中医提倡小儿要多进行

for infants so as to improve the tolerance to wind and cold. Otherwise, infants will be susceptible to diseases like the flowers in the greenhouse that cannot stand the wind. Therefore, change clothes on the basis of the weather. Keep the feet and hands warm but without sweats. The essentials are to keep head cool but back and feet warm. Don't wear too much. In TCM, it is called thick clothing approach. Of course, the approach needs to be performed step by step. In spring, take off clothes gradually so that infants can get accustomed to the cold.

室外活动,多见风日,提高对风寒的耐受能力。否则,就如温室内的花草,稍有风吹草动即会患病。要顺应天时寒温变化增减衣衫,令小儿冷热适度,以小儿的手足暖而不出汗为宜。保暖要点是头宜凉,背、足宜暖。小儿衣被忌厚热,平时穿衣不宜过多,并随季节减少衣服,中医称为"薄衣之法"。当然,施行"薄衣之法"也应循序渐进,至来春稍暖,须渐减其衣,不可随意卒减,使小儿慢慢适应寒冷刺激,避免伤中风寒。

(4) Vaccination: Vaccination is one of the most effective approaches to prevent infectious diseases. It can improve the immunity. With low immunity, infants are vulnerable to various infectious diseases. To guarantee the healthy growth of infants, infants under the age of 1 are required by the Ministry of Health according to *National EPI Regulations* to be vaccinated to strengthen the immunity to infectious diseases.

(4)预防为主,接种疫苗:预防接种是预防传染病发生的有效手段之一,可以提高人群的免疫水平。婴幼儿期体内免疫功能低下,对各种传染病都有较高的易感性。为了确保婴幼儿身心健康成长,必须按卫生部制定的《全国计划免疫工作条例》规定的免疫程序,为1岁以内的婴儿完成各种疫苗的基础免疫,以增强对传染病的免疫力。

1.2.3 Childhood

Childhood refers to the period from the age of 4 to 12. During this period, child will receive education in kindergarten and primary school as planned and also participate in various activities

1.2.3 儿童期

从4周岁到12周岁为儿童期,应有计划地进行幼儿园、小学教育,开展适于儿童特点的各种活动,做好预防

suitable for children. Meanwhile, prevention and health care need to be strengthened to prevent accidents. Cultivate virtues and initial capability of living independently. Exercise more.

保健工作,加强医护与教育,防止意外事故发生。要注意培养优秀品德及初步的独立生活能力。加强体育锻炼,使体格和智慧进一步发展。

(1) Early education and comprehensive development: Early education involves the cultivation of morality and healthy psychology, intelligence development, health education and aesthetics education. These four parts are mutual dependent and mutual support. Healthy mentality is inseparable to healthy body, and physical health inevitably influences the development of intelligence and causes inferiority, weakness, effeminacy and eccentric disposition. On the contrary, intelligence development will make children more confident, which is conducive to the increasing of the knowledge, morality and physique. Fine morality and personality can stimulate children to learn and become more conscious, dependable and assiduous. Aesthetic education can help shape the right view of life and world, make life more colorful and pleasant, thus promoting the development of intelligence and mental and physical health. Therefore, these four parts need to supplement each other and promote the harmonious development of mental and physical health all together.

(1) 早期教育,全面发展:早期教育包括德行教育与健康心理的培养、智力开发、健康教育和美学教育。德育、智育、体育、美育是相辅相成、相得益彰的。健康的心理寓于健康的身体,身体不好势必影响智力的发展,而且易形成自卑、软弱、娇气、孤僻等习气。智力的发展,能增加幼童的信心,有助于知识水平、思想品德和体质的提高。良好的品德与个性,可激发幼童学习、锻炼的自觉性和踏实刻苦的精神。美育可以促使正确人生观和世界观的萌发与形成,使生活丰富多彩,充满情趣和愉快,从而促进智力发展和身心健康。在教育的过程中,应当注意四者兼顾,相互促进,相互渗透,使孩子的身体与心理得以和谐发展。

(2) To avoid spoiling and advocate "long-raising": there are two meanings of long-raising. On the one hand, the raiser needs to well know the temper, personality and dietary habits of long and to master the training techniques. On the other hand, parents all hope their children become long,

(2) 溺爱为害,倡导"养龙":这里"养龙"包含了两层意义,其一,善养龙者,需熟知龙的性格脾气,饮食喜好,掌握驯养、驾驭龙的技艺;其二,养"龙"者,"望子成龙"之

which means to succeed and have a bright future. Therefore, long-raising is a program for raising and educating children. According to this objective, parents should not only care for children, but also discipline them. Going through hardships, children can grow into a man with strong body and mind.

"龙"。因此"养龙"是一种儿童养护和教育的成才目标。按照这样的目标,对儿童的养育既要有爱护,也要立规矩。要施以一定的苦难,经受适当的磨难,在爱的教育同时,也有挫折教育,培养坚强的躯体和心灵。

2 Adolescents

Adolescence refers to the period from the age of 12 to 24. It can be divided into puberty from the age of 12 to 18 and early adulthood from the age of 18 to 24.

2 青少年保养

青少年是指 12 岁至 24 岁这一阶段,统称青春期。又可分为青春发育期和青年期。从 12 岁至 18 岁为青春发育期,从 18 岁至 24 岁为青年期。

2.1 Physiological and Psychological Features

Puberty is the summit of growth and development. In this period, a child gains weight rapidly and matures into an adult body capable of sexual reproduction with clear physical differences of external sex organs. The body has well developed with full essence qi and harmonious qi and blood. With the development of physiology, the psychological behaviors also change. A teenager at this stage becomes vitalized with strong memory, illusioned with heterosexual pursuit, and rebellious with irritation. Young adulthood is the period which is essential to the physical, mental and intelligent development. However, a young adult is easily influenced by others, for the views of life and world haven't been shaped. If the natural rule of development is obeyed and the physical and moral education are emphasized, a solid foundation for lifelong health can be

2.1 生理和心理特点

青春发育期是人生中生长发育的高峰期。其特点是体重迅速增加,第二性征明显发育,生殖系统逐渐成熟,其他脏腑功能亦逐渐成熟和健全。机体精气充实,气血调和。随着生理方面的迅速发育,心理行为也出现了许多变化,表现为精神饱满,记忆力强,思想活跃,充满幻想,追求异性,逆反心理强,感情易激动,个体独立化倾向产生与发展。到了青年期,身体各方面的发育与功能都达到更加完善和成熟的程度。青春期是人生发育非常旺盛的阶段,是形体、心理

laid.

和智力发育的关键时期。但是，此时人生观和世界观尚未定型，易受外界影响，如果能按照身心发育的自然规律，注意体格的保健锻炼和思想品德的教育，可为一生的身心健康打下良好的基础。

2.2 Essentials

2.2.1 To Cultivate Psychological Health

Teenagers are at the psychological stage of weaning, presenting the complex mixing of childishness and maturation, dependence and independence. Therefore, they can be easily shaped. At this age, they are enthusiastic, positive and ambitious, but they always search for what is beyond their grasp with impulse and also quit easily. They have the ability to observe, analyze and judge. However, they are moody, emotional, poorly disciplined and sometimes biased. Although dependent on families, teenagers have an increasing access to other people and surrounding. Therefore, they desire for independence and less involvement from parents. However, with lack of experiences, they are easily influenced and can be directed into the other direction once parents and teachers neglect to give instructions. Targeting at the psychological features of teenagers, four aspects need to be emphasized in order to cultivate healthy mental status.

2.2 养生要点

2.2.1 心理素质的培养

青少年处于心理上的“断奶期”，表现为半幼稚、半成熟以及独立性与依赖性相交错的复杂现象，具有较大的可塑性。他们热情奔放、积极进取，却好高骛远，不易持久，在各方面会表现出一定的冲动性。他们对周围的事物有一定的观察分析和判断能力，但情绪波动较大，缺乏自制力，看问题偏激，有时不能明辨是非。他们虽然仍需依附于家庭，但与外界的人及环境的接触亦日益增多，其独立愿望日益强烈，不希望父母过多地干涉自己，却又缺乏社会经验，极易受外界环境的影响。师长如有疏忽，往往误入歧途。针对青少年的心理特征，培养其健康的心理素质极为重要，可从以下四个方面着手。

(1) To counsel and persuade patiently. Teachers and parents need to set good examples for teen-

（1）循循善诱，重在疏导：家长和教师要以身作则，

agers, respect their willingness for independence and protect their ego. Through persuasion and counseling, teachers and parents can make friends with teenagers, care for their studies and lives and attempt to enrich their activities. In addition, seniors can ask for teenagers' advice and follow the right one, gradually give more rights and create a pleasant environment in which teenagers are willing to talk. In this way, you can know the children and the surroundings of the friends, their mental status and emotions. Thus, targeted instructions can be given. Or some targeted questions can be proposed with consciousness for discussion. Through discussion, teenagers will make a clear distinction between right and wrong. Besides, parents have the responsibility to activate their interests and cultivate favorable hobbies, teach them to choose friends cautiously and advocate excellent publications. Group activities are encouraged to gradually shape right view on life and world. As for problems like mistakes and puppy love, do not compress or order violently. Instead, parents need to present reasons and persuade children patiently.

为人师表,给青少年以良好影响,同时又要尊重他们独立意向的发展,保护其自尊心,采用说服教育、积极诱导的方法,与他们交朋友,关心他们的学习与生活,并设法充实和丰富他们的业余生活。有事多与他们商量,尊重他们的正确意见,逐渐给他们更多的独立权利,为他们创造一个愉快的、愿意述说的环境,以便了解他们的交友情况及周围环境的影响,探知他们的心理活动与情绪变化,从而有的放矢地予以教导和帮助。可以有意识有针对性地提出问题交予他们讨论,通过辩论以明确是非观念,再向他们提出更高的要求。要从积极方面启发他们的兴趣与爱好,激发他们积极进取、刻苦奋斗的精神,培养良好的个性与习惯。要教他们慎重择友,避免与坏人接触。要向他们推荐优秀书刊,不接触不健康的读物。要鼓励他们积极参加集体活动,培养集体主义思想,逐渐树立正确的世界观和人生观,使他们有远大的理想与追求。对于他们的错误或早恋等问题,不能采取粗暴、压制及命令的方式,而是应摆事实,讲道理,耐心

(2) To be self-disciplined and highly-qualified. Although teenagers have almost grown into an adult physically, they are still poorly skilled in addressing problems and adapting. Under the guidance with teachers and seniors, teenagers should practice to be independent, strong positive, cautious about words and polite. Try to calm down when confronting something undesirable, respect the old and the young. Don't be emulative and learn to act like an adult.

(3) Sex education in a scientific way. The most distinctive feature of the whole puberty is the beginning and the finish of sex development. Teenagers begin to be aware of it. However, since teenagers are moody and poorly self-controlled, they can develop an unhealthy psychology under the influence of bad examples. As a result, they will fall into puppy love and get married too early and even quit school. Some even commit crimes. Therefore, sex education in puberty is of much importance.

细致地说服和劝导。

(2) 自我修炼，提高素养：青少年的身体发育虽已接近成人，可是对环境、生活的适应能力和对事物的综合处理能力仍然很差。青少年应该在师长的引导协助下，在自己所处的环境中，加强思想意识的锻炼和修养，力求养成独立自觉、坚强稳定、直爽开朗、亲切活泼的个性。遇事冷静，言行适度，文明礼貌，尊老爱幼，切忌恃智好胜，恃强好斗。要有自知之明，正确地对待学业问题，处理好个人与集体的关系，明确自己在不同场合所处的不同位置，善于角色变换，采用不同的处事方法，从而有利于社交活动，促进人事关系的和谐，有益于身心健康。

(3) 科学的性教育：贯穿于青春期的最大特征是性发育的开始与完成。其心理方面的最大变化也反映在性心理领域，性意识萌发，处于朦胧状态。由于青年人的情绪易于波动，自制力差，若受社会不良现象的影响，常可使某些青年滋长不健康性心理，以致早恋早婚，荒废学业，有的甚至触犯法律，走上犯罪道路。因此，青春期的性教育尤为重要。

Sex education includes two parts: knowledge and morality. Teenagers need to know the physiological changes during the puberty so as to satisfy the curiosity, deal with the confusion, shyness and nervousness caused by sex maturity in this period. Masturbation needs to be avoided. If the habit has been developed, try hard to quit it. Girls need to be cautious about hygiene. During the menstruation, segregate or eliminate the access to the filthy words, books, magazines, videos and networks. Guide them to healthy activities and focus on study. In addition, teenagers should be instructed with rules on behaviors between male and female to reveal the mysterious cover. Distinguish the friendship, love and marriage. Advocate late marriage and avoid puppy love. Knowledge about sound child rearing, family planning and sexual transmitted diseases (including AIDS) should be instructed.

青春期的性教育，包括性知识和性道德教育两个方面。要帮助青少年正确理解正常的生理变化，以解除性成熟造成的好奇、困惑、羞涩、焦虑、紧张的心理。要教育青年不要染上手淫习惯，如已染上者，则要树立坚强意志，坚决克服掉。女青年要做好经期卫生保健。要注意隔离和消除可能引起他们不良性行为的语言、书报、影视、网络等环境因素。安排好他们的课余时间，把他们引导到正当的活动中去，鼓励他们积极参加文体活动，把主要精力放在学习上。另外，帮助他们充分了解两性关系中的行为规范，破除性神秘感。正确区别和重视友谊、恋爱、婚育的关系。提倡晚婚，避免早恋，宣传优生、计划生育以及性病(包括艾滋病)的预防知识。

(4) Be strong. Since most teenagers are the only child in the family, they are spoiled, weak and dependent with poor communications and adaptation. Once confronted with defeats, they are terrified, confused, desperate and even suicidal. Therefore, children need to be taught strong, tough, independent and self-disciplined. With tolerance and endurance, they can take challenges and persistent. Be calm, decisive and brave. They need to savor the happiness of success and also the bitterness of fail-

(4) 培养坚强的性格：现在的青少年大多是独生子女，家庭的宠爱，容易导致心理脆弱，意志薄弱，养成依赖心理和养尊处优的不良习惯，表现为交往能力和适应能力较差，一旦挫折出现在他们面前时，就会惊恐万状，茫然无措，甚至容易因绝望而轻生。培养孩子坚强的性

ure, for life is filled up with obstacles. Thus, parents need to educate the children that failure is inevitable. Once facing up with failure, they need to treat it positively and analyze it objectively so as to lay a solid foundation for another success.

格对他们以后的人生道路有着重要的影响。所以,要培养孩子坚毅的性格,顽强的品质,自立的意识;要培养孩子的自我监控能力,使孩子养成自我教育的习惯,形成自我教育、自我管理的能力;要培养孩子的忍耐力和持久力,使他们勇于接受挑战,具有持之以恒、坚韧不拔的精神;进而培养沉着、果断、勇敢的积极心态。要让他们在享受成功的同时也品尝失败的滋味。因为人生不可能总是一帆风顺的,人生的道路上总会有许多的坎坷。所以,对孩子要进行失败教育和挫折教育,使他们充分认识到,任何时候,任何条件下,挫折总是难以避免的,培养他们正确认识与对待挫折,然后认真、冷静、客观地分析,为下一次的冲刺,为另一个成功的到来打下良好的基础。

2.2.2 To Regulate Diet

With quick development, teenagers need to take in nutrients comprehensively and properly, especially the proteins and energies. Carbohydrates and fats are the main source of energy. The former is mainly in staple foods. Proper fat also needs to be taken in. Girls shouldn't strictly control the intake of food due to weight lose, for it will result in malnutrition. Boys shouldn't take in excessive food or

2.2.2 饮食调摄

青少年生长发育迅速,代谢旺盛,必须全面合理地摄取营养,要特别注重蛋白质和热能的补充。碳水化合物、脂肪是热能的主要来源,碳水化合物主要含于主食之中,青少年应保证足够的饭量,增加粗粮在主食中的比

drink, either. For those with congenital weak constitutions, they should seize the opportunity to regulate diet and supplement the congenital insufficiency by cultivating the acquired root.

例，并摄入适量的脂肪。女青年不应为减肥而过度节食，以致营养不良。男青年也不可暴饮暴食，寒热无度。对于先天体质较弱者，更应抓紧在发育时期作好饮食调摄，通过培育后天以补其先天不足。

2.2.3 To Develop a Good Lifestyle

Teenagers shouldn't overwork. Schedules need to be made in a scientific way in which both study and outdoor activities are scheduled. Adequate sleep needs to be maintained. In this way, they can be energetic and healthy with increased effectiveness of study and work.

Good hygiene habits need to developed with the focus on oral sanitation. Try to keep a correct posture while reading, writing and standing so as to promote healthy development and prevent the diseases. Protect the throat and avoid smoking and alcohol drinking, for smoking and alcohol drinking harm the body and influence the psychological health.

Teenagers need to wear loose and plain clothes. Don't wear tight clothes, for they will affect the development of breast for female and testis for males. Don't wear tight pants, for they will cause ringworm of the groins and eczema.

2.2.3 良好生活习惯的培养

青少年不应自恃体壮、精力旺盛而过劳。应该根据具体情况科学地安排作息时间，既要专心致志地学习、工作，又要有适当的户外活动和正当的娱乐休息，保证充足的睡眠。如此方能保证精力充沛，提高学习、工作效率，有利于身心健康。

要养成良好的卫生习惯，注意口腔卫生。读书、写字、站立时应保持正确姿势，以促进正常发育，预防疾病的发生。变声期要特别注意保护好嗓子，应避免沾染吸烟、酗酒等恶习，吸烟、酗酒不仅危害身体，而且影响心理健康。如吸烟可使青年注意力涣散，记忆力减退，学习效率降低。

青少年的衣着宜宽松、朴素、大方。女青年不可束胸紧腰，以免影响乳房发育和肾脏功能；男青年不要穿紧身裤，以免影响睾丸正常的生理功能。夏秋两季男女青年穿紧身裤，容易引起腹股沟癣、湿疹等皮肤疾病。

2.2.4 To Actively Participate in Sports

Persistent sport exercise is essential to the growth of teenagers. Strengths, speed, stamina and agility should be considered. For strength, sprinting and weight lifting are necessary; for stamina, long-distant running and swimming are helpful; for agility, long jump, high jump and ball games are needed. These exercises can be chosen based on individuals.

2.2.4 积极参加体育锻炼

持之以恒的体育锻炼，是促进青少年生长发育，提高身体素质的关键因素。要注意身体的全面锻炼，选择项目时，要同时兼顾力量、速度、耐力、灵敏度等各项素质的发展。偏重力量的锻炼项目有短跑、举杠铃等；偏重耐力的锻炼项目有长跑、游泳等；偏重灵敏度的锻炼项目有跳远、跳高、球类运动等。可根据个体情况，选择锻炼。

Teenagers need to choose the duration, type and intensity of exercise according to their constitution and health condition. Do the one-hour exercise once or twice a day, one hour in the morning or after supper. Keep safe.

青少年参加体育锻炼，要根据自己的体质强弱和健康状况来安排锻炼时间、内容和强度。要注意循序渐进，一般一日锻炼 1～2 次，可安排在清晨和晚饭前 1 小时，每次 1 小时左右。锻炼前要做准备活动，要讲究运动卫生，注意运动安全。

3 The Middle-aged

3 中年保养

Middle age refers to the period between the age of 36 to 60.

中年是指从 36 岁到 60 岁这段时期。

3.1 Physiological and Psychological Features

3.1 生理和心理特点

This period is the turning point of life, for vitality begins to decline. Since the age of 30, physiological functions decline 1% with each year passing by. The middle-aged are stabilized in emotions. But

中年是生命历程的转折点，生命活力开始由盛转衰。人类在 30 岁以后，大约每增加一岁，功能减退 1%。中年

with the changes of physiological functions, psychological status also alters. With lack of knowledge on aging, someone tends to be suspicious about developing diseases of varying degrees and mistakes the developing charges as the signs of serions diseases. In addition, the middle-aged are under great pressure from society and family. Therefore, they live an irregular life with improper diet, indulgence, overstrain and excessive thinking. These are the main causes of aging and of many chronic diseases. Hence, health preservation is essential to the middle-aged. If it goes well, exuberant vitality can be maintained to delay aging, prevent diseases and prolong longevity.

是心理成熟阶段,情绪多趋于稳定状态。但随着脏腑生理功能的变化,心理也有相应的变化。有些人对生理逐步老化缺乏应有的认识和理解,常有不同程度的疑病倾向,错把衰老导致的退行性改变当作重病信号。中年又是"多事之秋",要承担来自社会、家庭等多方面的压力和重任,心理负担沉重。起居无常、饮食不节、嗜欲无度、操劳过度、思虑过多等是促使早衰的重要原因,也是许多老年慢性病的起因。中年的养生保健至关重要,如果调理得当,就可以保持旺盛的精力而防止早衰、预防老年病,可以延年益寿。

3.2 Essentials

3.2.1 Aloofness From Fame and Fortune

The middle-aged is a generation with burdens from society and family. Confronted with various conflicts from life, they tend to fall into depression, anxiety and nervousness. In a long run, essence qi must be consumed and mind impaired. As a result, senilism and diseases will occur. Therefore, the middle-aged need to be aloof from fame and fortune and avoid bothering by trifles. Apart from work, in their spare time, they can try to listen to the music, watch TV, talk with children, water flowers, keep fish, paint, practice calligraphy and also beautify themselves to vitalize themselves and enrich their lives. Besides, they can aloof themselves from ten-

3.2 养生要点

3.2.1 淡泊名利,精神畅达

中年是承上启下的一代,肩负社会、家庭的重担,加上现实生活中的诸多矛盾,易使思想情绪陷入抑郁、焦虑、紧张的状态。长此以往,必然耗伤精气,损害心神,早衰多病。所以中年人要精神畅达乐观,不要为琐事过分劳神。不要强求名利、患得患失。中年人的精神调摄,应注意合理用脑,有意识地培养良好的性格,寻找事业的精神支柱。工作、

sion and be emerged in the pleasant mental world by meditation. They can also reveal the anxiety and irritation to friends and relatives or participate in some activities to relieve the pressure.

学习之余，可以听音乐、看电视，与子女嬉笑谈心，共享天伦之乐。也可以浇花养鱼、作画习字、美化仪容仪表，使自己装束趋向年轻化，以振奋精神，增添生活乐趣；或者宁心静坐、百事不思，使大脑得以充分休息，使自己跳出紧张的状态，沉浸于愉悦舒缓的精神世界里。当忧虑焦躁、情绪不佳时，可对亲朋好友倾吐自己的苦闷，或适当参加文体活动，缓解心理上的压力。

3.2.2 Proper Balance Between Work and Rest

In the prime of the life, the middle-aged shoulders the responsibilities to support the old, raise the young and deal with the household chores. Therefore, long-term overwork should be avoided. Work and rest need to be properly balanced.

Multiple tasks need to be managed one by one based on priorities. Learn to steal a moment of leisure under pressure of a heavy job, such as doing work-break exercises, going upstairs and downstairs instead of taking elevators, riding and walking. Make a full use of time when waiting and taking buses by doing exercises like clicking teeth, swallowing saliva and contracting anus. Brainwork and

3.2.2 合理安排，劳逸结合

中年人年富力强，而被委以种种重任，又担负着赡养老人、抚养子女和安排家庭生活等多项工作，要注意避免长期“超负荷运转”，防止过度劳累，积劳成疾。在保证充分营养的前提下，要善于科学合理地安排工作，学会休息。休息的方式多种多样，适当地调节工作可谓是积极的休息方式。

对于繁多的事物，宜分清轻重缓急、主次先后，有节奏有步骤地逐一完成。要根据具体情况，规整生活节律，建立新的生活秩序。要善于忙里偷闲，利用各种机会进行适当运动。如工间操、上楼下楼、骑车走路、室内踱

physical labor can also be alternated. Or change the postures of working.

步等;利用等车、坐车时间,做一些叩齿、咽津、提肛等锻炼。也可以采用脑力劳动与体力劳动穿插,或改变一下作业姿势,如坐与站立交替。

Exercises are also positive ways to rest oneself, such as Taiji Quan, Eight-brocade Exercise (Ba Duan Jin), Five-animal Exercise (Wu Qin Xi), swimming, mountain climbing, playing chess and fishing. These exercises can both cultivate inner tranquility and also strengthen the body. Sleep is also important. The middle-aged needs to guarantee 6~7 hours' sleep every day. Don't stay up too late. It is irreversible that we rely too much on computers, but we need to rest our eyes frequently by closing eyes or watching the distant views.

体育锻炼、文娱活动同样是积极的休息方式,如太极拳、八段锦、五禽戏等传统健身方法,以及游泳、登高、对弈、垂钓等活动,既可怡情养性,又可锻炼身体,如能持之以恒,必有收益。睡眠是重要的休息方式,中年人必须保证6~7小时的睡眠时间,不可因工作繁忙经常熬夜,切忌通宵达旦地工作。现代人工作生活对于电脑的依赖,已经是无法改变的事实,应重视用眼不能过劳,经常采用瞑目、远眺的方法进行调节。

3.2.3 Abstinence for Preserving Essence and Cultivating Qi

3.2.3 节制房事,保精养气

With declined physical power, busy work and housework, the middle-aged should turn to abstinence. Frequent sexual intercourse will consume essence and impair kidney qi. Therefore, based on the condition, the frequencies should be reduced. According to ancient experts in health preservation, the 30s are advised to have sex every 8 days; the 40s, every 16 days; the 50s, every 20 days. Abstinence should be strictly abided by those with weak body so as to preserve essence and cultivate health.

人到中年体力下降,加之工作紧张,家务繁忙,故应节制房事。如果房事频繁,势必使精气过分消耗,损伤肾气。中年人应根据各人的实际情况,相应减少行房次数。古代养生家提出30岁8天一次,40岁16天一次,50岁20天一次的参考次数。尤其是身体较弱的中年人,要进一步减少行房次数，葆精以养生。

3.2.4 Proper Diet with Less Intake of Sweet and Fat Food

In this period, the body begins to decline with decreased constitution and body functions, reduced resistance and absorption. Improper diet will lead to various diseases. Therefore, the middle-aged should be cautious about diet and take in less sweet and fat food.

To be more specific, avoid preference for a certain flavor; light diet with less sugar, less salt and less oil is advised. Control the energies taken in to avoid obesity. The middle-aged should strictly control the intake of fat and properly supplement protein to maintain the functions of cells and repair the tissues, about 70 to 100 g a day with one thirds of fine protein, such as meat, fish, eggs and milk. Excessive intake of sugar needs to be avoided, for it will cause obesity and increase the burden of pancreas. Fresh vegetables and fruits are highly suggested to maintain supplement of vitamins and fibers, which will keep vitality and prevent constipation. Food rich in calcium such as milk, dried small shrimps and kelp can prevent osteoporosis. Control the intake of salt less than 6 g a day to prevent hypertension and cerebrocardiovascular diseases.

3.2.4 少食肥甘，合理膳食

中年人的身体从充满活力的青年阶段，开始转向衰退的阶段。体质状态和身体机能逐渐衰退，抗病能力和脾胃消化功能逐渐下降。中年若饮食不当，容易导致各种疾病。因此，注意节制饮食，少食肥甘之品，合理安排饮食是中年人养生的重要方面。

具体而言，中年人的饮食要五味不偏嗜，以少糖、少盐、少油的淡薄饮食为主，注意控制总热量，避免肥胖。人到中年要严格控制脂肪的摄入，适量补充蛋白质，一般每天摄入 70～100 克，其中至少 1/3 为优质蛋白，如肉、鱼、蛋、奶等，以维持细胞功能和修补体内的组织。糖类不宜过多，吃糖过多不仅容易肥胖，还会增加胰腺负担。要多吃新鲜蔬菜、水果，保证充足的维生素和纤维素的补充，可使身体保持活力，预防便秘。要多进含钙丰富的牛奶、虾皮、海带等，以防骨质疏松等症的发生。食要少盐，每人每日食盐少于 6 克，以免引起高血压和其他心脑血管疾病。

The middle-aged should take food regularly and properly to avoid digestive disorders, otherwise, obesity, diabetes, hypertension and cerebrocardiovascular diseases are developed.

中年人饮食要有节制,定时定量,以免引起消化功能紊乱而损害健康,如果进食不当、活动减少,很容易患肥胖症、糖尿病、高血压、心脑血管疾病等。

3.2.5 Exercises

3.2.5 运动锻炼,保持机能

In this period, the body begins to decline with decreased body functions. With lack of exercises, obesity is easily developed. With burdens of work and life, the middle-aged are frequently under tension, increasing the risk in getting diabetes, hypertension and hyperlipidemia. Exercises can relieve the tiredness and depression, keep vitality, improve the respiration and circulation, promote the qi movement, strengthen sinews and bones and delay the aging.

人过中年,身体生理机能由旺盛开始转衰,机体各组织器官的功能逐渐衰退。如果缺乏运动,则易引起发胖,再加上工作上肩挑重任,生活上有负担,精神上常处于紧张状态,增加了患糖尿病、高血压、高血脂的机会。体育锻炼,可培养人坚强刚毅开朗的性格,又可解除脑力疲劳和抑郁情绪,保持旺盛的工作精力,改善肺主呼吸和心主血脉功能,促进气血运行,强筋健骨,延缓衰老。

Exercises with proper intensity and low resistances should be chosen, such as table tennis, badminton, jogging, Taiji Quan and swimming. Choose the one you like and keep practicing at least twice a week. Spend more than 2 hours on exercises every week.

锻炼方法可根据每个人的体质情况和兴趣爱好,选择有适当运动强度、低对抗的项目,如乒乓球、羽毛球、慢跑、太极拳、游泳等。每周保持至少运动两次,每周总运动时间不少于 2 小时。

4 The old

4 老年保养

Those over 60 are the elder people.

人于 60 岁以后进入老年期。

4.1 Physiological and Psychological Features

With degeneration in physiological functions and morphology, the old is characterized with declined physiological functions of zang-fu organs, qi and blood and decreased stability in balancing yin and yang. Due to the changes of social status and roles, they also alter in psychology, presenting loneliness, depression, suspicion, irritation and anxiety. The old find themselves hard to adapt to new environments and regulate themselves. If confronted with unfavorable environment and stimuli, diseases will be triggered. Therefore, the old should adopt the approach of regulating the body and mind.

4.1 生理和心理特点

人到老年，机体会出现生理功能和形态学方面的退行性变化。其生理特点表现为脏腑气血生理机能的自然衰退，机体调控阴阳平和的稳定性降低。再加社会角色、社会地位的改变带来心理上的变化，常产生孤独垂暮、忧郁多疑、烦躁易怒等心理状态，其适应环境及自我调控能力低下，若遇不良环境和刺激因素，易于诱发多种疾病，较难恢复。老年养生保健应注意上述特点，有针对性地采用调养形神的方法保养身心。

4.2 Essentials

4.2.1 Be Content, Modest, Kind and Positive

The old need to be content, modest, kind and generous. They can calmly deal with different disagreements so as to maintain family and social harmony. They need to be wise and confident. Read frequently and learn some techniques. According to health condition, the old can also make some contribution to the society and enjoy the happiness of work and study.

4.2 养生要点

4.2.1 知足谦和，老而不怠

人至老年，处世宜知足常乐、豁达宽宏、谦让和善，从容冷静地处理各种矛盾，从而保持家庭和睦、社会关系的协调，有益于身心健康。老年人应明理智，存敬戒，生活知足少嗜欲，做到人老心不老，退休不怠惰，热爱生活，保持自信，勤于用脑，进取不止。经常读书看报，学习各种专业知识和技能。根据自己的身体健康状况，充分发挥余热，为社会作出新的贡献。如此可减慢功能的衰退，领略工作学习的乐趣。

寓保健于学习、贡献之中。

Meanwhile, avoid unfavorable stimuli. Based on the character and hobbies, the old can find something pleasant, such as meditation, talking with best friends, watching fish, listening to birds' singing in the woods.

同时，老年人应回避各种不良环境、精神因素的刺激。老年人应根据自己的性格和情趣，主动设法怡情悦志，如澄心静坐、益友清谈、临池观鱼、披林听鸟等，使生活自得其乐，有利康寿。

With diseases, the old needs to be optimistic and confident in fighting against diseases. They can participate in some meaningful activities and do some exercises to distract their attentions on the diseases. Besides, they should follow the instructions given by doctors and try to recover as soon as possible. Regular physical examination is needed, for it can help find some indications as early as possible and prevent or treat diseases in time.

老年人往往体弱多病，应树立乐观主义精神和战胜疾病的信心，参加一些有意义的活动和锻炼，分散自己的注意力。同时，应积极主动地配合治疗，可以尽快地恢复健康。还须定期进行体检，及早发现一些不良征兆，及时进行预防或治疗。

4.2.2 Diet Regulation with Focus on the Spleen and the Stomach

4.2.2 审慎调食，脾胃为重

The diet for the old should be nutritious, light and digestive.

老年人的饮食应该营养丰富、口味清淡、易于消化，适合老年生理特点。

(1) To be diverse: with declined essence qi, the old needs to take in diverse foods with proper combination of grains, fruits, meat and vegetables. This will guarantee rich and comprehensive nutrition which can supplement essence qi and delay aging. Therefore, the old shouldn't strictly control or indulge the intake of one food. Deficient nutrients should be supplemented.

（1）食宜多样：年高之人，精气渐衰，应该摄食多样饮食，使谷、果、畜、菜适当搭配，做到营养丰富全面，以补益精气，延缓衰老。老年人不要偏食，不要过分限制或过量食用某些食品，又应适当补充一些机体缺乏的营养物质，使老年人获得均衡的营养。

For example, with declined psychological functions, calcium metabolism will fall into negative

例如，老年人由于生理机能减退，容易发生钙代谢

balance, causing osteoporosis, decalcification and fracture. Meanwhile, due to decreased gastric acid, the calcium absorption will be affected. Therefore, calcium-rich food, such as milk, milk product, bean, bean products, celery, Shan Zha (*Fructus Crataegi*) and Yan Sui(*Herba Coriandri*), should be frequently taken.

的负平衡，出现骨质疏松症及脱钙现象，也极易造成骨折。同时，老人胃酸分泌相对减少，也会影响钙的吸收和利用。故在饮食中选用含钙高的食品，适当多补充钙质，对老年人具有特殊意义。乳类及乳制品、大豆及豆制品是较好的食物钙来源，芹菜、山楂、香菜等含钙量也较高。

Due to deficient kidney qi and declined functions of spleen and stomach, those for supplementing spleen and kidney, such as Lian Zi, Shan Yao, Ou Jie (*Rhizomatis Nodus Nelumbinis*), He Tao Ren, Hei Dou(*Semen Sojae Nigrum*), are helpful. Or herbal diet is also necessary.

针对老年人肾气亏虚，脾胃功能减退的特点，可经常食用莲子、山药、藕粉、菱角、核桃、黑豆等补脾肾益康寿之食品，或辅食药膳进行食疗。

(2) To be light: Since the old has deficiency of spleen and stomach, the diet needs to be light. Fish, lean meat, bean products and fresh vegetables and fruits are necessary. Heavy, fatty or salty foods are not advisable. Vegetable oil instead of animal fat is necessary. According to modern nutriology, food rich in proteins, vitamins and fibers and with less sugar, fat and salt are the light ones.

(2) 食宜清淡：老年人之脾胃虚衰，受纳运化力薄，其饮食宜清淡，多吃鱼、瘦肉、豆类食品和新鲜蔬菜水果，不宜吃浓浊、肥腻或过咸的食品。要限制动物脂肪，宜食植物油。现代营养学提出老年人的饮食应是“三多三少”，即蛋白质多、维生素多、纤维素多；糖类少、脂肪少、盐少，正符合“清淡”这一原则。

(3) To be warm and soft: With declined yang qi, the spleen and the stomach adore the warm and dislike the cold. Therefore, warm foods are advised to protect the spleen and stomach. Due to the deficiency of spleen and stomach, and as well as loose

(3) 食宜温热熟软：老年人阳气日衰，而脾胃又喜暖恶冷，故宜食用温热之品护持脾胃，勿食或少食生冷，以免损伤脾胃，但亦不宜温

teeth, soft food instead of hard one are suggested. According to *Introduction to Medicine* (Yi Xue Ru Men) by LI Yan in Ming dynasty, porridge is advocated for the old, for it is digestible and can benefit the stomach and generate the liquids.

热过甚,以"热不炙唇,冷不振齿"为宜。老人脾胃虚弱,加上牙齿松动脱落,咀嚼困难,故宜食用软食,忌食黏硬不易消化之品。明代医家李梴于《医学入门》中提倡老人食粥,因为粥不仅容易消化,且益胃生津,对老年人的脾胃尤为适宜。

(4) To eat less and slowly: the old should take food properly. *A Book for Supporting the Old* (Yang Lao Feng Qin Shu) suggests that the old needs to take less food but more frequently, for it can guarantee the nutrition without harming the stomach. In addition, eating slowly can not only help digestion and absorption, but also avoid swallowing, choking and coughing.

(4) 食宜少缓:老年人宜谨记"食饮有节",不宜过饱。《养老奉亲书》主张老人少量多餐,既保证营养供足,又不伤肠胃,颇值得借鉴。进食不可过急过快,宜细嚼慢咽,这不仅有助于饮食的消化吸收,还可避免"吞、呛、噎、咳"的发生。

4.2.3 Proper Lifestyle with a Balance Between Work and Rest

4.2.3 谨慎起居,劳逸适度

With deficiency of qi and blood, the old often have deficient defensive qi. As a result, they easily catch a cold. Living a relaxed, routine and reasonable lifestyle is a key to health preservation for the old.

老年人的气血不足,护持肌表的卫气常虚,易致外感,当谨慎调摄生活起居。老年人的生活,既不要安排得十分紧张,又不要毫无规律,要科学合理,符合老年人的生理特点,这是老年养生之大要。

Clean, quiet and convenient living environment with ventilated air, ample sunlight and proper humidity is advocated. For the old, proper sleep should be guaranteed. Don't sleep for a long time, for it will impair spirit and also influence the circulation of qi, blood, nutritional qi and defensive qi. Sleep early,

老年人的居住环境以安静清洁、空气流通、阳光充足、湿度适宜,生活方便为好。在起居习惯方面,首先要保证良好的睡眠,但不可嗜卧,嗜卧则损神气,也影响人体气血营

and get up early. It is proper to sleep with the right side rested on the bed and legs bent.

卫的运行。宜早卧早起,以右侧屈卧为佳。注意避风防冻,但忌蒙头而睡。

Keep chest, back, legs, waist and feet warm and changes clothes on the basis of seasons.

老年人应慎衣着,适寒暖。要根据季节气候的变化而随时增减衣衫。要注意胸、背、腿、腰及双脚的保暖。

Due to declined kidney qi, have less sex. For the old with weak body, sex needs to be avoided.

老年人的肾气逐渐衰退,房室之事应随龄增而递减。年高体弱者要断欲独卧,避忌房事。体质刚强有性要求者,不要强忍,但应适可而止。

Because of declined body functions, the old frequently feels tired. Therefore, try to do something within reach. Don't overstrain yourself.

老年人机体功能逐渐减退,较易疲劳,尤当注意劳逸适度。要尽可能做些力所能及的体力劳动或脑力劳动,但要量力而行,做到行不疾步、耳不极听、目不极视、坐不至久、卧不极疲,切勿过度疲倦,以免过劳致病。

It is necessary for the old to develop a fine hygienic habit. Frequently wash face, comb hair and brush teeth. Bathe feet with warm water before sleep. Defecate regularly and eliminate the factors that may cause constipation in time so that the diseases resulted from irregular defecation and urination can be warded off.

老年人应保持良好的卫生习惯。面宜常洗,发宜常梳,早晚漱口。临睡前,宜用热水洗泡双足。要定时排便,经常保持大小便通畅,及时排除导致二便障碍的因素,防止因二便失常而诱发疾病。

4.2.4 Proper Exercises to Promote Blood Circulation

4.2.4 适度运动,行血活络

Due to deficient essence qi and slow circulation of qi and blood, the old are characterized with stasis and stagnation. Exercise can promote the circulation of qi and blood, smooth sinews and delay aging. Most importantly, exercises can generate a vir-

年老之人,精气虚衰,气血运行迟缓,故又多瘀多滞。积极的体育锻炼可以促进气血运行,舒筋活络,延缓衰老,并可产生一种良性心理

tuous stimulus, making people vitalized. They also play a role in eliminating solidarity, depression, suspicion, irritation and anxiety.

刺激,使人精神焕发,对消除孤独垂暮,忧郁多疑,烦躁易怒等情绪有积极作用。

The old need to choose the suitable exercises and do it properly, gradually and persistently. Before exercises, you'd better have a comprehensive examination. Under the guidance of the doctor, the old should choose the proper exercises with slow and small-ranged movements, such as Taiji Quan, Wu Qin Xi, breathing exercises, martial arts, Ba Duan Jin, jogging, walking, swimming, table tennis, badminton and special gymnastics for the old. Keep practicing once or twice a day in the morning after sunrise or one and a half hour after supper.

老年人运动锻炼应遵循因人制宜、适时适量、循序渐进、持之以恒的原则。参加锻炼前,要请医生进行全面检查,了解身体健康状况及有无重大疾病。在医生的指导下,选择恰当的运动项目,掌握好活动强度、速度和时间。老年人之运动量宜小不宜大、动作宜缓慢而有节律。适合老年人的运动项目有太极拳、气功、武术、慢跑、散步、游泳、乒乓球、羽毛球、老年体操等。锻炼时要量力而行,力戒争胜好强,避免情绪过于紧张或激动。运动次数每日一般宜 1～2 次,时间以早晨日出后为好,晚上可安排在饭后一个半小时以后。

Don't do exercises in midsummer in the sunlight or in snowy days, otherwise the old will get sunstroke and cerebrovascular attacks, or even fall.

老年人切忌在恶劣气候环境中锻炼,以免带来不良后果。例如盛夏季节,不要在烈日下锻炼,以防中暑或发生脑血管意外;冬季冰天雪地,天冷路滑,外出锻炼,要注意防寒保暖,防止跌倒。雾霾、大风大雨天气,不宜外出运动。

When feeling uncomfortable, they should discontinue the exercises. After three months' exercise, they'd better to make a self-conclusion for the

老年人应掌握自我监护知识。运动时,要根据主观感觉、心率及体重变化来判断运

sleep, defecation and urination, appetite, heart rate and rhythm. Once something is felt wrong, visit the doctor immediately and regulate the program.

动量是否合适,酌情调整。必要时可暂时停止锻炼,不要勉强。锻炼3个月以后,应进行自我健康小结,总结睡眠、二便、食欲、心率、心律正常与否。一旦发现情况,应及时就诊,调整运动方案。

4.2.5 Take Medicines Properly

Due to the degenerative changes in physiology and declined body functions, medicines for the old, not only for treatment and but also health care, are different from those for the young. Generally speaking, take more medicines for supplement and less ones for dredging. Herbs should be moderate and small-dosed. When supplementing, five zang-organs should be considered with the focus on the spleen and the kidneys; to regulate yin and yang, constitutions should be differentiated for supplementing; when taking medicines, seasonal changes need to be considered; dosage forms like pills, powders and plasters are better than decoctions; medicines should be combined with diet. Only in this way, the yin and yang can be balanced to prolong longevity and ward off diseases.

4.2.5 合理用药,补偏救弊

老年人由于生理上退行性改变,机体功能减退,无论是治疗用药,还是保健用药,都不同于中青年。一般而言,老年人保健用药应遵循以下原则:宜多进补少用泻;药宜平和,药量宜小;注重脾肾,兼顾五脏;辨体质论补,调整阴阳;掌握时令季节变化规律用药,定期观察;多以丸散膏丹,少用汤剂;药食并举,因势利导。如此方能收到补偏救弊,防病延年之效。

Section 2 Health Preservation Based on Genders

第2节 辨性别施养

1 Males

1.1 Physiological and Psychological Features of Males

1.1.1 Masculine Males

Female belongs to Yin, while male to Yang.

1 男性保养

1.1 男性生理和心理特点

1.1.1 男性为阳刚之质

女子属阴,而男子属阳。

Males are strong and masculine with robust muscles and nimble body. They are brave, aggressive, apt to movement against staying still, decisive, daring to speak and act, and open-minded. In social and family life, males are strongly enterprising and self-respected. But compared to females, they are over-unyielding and lack of flexibility and the ability to deal with details and control the over-excited emotion.

男性具有强悍阳刚之质，形态表现为肌肉筋骨强健隆起，肢体运动敏捷有力；心理上具有主动勇敢、争强好胜、喜动恶静的特征；具有处事果断刚毅、敢想敢说敢为、做事干脆利落的气质。心胸较为开阔，坦诚大度，感情粗犷，性格豪放。男性进取心较强，在社会交往、家庭生活和事业上都表现出较强的好胜心和自尊心。然较女性而言，刚强有余而柔韧不足，对事情的细节处理和自制能力相对较弱，易出现亢奋的情绪变化。

1.1.2 Males Live on Essence and Blood

Essence and blood is the indispensable matter to human life. Males live on essence while females live on blood. In sexual life, males satisfy themselves through spermiation, which remind the males restrict their sexual desire in case the damage of essence. If not, males may suffer from slowness of thought, gloomy eyes, soreness and weakness of waist and knees, dizziness and tinnitus, forgetfulness and fatigue, impotence and premature ejaculation, and spermatorrhea.

1.1.2 男子以精为主

精血是人类生命活动不可缺少的基本物质，相对而言，男子以精为基础，女子以血为基础。男子在性生活中，通过排精，消耗相当数量的精液，以满足生理和心理上的需求。男性这种独特的排精功能，决定了男性易于精亏的生理特点，所以要适当节制性欲和性行为，尤其不能纵欲。房事不节的男子，常常出现思维迟钝、两目无光、腰膝酸软、头晕耳鸣、健忘乏力、阳痿早泄、遗精滑精等症状。

1.2 Essentials

1.2.1 To Restrict Sexual Desire and Preserve Essence

Kidney essence is of vital importance to males.

1.2 男性养生要点

1.2.1 节欲保精

肾精在男性健康中具有

Therefore, the daily health preservation for males relies on the preservation of kidney essence. To restrict sexual desire means to avoid over frequency of sexual life, not to avoid sex. The youngsters must have sex after grow up to be mature, and the married men should restrict sexual life in case the exhaust of kidney essence.

十分重要的作用。因此，男性日常保健重在顾护肾精。节欲，即节制过频的性生活，并非禁止性生活。男性肾精亏耗，多由房事不节所致。少年男子应晚近女色，待身体生长盛壮之后再论婚育，不可过早，以免耗伤肾精，对身体造成伤害。已婚男子应节制房事，切忌纵欲，以免精液屡泄，而致精竭气衰，神疲形损。

1.2.2 To Regulate Mind and Essence

Ever since ancient times, Chinese medicine lays stress on essence and energy, the former one being the foundation of the latter one, and disposing it. Energy is nourished by essence and defense essence at the same time. They depend on each other to reserve life. Therefore, males are ought to pay attention to moral cultivation for the spiritual tranquility. Less desire and tranquility of spirit lead to steady essence and energy. The distracting thoughts and excessive desire ends in loss of spirit and exhaust of energy.

1.2.2 调神养精

自古以来，中医学非常重视精与神的关系，认为精是神产生的物质基础，而神对精又有支配作用。精可养神，神可御精，积精可全神，宁神可保精，二者相互为用，维持正常的生命活动。因此，男子应注重自身的道德修养，增强心神的安定性，以期神清情静。只有收心养心，思想清静，少思寡欲，戒除杂念，情绪安宁，精气才能内守，不易外泄。若心神不宁，神驰于外，或思虑过度，所欲不得，则精易走失或暗耗。

1.2.3 To Conserve Yang Qi

Yang qi is the power of life. As the master of masculine, yang qi ensure the health of males. Cold, belonging to yin evil, is against yang qi. When the temperature descends, males must keep

1.2.3 养护阳气

阳气是生命活动的动力，男性为阳刚之质，阳气所主，男性的强健与否，在很大程度上取决于阳气是否旺

warm against cold. In hot summer, males must prevent from too much cold food and cold environment. In early spring, when the nature wakes up and yang qi ascends, males should better wear clothes appropriately towards the temperature in case that yang qi been hurt by cold.

盛。寒为阴邪，最易伤人阳气。故气温较低，气候寒冷时，男子更应注意防寒保暖，以免为寒气所伤。气候炎热时，也不应贪食寒凉，乘风露宿。春季之时，自然之阳气升发，万物生机盎然，此时顺时保养，衣着宜捂，不可顿减，以免寒气伤阳。

1.2.4 To Quit Smoking and Limit Drinking

An increasing study tend to prove that smoking do harm to males in the hypothalamic-pituitary-gonad axis and the quality and number of sperms. The Nicotine and multiring hydrocarbon compound may develop spermophlebectasia, lead to testis atrophy, Sperm production disruption and end in infertility. Apart from that, smoking is one of the most important reasons for lung cancer and liver cancer. Therefore, non-smoking is important for males' health.

1.2.4 戒烟限酒

吸烟对男性健康的危害愈来愈清楚地被科学研究所证实，吸烟可以干扰丘脑－垂体－性腺轴功能，降低男子精液质量，导致少精子症和弱精子症，使精子数目减少，还可诱发精索静脉曲张，导致不育。烟草中的尼古丁和多环芳香烃化合物对多种实验动物均可造成睾丸萎缩、精子生成中断，形态改变。有研究证实男性多发肺癌、肝癌的原因之一就是吸烟。因此，不吸烟是男性健康生活的重要方面。

Wine bears the essence of grain and water, and five flavors. Appropriate drink will help keep fit, that is why generations of medical practitioners, specialists of regimen and men of letters sing high praise for wines. Some medical wines are regarded as medicine to prolong life. But excessive drinking, as recorded in GONG Tingxian's *Harm of Alcoholism* (Yin Jiu Shang Shen Lun) and LUO Tianyi's *Harm on Spleen and Stomach* (Yin Shang Pi Wei),

酒为水谷之精气，五味之精华，如饮用得当，对于强身健体，颇为有益，故历代医学家、养生学家以及文人墨客对酒大加赞誉，许多药酒更是祛病延年的佳品。但嗜酒过饮则有诸多危害，龚廷贤有《嗜酒伤身论》，罗天益有《饮伤脾胃论》，认为多饮

will harm essence and energy, qi and blood and longevity. Modern studies demonstrate that wine damages the membrane of sperms, distorts or inactivate sperms and induces prostatic congestion and prostatitis. Males must drink appropriately and avoid alcoholism, especially having sex after drinking wine.

酒会动精伤神，耗气伤血，影响寿命。现代研究认为，酒能破坏精子膜结构，使精子发生畸变或活力减弱，说明酒对男性生殖有不利影响，过量饮酒，会使前列腺充血，容易诱发和引起前列腺炎。所以，男性饮酒要把握适量的原则，不要酗酒，酒后行房更为养生大忌。

1.2.5 To Regulate and Nourish with Diet

Kidney contains congenital essence, but maintains the normal function with essence of grain and water. Therefore, the daily diet must keep regular eating and balance meat and vegetables.

1.2.5 饮食调养

肾所藏的先天之精，须赖后天饮食水谷精微不断化生，才能泉源不竭，行使其正常的生理功能。所以饮食上应做到饥饱适度，荤素结合，膳食平衡，不可过饥过饱。

The essence of food produces the essence of human body. Especially some resources from animals, like duck's meat, lamb, sea cucumber, turtle, tortoise, shrimp and so one, are good for human health.

饮食精气能化生人之精气。特别是血肉有情之品，如鸭肉、羊肉、海参、甲鱼、乌龟、虾等，适量食用，可有益精填髓，强身健体。

Healthy diet enhances Yang qi. Some food which are warm, acrid and sweet can assist Yang qi. For example, scallion, ginger, garlic, date, peanut, lamb and so on are warm against yin cold. Some average dishes and snacks, like Sheng Jiang porridge, lamb porridge, boiled chicken with Dang Gui, stir-fried leek with walnut are beneficial for masculine and health.

饮食可生阳。饮食中辛甘温热之品，大多有生阳助阳之功。诸如葱、姜、蒜、枣、花生、羊肉之类食物，皆能助人阳气，祛散阴寒。许多民间传统小吃和菜肴，都有生阳的作用，如生姜粥、羊肉粥、当归炖鸡、核桃仁炒韭菜等，男子若经常合理食用，能资助阳气，增进健康。

1.2.6 To Regulate and Nourish with Chinese Medicine

Generations of specialists of regimen, like

1.2.6 药物调养

药物补精为历代养生家

ZHANG Jinyue in Ming Dynasty, advocate that cooked rehmannia is a good choice for enhance essence. Besides, Lu Jiao Jiao (*Colla Corni Cervi*), Gui Ban Jiao (*Testudinis Carapapacis Et Plastri*), bovine spinal cord, Zi He Che (*Placenta Hominis*) and so on are helpful to supplement the kidney and boosts essence.

所倡导，如明代张景岳认为熟地乃补精填精之佳品，清代名医叶天士主张用血肉有情之品补精，如鹿角胶、龟板胶、牛骨髓、紫河车之类，都具有较好的补益肾精的作用。

Some medicines are very functional for males. Ren Shen (*Radix Ginseng*), Huang Qi (*Radix Astragali seu Hedysari*), Bai Zhu (*Rhizoma Atractylodis Macrocephalae*), Shan Yao (*Rhizoma Dioscoreae*), Gan Cao (*Radix Glycyrrhizae*), and Feng Mi (*Mel*) are useful to enhance qi; Lu Rong (*Cornu Cervi Pantotrichum*), Ba Ji Tian (*Radix Morindae Officinalis*), Xian Mao (*Rhizoma Curculiginis*), Yin Yang Huo (*Herba Epimedii*), Du Zhong (*Cortex Eucommiae*), and Tu Si Zi (*Semen Cuscutae*) are useful to supplement Yang. What to mention is to take the medicine with appropriate time and dose, for example, Jingui Shengqi wan (Golden Coffer Kidney Qi4 Pill), You Gui Wan (Right-Restoring [Life gate] pill), Lu Jiao Bu Shen Wan (Deerhorn-Restoring [life gate] pill). The excessive use of the medicine will do harm to health of the bigots.

另外，补气助阳药物在男性保健中发挥着重要作用，诸如人参、黄芪、白术、山药、甘草、蜂蜜等补气药，鹿茸、巴戟天、仙茅、淫羊藿、杜仲、菟丝子等补阳药均作用可靠。益气补阳的中成药，如金匮肾气丸、右归丸、鹿龟补肾丸等，服用方便，疗效确切。需要注意的是，服药不可过量过久，不能迷信药物的作用，而恣情纵欲，不加节制，最终都将损害健康。

2 Females

2 女性保养

2.1 The Physical and Psychological Features of Females

2.1 女性生理和心理特点

Females have uterus in terms of anatomy, and menstruation, pregnancy, parturition, and nursing in terms of physiology, which are different from males in these organs and in the circulation of qi and blood. Males rely on essence, while females rely on blood.

妇女在解剖上有胞宫，在生理上有月经、胎孕、产育、哺乳等特点，其脏腑经络气血活动的某些方面与男子有所不同。男子“以精为主”，而女子“以血为本”。

Females, sentimental and emotional, are more cater to loose qi and blood, thus to be suffered from illness and senilism. Therefore, health care maintenance is of special meaning to females. The health of females is important to not only their own health but also the constitution and mentality of the descendents.

妇女又具有感情丰富、情不自制的心理特点，气血容易耗损，情志容易受伤，相对更易患病早衰。做好妇女的卫生保健，有着特殊重要的意义。他们的健康不仅影响自身寿命，还关系到后代的体质和智力发展。为了预防并减少妇女疾病的发生，保证妇女的健康长寿，除了注意一般的卫生保健外，尚需注重经期、孕期、产褥期、哺乳期及更年期的卫生保健。

2.2 Essentials

2.2.1 Health Preservation During Menstruation

Menstruation, periodical blooding of uterus, is the special physiological phenomenon of females. Regular menstruation indicates that females are mature to give birth to babies. Generally the period is of no difference from other days, except some females feel lack of strength and the lower abdomen or back bearing down for a few days before those non-c feelings disappear naturally.

Kidney governs storage, while liver govern free coursing, the mutual effect of which result in the regular period of menstruation. For the preservation of menstruation, it is important to maintain appropriate blood excretion in time and to regulate diet, emotion and daily life.

(1) Sanitation: During the period, since

2.2 女性养生要点

2.2.1 经期养生保健

月经是女性周期性子宫出血的生理现象。正常而有规律的月经是女性生殖机能成熟，具备孕、产能力的重要标志。一般经期无特殊症状。某些妇女在月经期出现乏力、少腹或腰脊下坠等不适症状，经后自然消失，不影响正常生活，一般不以病态论。

肾主封藏，肝主疏泄。月经的周期性变化，是肾、肝两脏藏、泄相互为用的结果。月经期保健应以保持经血按时而下，泄而有度为主。应当于饮食、精神、生活起居各方面谨慎调摄。

（1）保持清洁：行经期

females' blood chamber is open, they are catering to be attacked by pathogenic factors. Therefore, females must keep vulva clean, underwear sun-dry, sanitary towel regularly changed, use shower instead of tub bath and swimming, avoid sex and examination per vagina without sterilization.

(2) Appropriate temperature: Menstrual bleeding, stagnate in coldness and frenetically moving in hotness, is freely moving in warmness. Coldness may obstruct qi and blood in channels and lead to menstrual pain and block; hotness forces blood move frenetically and lead to advanced menstruation, prolonged menstruation and flooding and spotting. Hence during the period, females are ought to change clothes according to the changes of the seasons, adjust the room temperature in case coldness and hotness, avoid summer heat, getting soaked in rain or wading, bathing with cold water, sitting or lying on wet ground, work in cold water and so on, so as to protect themselves from the pathogenic factors.

(3) Rational diet: During the period, menstrual bleeding sometimes brings about exuberance of liver and deficiency of spleen, manifesting as breast distending pain, detention in lower abdomen, and decreased food intake and loose stool. In that case, it is better to choose the mild and nutritious food, not too hot or cold, to supplement blood. Cold food may damage Yang qi and obstruct blood in blood vessels and lead to menstrual pain and block; hot

间，血室正开，邪毒易于入侵致病，必须保持外阴清洁，内裤勤洗勤换，最好置于日光下晒干。月经用卫生巾要选择柔软、透气、吸水性好的产品，并及时更换，保持清洁。洗浴宜淋浴，不可盆浴，不得游泳。严禁房事和阴道检查，如因诊断必须做阴道检查者，应在消毒情况下进行。

（2）寒温适宜：经血贵在行而有度，血得温则畅行，遇寒则凝涩，逢热则妄行。若经行之际感受寒邪，寒行凝滞，经络气血阻滞，常可发生痛经、闭经等；若感受热邪，热扰血海，迫血妄行，多发为月经先期、经期延长、崩漏等。所以，月经期应根据气候的变化适时增减衣物，调节室内温度，防止过寒过热引起经气不调而为患。注意避免炎暑高温、冒雨涉水、冷水洗浴、坐卧湿地、水中作业等，以防六淫邪气侵犯。

（3）合理饮食：月经期间，经血溢泄，常有乳房胀痛，少腹坠胀，纳少便溏等肝强脾弱现象，饮食一般应取寒温平和、易于消化而富有营养之品，以补充消耗的经血。不可多食生冷酸物、辛辣的食品。多食生冷酸物则容易损伤阳气，凝滞血脉，使

food may damage Ying qi and left Yang qi overactive, forces blood move frenetically and lead to advanced menstruation, prolonged menstruation and flooding and spotting. Females can choose food according to menstruation based on pattern identification as the basis for determining treatment. Those who have a higher volume of menstrual blood loss than average level may choose cold food to cool down excessive heat, for example, lotus root, root of rehmannia, phragmites shoot and so on. Those who have insufficient Yin blood may have dates, longan flesh, lotus fruit, chestnut, walnut, dried grape and so on to regulate Ying blood. Or those who need to supplement qi and blood can eat chicken's meat, duck's meat, fish, other meats, milk, eggs and so on.

气血运行涩滞而引起痛经、月经量少、甚或闭经；多食辛辣热之品则容易助阳耗阴，致血分蕴热，迫血妄行，令经期延长或经量增多。也可以根据月经具体情况，在辨证的基础上，有针对性地选用合适的食品。经血量多属实热者，宜用清热降火，凉血止血之品，如莲藕、生地、芦笋等；阴血不足者可适当进食大枣、桂圆、莲子、栗子、核桃、葡萄干等以调补阴血，或选用鸡、鸭、鱼、肉类、乳类、蛋类等血肉有情之品以益气养血。

(4) Emotion regulation: Females may have unsteady emotion before menstrual bleeding starts, like vexation and irascibility, gloom, depression and sadness. During the period, along with bleeding, the insufficient Yin blood and exuberant Liver qi may bring about tension, depression, vexation, irascibility, breast distending pain, aching lumbus, fatigue, detention in lower abdomen and so on. Meanwhile, emotion disorder is one of the most important reasons of menstruation disorder. Therefore, before or during the period, females must regulate emotion against excessive seven emotions. Otherwise, it will cause the malfunction of zang-fu viscera and disorder of qi and blood, which may result in discomfort or even amenorrhea and sterility.

（4）调和情志：女性在行经前气血郁而未达，常常伴随不同程度的情志变化，如心烦易怒，闷闷不乐，抑郁忧伤等。月经期间经血下泄，阴血偏虚，肝气偏盛，此时情绪易于波动，每每紧张忧郁、烦闷易怒，伴乳房胀痛、腰酸疲乏、少腹坠胀等。同时，情志失常又是女性月经失调的重要原因。因此，在经前和经期都应保持心情舒畅，避免七情过度。否则，会引起脏腑功能失调，气血运行逆乱，轻则加重经间不适感，导致月经失调，重则出现闭经、不孕等症。

(5) Appropriate physical exercises: Menstrual

（5）活动适量：经期以溢

bleeding relies on free activity of qi and blood. Appropriate physical exercises are helpful to soothe the abdomen pain. But excessive labor and acute movement may lead to menorrhagia, prolonged menstruation and even flooding and spotting.

泄经血为主,需要气血调畅。适当活动,有利于经行畅利,减少腹痛,但不宜过劳,要避免过度紧张疲劳、剧烈运动及重体力劳动。若劳倦过度则耗气动血,可致月经过多、经期延长、崩漏等症。

2.2.2 Health Preservation of Pregnancy

During pregnancy, menstruation stops to accumulate yin blood to cultivate fetus. The expectant mother's emotion and diet, which highly influence the exuberance and debilitation of qi and blood, not only affect the health of her own but also the development of the fetus. Health preservation of pregnancy is an important step for prepotency.

2.2.2 胎孕期养生保健

胎孕期月经闭止,阴血聚以养胎,孕妇的情志变化、饮食起居各方面不仅影响自身的健康,而且母体脏腑气血之盛衰直接影响着胎儿的生长发育。因此,妊娠期摄生调护是保证母子身心健康、实现优生优育的重要环节。

(1) To regulate emotion against anger: Free flow of qi in mother's body ensures the safety of the fetus, while counter flow of qi do harm to the fetus. Hence pregnant women must keep emotion steady and relaxed away from the stimulation of unhealthy emotions. Liver is the foundation of females' health. Counter flow of liver qi is catering to stimulate anger. At the beginning of pregnancy, channels are closed and the counter flow of liver qi leads to vomiting. Therefore, anger is the first unhealthy emotion to resist during pregnancy.

(1) 调情志,戒恼怒:气调则胎安,气逆则胎病。故孕期保健首重调畅情志以舒达气机。孕妇宜情志舒畅,情绪稳定,避免各种不良情志的刺激。女子以肝为先天,肝在志为怒,怒则气逆。特别是妊娠之初,经脉内闭,逆气上冲,食饮辄吐。所以,在各种不良情志之中,尤当戒除恼怒。

(2) To soothe the emotion for fetus training: Forbears consider that emotional tranquility is the top technique to nourish the fetus. The pregnant women should remain serene and gentle and well-preserved. Kind words and beautiful things are inner power for the overall health of fetus. While the

(2) 怡心神,施胎教:古人将安闲宁静、怡养心神视为养胎第一妙法。妊娠期实施胎教,不仅要心情宁静,性情温和,还要注意加强修养。应言行端正,多接触美好的

evil scene, sound and words should be banned. The room for the pregnant women, if necessary, can be painted into a new gentle color with pictures of beautiful views or lovely babies, handsome men or women, and some other decorations in accordance with the pregnancy.

事物，以期外感内应，促使胎儿的身心发育。尽量避免各种恶性刺激，做到目不视恶色，耳不听恶声，口不出恶言，目的是为胎儿生长提供良好的环境。也可以将居室进行特殊装饰，使颜色柔和、温馨，墙壁可贴挂秀美的风景、俊美的男女、可爱的婴儿的图像，或孕妇喜欢而且健康的挂饰，以愉悦身心。

(3) To avoid sex and keep gentle sports: The ancient doctors in China insist that sex is the top taboo of pregnancy because sex consumes kidney essence and disturbs, or even kills the fetus. Therefore, pregnant women, especially in the first three months, must limit desire and rest in a different room to avoid the damage of sex to the thoroughfare and controlling vessels which protect human body from evil qi. After pregnancy, blood nourishes and qi protects fetus. Appropriate sports keep qi and blood in harmony and flowing freely in all the vessels, which benefit fetus and parturition. Slight wrenching and contusion do no harm to the fetus, but exhaustion do harm to the fetus. Moderate activity and rest is important to pregnancy. Long-time sitting or lying will lead to malposition of the fetus because of the stagnation of blood and qi; while exhaustion usually results in abortion.

（3）戒房事，小勤劳：古代医家认为保胎以绝欲为第一要策，妊娠期应清心寡欲、分房静养。因房事触动欲火易伤损肾精肾气，引起胎动不安或胎堕、小产。在孕期前三个月内及最后 3 个月，应谨戒房事，以免损伤冲任、胞脉，导致病邪内侵。妇人孕后，血以养胎，气以护胎。适度活动使气血调和，百脉流畅，有利于分娩和胎儿的生长、发育，虽微有闪挫不致堕胎。过劳伤胎，微劳宜胎，孕期讲究劳逸适度。若过度安逸，久坐久卧，气血凝滞，常致胎位不正、难产；过劳气衰，则易堕胎、小产等。

(4) To resist outside evil factors with appropriate temperature: Vital qi of the pregnant women usually becomes weak for the fetus consumes much qi and blood of the mother. Without careful protection, pregnant women are catering to be attacked by

（4）避外邪，慎寒温：妊娠之后，气血聚以养胎，正气暂虚，若不慎调护，易受虚邪贼风。感冒外邪，郁热不解，多致小产、堕胎。尤其是妊

evil qi and bandit wind. Coldness usually causes fever and is inclined to result in abortion. The infection of pathogenic factors brings about malformation of the fetus. Hence pregnant women must wear clothes according to the change of the seasons and temperature. One thing to mention that pregnant women generally have a higher body temperature than average people, so too much clothes may heat the orifices open and bring the wind-pathogen into the body. Besides, electromagnetic radiation and radioactivity are vital to fetus, hence to be avoided.

娠早期染伤时邪,还可影响胎儿的生长发育,导致先天畸形。因此孕期要顺应四时气候之变化,及时增减衣物,避免外邪侵袭。由于孕妇体质偏热,所以,受孕之后特别要注意衣勿太暖,因为暖则窍开,易招风邪。胎孕期尤其要注意避免各种电磁辐射、放射性物质等有害物质的影响,保证胎儿的健康发育。

(5) To keep diet and choose medicine cautiously: Generally speaking, pregnancy reaction appears at the early stage of pregnancy, so pregnant women should choose light and nutritious diet and eat less each meal but eat more often than before. Those who have serious vomiting may have some cookies and dry fruit as snacks. No soup at breakfast for less stimulation to stomach but olive, orange, loquat, Sheng Jiang, Yan Sui, which can soothe stomach and Shan Zha, rice vinegar, water chestnuts for better digestion. For those who fiercely vomit need to drink water frequently and have some food to protect yin essence, for example, tomato, watermelon, malt sugar, Feng Mi, Ou(*Nelumbinis Rhizomatis Nodus*), and milk.

(5) 节饮食,慎用药:妊娠早期一般会有不同程度的妊娠反应,此时进食应少量多餐,给予清淡易于消化且富有营养之品。呕吐较重者,可给予饼干、干果等,作为零食。早餐少给汤饮,以减少对胃的刺激。理气安胃之橄榄、柑橘、枇杷、生姜、香菜,以及消导和胃之山楂、米醋、荸荠等均可适量选食。呕吐剧烈者,多有伤津耗液,宜多饮水,并食用滋润生津之番茄、西瓜、饴糖、蜂蜜、莲藕、乳类等以顾护阴液。

Pregnant women need more nutrients for fetus, so the diet is extremely important. Pregnant women need various and digestive food with rich nutrient. Meat, eggs, beans with rich protein and vegetables and fruits with rich vitamins and cellulose are preferable. However, excessive diet also do harm to fetus. *Quiet the fetus* of *Female Division of Bamboo Forest* (Zhu Lin Nü Ke Zheng Zhi) makes a list of

妇女怀孕之后需要更多的营养以供胎儿生长发育之需,因此,妊娠期间要特别重视饮食的调摄。饮食宜营养丰富,易于消化,品类多样。选择含有高蛋白的肉类、蛋类、豆类及含大量维生素和纤维素的蔬菜、水果等。但

food for pregnant women, like lotus seed, euryale (seed), pine nut, cooked lotus root, dioscorea (root), duck, golden carp, sea perch, eel, icefish, sea cucumber, mussel, pig's meat, pig's stomach, asparagus, sesame oil, bean curd skin and so on.

饮食应有所节制,过量饮食也有碍胎产。《竹林女科证治》列举了一些适合孕妇食用的食品,如莲子、芡实、松子、熟藕、山药、鲫鱼、鸭、鲈鱼、鳗鱼、银鱼、海参、淡菜、猪、肚、笋、麻油、腐皮等,可酌情使用。孕妇不可过食生冷、暴饮暴食,以防损伤脾胃。应戒烟忌酒、勿食辛辣炙煿与肥甘厚味,以防化热伤阴动血损及胎元。

During the pregnancy, all the foods that are drastic precipitant, water-expelling, stasis-dispelling, oxytocic, blood vessel-freeing, qi-breaking, orifice-freeing, extremely hot and toxic should be banned or taken cautiously in case the bad effect on pregnant women and fetus. If necessary for the diseases, they must be taken with strict dosage and method of administration based on specific patterns and the constitution of the pregnant woman.

妊娠期间,凡峻下、逐水、祛瘀、催胎、通利、破气、通窍及大辛大热有毒之品应禁用或慎用,以避免药物对孕妇和胎儿的不良影响。若确系病情需要,须本着中病即止的原则,结合孕妇体质之状况,严格掌握适应证、用量和服法。

(6) To keep clean and wear comfortable clothes: Pregnant women must keep body clean by frequent shower and changing underwear. Loose clothes are more suitable for them instead of tight ones in case block qi and blood and do harm to fetus.

(6) 讲卫生,宽服饰:孕妇应讲究卫生,经常洗澡,换洗衣裤。衣着宜宽大柔软合体,忌胸腹束缚过紧,以免气血营运不畅,影响胎儿的发育。

At the same time, regular examination is necessary to know about the condition of pregnant women and fetus, so when emergencies happens doctors will dispose them to preserve the health of the expectant mother and the fetus.

此外,孕期应定期进行产前检查,随时了解孕妇及胎儿情况,若出现异常情况,应及时处理,以确保孕妇的健康及胎儿的正常发育。

2.2.3 Health Preservation of Puerperium

2.2.3 产褥期养生保健

The 6-8 weeks after is regarded as puerperium

产后 6～8 周时间内属

of the mother. The mother's constitution reveals vacuity and stasis because loss of blood and qi, breast-nursing of the bay and wound on uterus. Without appropriate health care some diseases will develop. Appropriate health care benefits both the mother's recovery and the baby's breast nursing.

产褥期。由于分娩时耗气失血,又分泌乳汁以哺育婴儿,产后子宫尚未复旧,其体质特点是多虚多瘀。若调摄不慎,易发生产后诸疾。合理的产后调摄可以促进产妇身体恢复,保障婴儿正常哺乳,对母子的身体健康均具有积极意义。

(1) Appropriate rest and activity: With bleeding during delivery, primordial qi is impaired. Thus, the mother should have a good rest to restore primordial qi and to feed baby. Having ample sleep, especially during the 24 hours after labor, can relieve the exhaustion and restore the tensions of muscles in pelvic floor. In addition, do not work or bear load too early, otherwise lochia, prolapse of uterus and hypogalactia will occur.

(1)新产静养,劳逸适度:临产用力失血,多致元气虚损,故产后宜静养以恢复元气,也利于哺育婴儿。保证睡眠充足,特别是产后 24 小时必须卧床休息,以缓解分娩时的疲劳及恢复盆底肌肉的张力。新产不宜过早操劳负重,避免发生产后恶露不绝、阴挺下脱、缺乳等病。

There are stasis of qi and blood in puerperium, so the mother lying on bed should change posture frequently and get up after 24 hours to do appropriate exercises except for difficult delivery and surgical delivery. It is helpful for qi and blood to circulate freely, lochia eliminate from uterus and avoid fecal and urinary stoppage.

产后气血常有瘀滞,卧床休息时要经常变换卧位,但不必完全卧床。除难产或手术产外,一般顺产可在产后 24 小时起床活动,并且逐渐增加活动量,进行适量的轻微运动。产后适当下床活动,可以畅通气血,不仅有利于恶露的排出和子宫的恢复,也可以令二便通畅,避免产后二便不通等病。

Therefore, after giving birth to a baby, the mother need appropriate rest and activity to help recover the physiological function and avoid diseases.

因此,产后既要充分休息,又应适度活动,劳逸适度不仅有利于生理功能的恢复,同时也可免生产后诸病。

(2) Appropriate temperature: Childbirth exhausts qi, blood and vessels, so the constitution of the mother reveals vacuity and coldness. The loose interstices and insecure construction and defense is catering to be attacked by external evil. That is why the mother must wear appropriate clothes to keep warm against cold wind in case postpartum body pain. Especially in winter and summer, the mother must wear appropriate clothes to avoid catching cold in winter or summer, or attacking by heat strike in summer.

(2) 调适寒暑，避受风寒：产后气血俱损，百脉空虚，故多见虚寒之象。而且腠理疏松，营卫不固，易受外邪侵袭。所以，产妇的生活环境必须清洁卫生，温暖舒适，空气新鲜，特别强调避风寒、保温暖，不宜当风而卧，以免外邪侵袭而患产后身痛等。冬季尤当注意保暖，防止触冒风寒。但产妇着衣厚薄要适宜，夏季不宜厚衣密室，以免发生中暑；亦不可过于贪凉，凉水洗浴，以免感冒。

(3) Light diet and no consumption of raw or cold foods: The mother is weak after giving birth to the baby for the loss of blood and breast nursing, so nutritious food is helpful for the recovery of the mother and sufficient breast milk for the baby. However, because of the physical fatigue, vacuity of qi and blood, and deficiency of spleen and stomach's function of moving and transforming, the diet must be light.

(3) 新产清补，忌食生冷：产妇因分娩气血的耗损和产后哺乳的需要，多有虚弱之象，所以，通过饮食补益以加强营养，可以促进产妇身体的恢复，使乳汁分泌充足。但是一般产后一周内由于体力消耗较大，气血骤虚，脾胃运化功能相对不足，不可大补。

Light supplement, the nutritious and digestive food, is appropriate for the women who have just given birth to a baby, for example, bean soybean milk, brown sugar soup, milk, millet porridge, chicken soup, egg thick soup, broth, fish soup, and so on. Two weeks after the birth, it is better to have some food to warm and supplement qi and blood and quicken the blood and transform stasis, for example, ginger lamb soup (Dang Gui Sheng

所以，新产妇应以清补为主，可多饮汤汁丰富，味道清淡，富含营养，且又容易消化的食物，如豆浆、红糖水、牛奶、小米粥、鸡汤、蛋羹、肉汤、鱼汤等。分娩两周以后，多偏于虚寒之象，可予以温补，如当归生姜羊肉汤或益母草红糖水等，以温补气血，

Jiang Yang Rou Tang) or leonurus brown sugar soup. It is better to have meals 4-5 times a day, not too hungry or too full. The diet for the mother must be nourishing but not to hamper the function of stomach, supplementing the vacuity but not to develop stasis. Warm food is preferable, instead of the cold ones, which may decrease breast milk and render baby's running belly and hot ones, which damage the liquid and stir the blood to result in difficult defecation and lochiorrhagia.

活血化瘀。产妇饮食宜少量多餐，每日可进餐4～5次，不可过饥过饱。依据产后多虚、多瘀的体质特点，产后食补以滋补不碍胃、补虚不留瘀为原则。产妇进食宜选择温性食品，若过食寒凉食物，一则影响泌乳，且易使乳儿腹泻。忌食过于生冷油腻之品，以防损伤脾胃、恶露不下或乳汁郁积不通，也不宜吃辛热伤津动血之物，以防大便困难和恶露过多。

(4) Emotion regulation against depression: A woman takes more responsibility and psychological stress after becoming a mother. Without emotion regulation, some psychological diseases may develop to hurt the mother, like depression, anxiety, and panic. Therefore, the mother should be prepared psychologically to difficulties in becoming a mother. At the same time, her families should look after her carefully with nice words, so as to make her mind pleasing and qi and blood in harmony.

（4）调畅情志，预防抑郁：产妇分娩后，突然转换成母亲的角色，需担负更多的责任，因此在心理上会承受较大的压力，如果不能很好地进行心理调适，会出现各种情志病变，表现为烦躁抑郁、焦虑不安、惊悸恐惧等情志症状。因此，产妇自身要做好母亲的角色转换，调整心态，对产后的身体状况和照料孩子的困难有充分的思想准备。家人对产妇需给予关心体贴，好言相对，令其情怀舒畅，精神愉悦，使气血平和。

(5) Sanitation and sex delay in sex: During the perineum, since blood chamber is open, and lochia and sweat are discharging, the mother is catering to be attacked by evil and toxin. Therefore, frequent shower is good to keep clean, but no tub bath in the 4 weeks after giving birth to baby in case vaginal

（5）注意清洁，忌早入房：产褥期血室正开，恶露排出，产后汗液较多，易感邪毒而致病，故宜经常洗浴，保持皮肤清洁。产后4周不能盆浴，以防邪毒内侵而导致带

discharge symptoms, postpartum heat, postpartum abdominal pain, and postpartum blooding. The vulva must be cleaned with warm water daily and the under wears must be changed and sun dried. The wound must be sterilized or cleaned by liquid medicine. No sex within the three months in case various diseases.

下病、产后发热、产后腹痛及产后血崩等。要特别注意外阴清洁，每天宜用温开水洗涤外阴，及时更换会阴垫，内衣裤要常洗晒。有分娩创伤者，应使用消毒敷料，亦可用药液熏洗。产后 3 个月内，不可行房事，否则会导致多种产后疾病。

2.2.4 Health Preservation of Breast Nursing

Breast nursing, a stage for the recovery of the mother, usually lasts one year. Health care during the stage of breast nursing help the mother recover and produce rich breast milk.

(1) Sanitation of breast: The mother should breast the baby within half an hour after the bay is born, the earlier, the better. Before the first time to breast nurse, the nipples must be cleaned and smeared with vegetable oil to soften the skin and cleaned again before nursing the baby. At the beginning, the breast milk usually gathers to block the mammary gland and the mother may feel distending pain. At this stage, it is better to breast nurse the baby frequently, give a hot-wet compress to the breast, give a massage to the breast from the root of the breast to the nipple, or use Chinese medicine Tong Quan Xia Ru San to help the milk run smoothly. Those who have rich milk and distending pain should not have too much soup.

Each time before breast nursing, the mother

2.2.4 哺乳期养生保健

哺乳期是产妇以乳汁哺育婴儿、产后机体逐渐康复的阶段，一般一年左右。哺乳期合理保健可以使乳母身体得以恢复，乳汁分泌充沛，对母子健康都有重要意义。

(1) 注意乳房卫生：产后应尽早让婴儿吸吮乳头，要帮助乳妇在产后半小时内开奶。初次哺乳前要洗净乳头并涂抹植物油，使乳头的积垢及痂皮变软，然后用肥皂和清水洗净。开始哺乳时，可出现蒸乳反应，乳房往往胀硬疼痛，乳汁排出不通畅，可频繁哺乳，尽量将乳汁排空；也可作局部湿热敷，或用手由乳房四周向乳头方向轻轻按摩乳房，以疏通乳络，使乳汁得行；也可用中药下乳涌泉散等促其通乳。已经有乳房胀痛症状而乳汁分泌充足者要减少汤类饮食的摄入。

每次哺乳前，乳母要洗

must clean her hands and the nipple with warm boiled water. After breast nursing, the nipples must be cleaned again and the breast milk sucked out in order to boost the secretion of breast milk and avoid acute mastitis. If it happens, go to the doctor immediately. Regular breast nursing not only avoid indigestion of the baby but also give the mother more time to rest.

手,用温开水清洗乳头。哺乳后也要保持乳头清洁,如仍有余乳,可用手或用吸奶器将乳汁挤出、吸空,以促进乳汁分泌旺盛,并防止乳汁淤积而发生乳痈。若出现乳头皲裂或乳痈,应及时医治。要定时哺乳,既可预防婴儿消化不良,也有利于乳母休息。

(2) Nutritious food: Breast milk comes from food. The mother should have more nutritious food and soup to enrich the milk. No matter vacuity or repletion, those who lack of breast milk must improve the function of spleen and stomach and enhance qi and blood. Some food are functional to promote lactation, like shrimp, pig's totter, hen, peanut, soybean, day lily, golden carp, soybean curd, etc. Insufficient qi and blood can be improved by fish soup, chicken soup and pig's totter soup, if necessary, with Dang Gui and Huang Qi root. Blocked qi, blood and vessels can be freed by Lou Lu(*Radix Rhapontici*), Chuan Shan Jia (*Squama Manis*), Wang Bu Liu Xing(*Semen Vaccariae*) and so on. Zhi Ma, infested ear of wild rice, pig's totter, pig's intestines, Chinese waxgourd peel, common floweringqince fruit, red bean and so on, based on the mother's taste. The food for the mother should better be light and nutritious instead of restorative, raw, cold, or salty. The restorative food may worsen the stagnation of phlegm-damp and lead to obesity of the mother, even worse, may reduce the breast milk.

(2) 增加饮食营养:乳汁化源于饮食水谷,所以乳母应增进营养,强健脾胃,多喝汤水,以保证乳汁充沛。产后缺乳虽有虚实之别,但总以调养脾胃,滋补气血为主。虾肉、猪蹄、母鸡、花生、黄豆、黄花菜、鲤鱼、鲫鱼、豆腐等均有生乳、催乳之功。对于气血不足之缺乳,可多喝鱼汤、鸡汤、猪蹄汤等,必要时加用当归、黄芪煲汤食用。气血壅闭,经络不通者可用漏芦、穿山甲、王不留行等疏通气血。芝麻、茭白、猪蹄、猪肠、冬瓜、丝瓜、木瓜、赤豆等均系通乳之品,可依据产妇口味加以选食。饮食宜清淡而富有营养,勿滥用补品,勿过食生冷,也不可过咸。忌食辛热刺激性食品。痰湿体质者若滥用滋补,则痰湿凝滞,不仅容易导致乳母形体肥胖,而且可以影响乳汁分泌引起缺乳。

(3) Emotion and daily life: A good mental status, sufficient sleep, and regular life are the foundation for the recovery of the mother and breast secretion. Therefore, the mother must try to keep relaxed in mind, regular life, appropriate rest and labor and avoid pregnancy again.

(3) 调理情志起居：良好的精神状态，充足的休息睡眠，有规律的生活，是产妇身心得以恢复、乳汁得以正常分泌的必要条件。所以，乳母必须保持心情舒畅，避免情绪激烈波动，尽可能做到起居有时，劳逸适度，并及时避孕。

(4) No drug abuse: Many medicines affect the excretion of breast milk, and finally through the milk affect the health of the baby. If take the medicines in a long term, the milk is probably poisonous to the baby. For example, Malt can terminate lactation, Rhubarb lead to diarrhea of the baby, and so on. Hence the mother must be cautious when take medicines.

(4) 不可滥用药物：许多药物影响乳汁分泌，或经过乳母的血循环进入乳汁影响婴儿的身体健康。如长期或大量服用，不利于哺乳或使婴儿中毒。例如，乳母服麦芽可导致回乳，服用大黄可使婴儿泄泻。因此，乳母于哺乳期应慎服药物。

2.2.5 Health Preservation of Climacteric Period

Climacteric period, or near menopause, refers to the changing period of women from child-bearing period to the period of aging, approximately 45-55. Along with the debilitation of kidney qi and Chong-Ren vessel, the function of Ying and Yang and Zang-fu viscera disordered and climacteric syndrome appears, like sweating, dizzy, headache, tinnitus, palpitation, insomnia, agitation, depression, and menoxenia, etc. Health care of this stage may delay aging, avoid the above syndrome or shorten the time of this stage.

2.2.5 更年期养生保健

更年期，或称“围绝经期”，是妇女由壮年的育龄期步入生殖功能衰退的老年期的过渡时期，一般在 45～55 岁之间。由于肾气渐衰，冲任二脉虚衰，可致阴阳失调，脏腑功能紊乱，一部分妇女会出现烘热汗出、头晕目眩、头痛耳鸣、心悸失眠、烦躁易怒、忧郁悲伤、月经紊乱等症状，称为更年期综合征，或称“经断前后诸证”，表现的轻重因人而异。如果调摄适当，可减缓衰老，避免或减轻更年期综合征，或缩短反应时间，对整个老年期的健康都有重要作用。

(1) Optimistic and steady mood: Females in climacteric period are inclined to be out of mood for lack of Kidney yin and menstruation, mainly manifested as effulgent heart-liver fire for yin vacuity and yang hyperactivity, clinically, insomnia, vexation and agitation, irascibility, depression and grief. Women would better try to relax from the negative mood like stress, anxiety, horror, etc., with more social life. Hobbies and interests are good to cultivate temperament and distract attention. Optimism and open-mindedness ensure females live through the climacteric period.

(1) 情绪稳定乐观：更年期情志变化的机理多由于肾阴不足、癸水减少，阴虚则阳亢而火旺导致，故一般以心肝火旺为主，常出现一系列精神情志的改变，如失眠、烦躁、易怒、忧郁、悲伤等。女性应当正确认识这一阶段的生理变化，解除思想顾虑，尽量避免不良的精神刺激，消除紧张、焦虑、恐惧等消极心理。注意增加社会交往，使不良情绪得到及时宣泄。根据自己的性格爱好培养良好的兴趣以怡情养性，转移注意力。保持情绪乐观稳定，开阔胸怀，以舒缓心理压力，顺利度过更年期。

(2) Diet: In climacteric period, females' kidney qi, Chong-Ren and menstruation are desiccated, so more food to strengthen kidney essence is required. At the same time, take less greasy food to protect spleen and stomach, the foundation to produce qi and blood, and to ward off obesity. No smoking, less wine and irritating food, like coffee, thick tea, pepper, etc., and more vegetable, fruit and yams to keep bowels open and ward off heart-liver fire and more serious climacteric symptoms.

(2) 注重饮食调养：更年期妇女肾气渐衰，冲任不足，天癸渐竭，故应食用强肾益精之品以调养之。天癸既绝，养在太阴，应顾护脾胃，以助气血生化之源，少食油腻之物，以防止滞碍脾胃，导致运化乏力，痰湿内生，出现肥胖。禁烟并限制饮酒，少吃辛辣刺激性食品，如酒、咖啡、浓茶、胡椒等，多吃蔬菜水果及薯类食物，保持大便通畅，以免助长心肝火旺的病理，使更年期症状加重。

(3) Physical exercises: Sufficient sleep and rest are necessary, but sleep for too long time do harm to health. Work as usual and do physical exercises according to the physical condition, for example, Taiji Quan, Taiji sword, Eight-brocade Exercise (Ba Duan Jin) and so on. Moderate exercises regulate qi and blood, improve sleeping, help keep fit, make you happy and improve health.

(3) 适量体育活动:更年期妇女应保证睡眠和休息,但要注意过分贪睡反致懒散萎靡,不利于身心健康。只要身体状况许可,就应坚持正常工作。还应选择适合自己的运动方式,如太极拳、太极剑、八段锦等传统运动体育活动,适当运动可以调节气血运行,改善睡眠,避免体重过度增加,愉悦身心,改善健康状况。

(4) Regular physical examination: Females in climacteric period are inclined to have tumors since menstruation becomes irregular, so physical examination at least every half a year is quite necessary. The increase of vaginal discharge, bleeding after menopause, masses in breast or abdomen, etc., calls for urgent diagnosis, especially for those who have climacteric syndrome, it is necessary to have medicine besides diet.

(4) 定期检查身体:女性更年期常有月经紊乱,也是生殖器官肿瘤的好发年龄,应每隔半年至一年做一次体检。若出现白带增多、绝经后阴道出血、乳房或少腹部包块,需及时就医诊治。对于更年期综合征患者,除了饮食起居方面的调护外,症状严重者配合药物可以改善症状,以免贻误和加重病情。

Section 3 Health Preservation for Different Professions

第3节 辨职业施养

Different occupations have different working environment, modes, and labor intensity that influence people's health on different levels, hence to take different measures for health preservation. Despite of the variety of professions, this section dis-

不同职业的工作环境、工作方式和劳动强度均不同,职业对健康的影响也有差异,因此,养生要考虑到不同职业间的这种差异,研究

cusses manual workers and mental workers.

不同职业类别养生的特殊性，有针对性地采用适合的措施和方法，提高养生的效果。目前职业的种类非常多，限于篇幅，本书仅举体力劳动者与脑力劳动者为例。

1 Essentials for Health Preservation of Physical Laborers

1 体力劳动者保养要点

The health of manual workers is tightly related to working condition, environment, gesture, labor intensity, and length. The manual workers with muscles and that consume a large quantity of energy and accelerates metabolism. Some workers have to keep a fixed gesture, which may strain specific muscles and bones. They need better working environment and diet and keep balance of labor and rest against taxation detriment. Those who work in harmful environment must take precautions against occupation disease accordingly, for example to control noise, radiations, too low or high temperature and some other poisonous or pathogenic matters, like lead, mercury, benzene, organophosphate, and dust etc.

体力劳动者的健康，与劳动条件、劳动环境、劳动姿势、劳动强度和持续时间有着密切的关系。体力劳动者以筋骨肌肉活动为主，其特征是消耗能量多，体内物质代谢旺盛。不同工种的劳动者在进行生产劳动时，身体需要保持一定体位，采取某个固定姿势或重复单一的动作，局部筋骨肌肉长时间地处于紧张状态，负担沉重，久而久之可引起相关肌肉关节劳损。体力劳动者的养生应注意不断改善生活劳动条件和劳动环境，安排合理的饮食起居，劳逸结合，预防各种劳损。对于某些职业损害，应根据不同工种，因人因地制宜，采用相应的方法进行积极防护。如设法控制噪声、放射性物质，低温和高温以及铅、汞、苯、甲醇、有机磷、粉尘等职业危害因素，防止职业病的发生。

1.1 Diet

The large sum of energy consumed by daily physical work must be made up by grain and water qi and clear yang from diet. That is why manual workers must take in enough beef, pork, chicken, duck, fish and eggs, as well as some vegetables and fruits for overall nutrients. At the same time, diet may help reduce the negative effects by work, for example, mung bean and lily bulb decoction resolves heat for those working in summer or by the side of boiler. If sweet lost too much, they must have some salty drinks.

Those who work in cold region or refrigeration house may have some warm-natured food, like scallion, ginger, garlic, Chinese leek, and sward bean pod with appropriate moderate wine to warm yang, quicken the blood and dissipate cold. Those who work in the cold and wet places like under mine, in tunnel and water may choose some pepper, zanthoxylum, and fennel fruit to transform dampness and dissipate cold.

1.1 饮食调养

体力劳动者每天要消耗大量能量，这就需要从饮食中补充足够的水谷之气，通过水谷精微化生的清阳，充实四肢关节肌肉，维持其强健有力的状态。所以，体力劳动者每天要保证充足的牛肉、猪肉、鸡鸭肉、鱼肉和禽蛋的摄入，米面主食之外要搭配适量的蔬菜和水果，保证营养的全面供给。此外，尚需根据不同工种，选择相应的食物，可在一定程度上减轻或解除有害因素的危害。如从事暑天室外、锅炉旁等高温作业的工人，可经常饮用绿豆百合汤解热降温，因出汗甚多，体内损失的无机盐和水分多，还要注意补给含盐饮料。

在寒冷地区、冷库等低温环境下的体力劳动者，可适当选用牛羊肉等温热性质的食品，以及葱、姜、蒜、韭菜、刀豆等温性的蔬菜，少量饮用低度酒，以达到温阳、活血、散寒的作用。如对于在矿井、地道、水下等阴冷潮湿环境下作业的人员，除上述温热饮食外，可酌情选用辣椒、花椒、小茴香等具有化湿驱寒作用的食物。

1.2 Physical Fitness Activities

Physical fitness activity cannot be replaced by physical work for it does not aim at fitness but repeat one or two fixed gestures with a part of muscles active but the others inactive, which may lead to unbalanced development of muscles and strain of those active joints. Therefore, physical fitness activities improve function of Zangfu, boost the circulation of qi and blood, and improve energy and health for the manual workers to work more efficiently. The manual workers can do exercises by walking, jogging, boxing, leg swing, gymnastics, and ball games, etc.

Clock assemblers, sculptors, and typists who do sedentary work for a long time may pick up general movements, especially balls games to improve the sensitivity of fingers and fists, and wittedness of min by sufficient nutrients for limbs.

Manual worker would better do the moderate physical exercises rather that exhausting ones, like jogging, gymnastics, etc. to relax muscles.

1.2 健身运动

体力劳动从运动量而言,也是一种运动,但它不能代替健身运动。因为,体力劳动的动作的方式、持续的时间、负荷的重量均不是以健身为目的,而往往采用1～2种固定姿势或一定的体位进行重复动作,身体某一部分肌肉持续运动,而另一部分肌肉处于相对静止状态,身体的肌群不能得到均衡发展,负重的关节容易劳损。因此,需要选用针对性的运动,来改善这种不平衡的状况,同时,通过健身运动,提高脏腑功能,促进气血运行,增进健康,增加体力,能更从容地应对体力劳动。体力劳动者应结合本身劳动强度和工作特点,适当选择运动方式和运动量,如散步、慢跑、打拳、摆腿、体操、球类等活动。

钟表装配工、雕刻工、打字员等,长时间地静坐工作,可选择全身性活动,特别是球类运动,有助手指、手腕的灵巧、敏感,并可健脑益智,改善局部肢体气血营养的供给。

从事强度较大的体力劳动者,不宜进行剧烈的体育活动,可进行一些强度较小的体育活动,如慢跑、健身操等,使参与劳动的肌肉得到

Chaffeur, tailor and transfer line worker have to work in a complicated environment in which they use their energy and mind to extreme, thus prone to suffer from insomnia, headache and neurogenic hypertension, etc. It is better for them to chose moderate sports, like Taiji, qigong and the like to rest the breath, quiet the mind, and activate the body so as to relax the mind, move qi, soothe the sinews, and quicken the blood.

充分放松和休息。

司机、缝纫工人及连续流水作业工人，其劳动技术性强，既耗体力又费脑力，他们的劳动环境复杂，大脑神经高度紧张，易患失眠、头痛、神经性高血压等病，宜选择运动量小、动作柔和的运动，如太极拳、医学气功等中国传统健身功法。这些功法都要求静息、安神、动形，既可放松精神，又可行气、舒筋、活血。

1.3 Daily Routine

1.3.1 Safety Precautions

Manual workers must abide by the regulations to protect themselves from occupational diseases and accident. Those working in noise please wear ear defender; in radiations observe the regulations to wear protective clothing and appliances; in high temperature wear loose and ventilate clothes and strengthen heat insulation and radiation; in low temperature keep warm; and in poisonous environment take precautions to decrease the volume of poisons absorbed in human body.

1.3 科学作息

1.3.1 注意劳动防护

体力劳动者应认真执行劳动保护措施和工作操作规程，预防职业病和工伤事故的发生。在噪声环境下工作应坚持使用护耳器，降低噪声。放射工作人员应严格遵守操作规则，避免放射性物质的污染，工作前必须穿戴好个人防护用具。高温环境下工作，应穿宽松、透气的工作服，工作环境应加强隔热散热。低温环境下的劳动者应注意保暖。接触有害物质的工人应坚持正确使用劳动防护用品，减少对毒物的吸收。

1.3.2 Timeout

The ways to take timeout depends on different environments and working schedules. For those who

1.3.2 实行工间休息

不同工种的劳动者可根据工作条件和工作时间采取

work in noise and dust it is better to leave the environment they work, who stand for a long time to relax the legs preventing varicosity, and who work on production line relax muscles and brain.

不同的休息方式。在噪声、粉尘等环境下的劳动者应在工间休息时间暂时离开劳动场所。长期站立的工人，休息时要活动下肢，减轻腿部疲劳，预防静脉曲张。在生产线上工作的工人应作放松性运动，缓解肌肉疲劳和精神紧张。

1.3.3 Regular Physical Examination

Some environments may do harm to the health of manual workers, so some specific examinations besides basic ones according to different kinds of work must be applied. For example, specific ear check-up and precautions are necessary for those working in noise. Examinations on skin, blood, and nervous system every 6-12 months are for those who work in radiation environment, any anomalies appearing change the job immediately. Regular examinations on blood, urine, and liver and kidney functions every quarter of year, half a year, or every year are for those working with poisonous chemicals according to the concentration in the working environment. All such workers must accept progressive observations on health with documents recorded on personal monitoring cards.

1.3.3 定期健康检查

由于体力劳动者的某些工作环境可能影响其生理功能，损害健康，因此，除常规的健康体检外，体力劳动者应根据工种定期进行特别项目的检查。如长期在噪声环境中的劳动者可能发生噪声性听力损伤和噪声性耳聋，应定期检查听力，采取相应保护措施。而从事放射工作人员应每隔 6～12 个月检查一次身体，尤其要注意皮肤、血液、神经系统等的变化，如发现异常，应及时处理，严重者应调换工作。接触有害化学物质的劳动者应视接触化学物质的浓度情况分 1 季度、半年、1 年定期体检血、尿、肝肾功能等相关化验指标，建立健康监护卡，记录检查结果，进行长期健康观察。

1.3.4 Reasonable Use of Brain

Ancient experts on health preservation claimed reasonable mental work is necessary for longevity.

1.3.4 合理用脑

古代养生家认为，适度脑力活动是保证人体健康长

All the human organs remain healthy when used reasonably and vice versa, so manual workers must ensure the activity of mind for health and longevity. Cultivate interests and choose different curricular based on one's occupation, like gardening, cooking, sewing, painting, etc. Try to improve memory by reading papers or some games, like chess, riddles, etc.

寿不可缺少的一个方面。人体脏腑器官都是用进废退，要保证大脑活力，健康长寿，体力劳动者也要勤用脑。要培养自己的学习兴趣，结合职业特点选修不同的课程，如学习园艺、烹调、缝纫、编织、绘画等，并有意识地锻炼记忆力，下班后多读书看报，也可以参加一些动脑筋的游艺活动，如棋弈、猜谜语等。

2 Essentials for Health Preservation of Mental Workers

2 脑力劳动者保养要点

Mental workers use brain a lot, which often leads to sub health. For instance, excessive thought and preoccupation do harm to spleen, which results in loss of appetite and discomfort in stomach; overuse of heart spirit damages yin blood, leading to heart throb and anxiety; fast speed and high pressure of work block the liver qi, leading to depression, insomnia, and declination of memeory; lack of physical exercises brings about inhibited qi and blood which finally results in cold limbs, anchylosis, obesity, fatty liver, and hyperlipidemic, etc.; sedentary work exhausts joints of neck and back; overuse of eyes results in dry eyes, blur vision, and impaired vision, etc.

脑力劳动者是从事以思维活动为主的工作，其职业特点决定了这类人群容易出现亚健康的状况。如过多思虑，思虑伤脾，导致食欲不振，胃脘不适；心神过用，耗伤阴血，常见头晕心悸、心烦焦虑；工作节奏快压力大，导致肝气郁结，引起情绪低落、失眠多梦、记忆力下降；缺少运动，筋脉骨肉得不到应有的锻炼，气血运行不畅，日久痰瘀停留，易见手足不温，关节僵硬不柔和，以及身体肥胖、脂肪肝、高脂血症等；长期坐姿，腰背肩颈关节容易劳损；用眼过度，导致眼睛干涩，视物模糊甚至视力下降等。

Therefore, for mental workers, health preser-

因此，脑力劳动者养生

vation aims at preventing sub health conditions listed above and improving health with the four tips below.

的目的就是要预防上述亚健康状况甚至疾病的发生，采取有效措施，提高该类人群的健康水平。其养生要点有以下 4 个方面。

2.1 The Balance of Work and Rest

Evade long-time concentration on mental work and try to keep balance between work and rest. Do not work continuously for too long time, two hours being the maximum length, and then have a rest. Change the scopes of work alternatively, for example, after abstract though, read foreign languages, music or read pictures, which uses left and right side of brain for keeping balance. A reasonable pace of work and rest protects brain, remains sufficient energy, and improves memory and efficiency.

Modern mental workers, highly relying on computer must avoid long-time work with computer. Set the schedule of one-hour work and then remind yourself of a rest. Leave the computer, stand up, and if possible, go outside to breathe in fresh air.

2.1 工作节奏，张弛有度

脑力劳动者要避免精神持续性的高度集中，应该合理安排工作内容和工作时间，做到有张有弛。连续工作的时间不宜过长，一般说来，不应超过 2 小时，应适当休息以使高度集中的思想得以放松。连续用脑时，还应注意更换工作内容，如高度抽象思维之后，可替换读外语、听音乐、看图像，以利左右脑活动的平衡。有节奏地工作和学习，不仅有助于保护大脑，保持饱满的精神状态，而且还可以提高记忆力，收到事半功倍的效果。

现代脑力劳动者对电脑的依赖程度比较高，要避免长时间在电脑前工作，可设定 1 小时左右的时间，提醒自己离开电脑，替换为站位工作的内容或适当休息，有条件的情况下，可到室外舒展肢体，呼吸新鲜空气。

2.2 Regular Life

Overtime, staying up late, improper diet are mistakes many mental workers make to result in anxiety, agitation, dispiritedness, distraction, and

2.2 生活规律，起居有常

加班、熬夜、饮食无常是许多脑力劳动者的通病，因而容易出现烦躁、激动或精

degrading memory, which seriously influence work efficiency and do harm to health. Hence, it is obligated to cultivate good habits, like no smoking and heavy drinking, regular meals and defecation, early bed and early up for enough time to sleep, etc. Overtime should stop no later than 12:00 am. No fierce sports, coffee or heavy tea may excite the mind before going to bed. Regular life helps remain sufficient energy, improves concentration, thinking ability health and efficiency.

神萎靡、注意力分散、记忆力减退等症状，严重影响脑力劳动者的工作效率，对健康造成损害。故此应当养成良好的生活习惯，不吸烟、酗酒，定时三餐，定时大便，早睡早起，保持充足的睡眠时间。如因工作需要而不得不加班时，最晚也应在子时前（零点）入眠。临睡前避免剧烈运动、喝咖啡、浓茶，避免接触引起精神兴奋的事物。有规律的生活起居，可以使人保持比较充沛的工作精力，注意力容易集中，提高思考能力，提升工作效率，既有利于自身健康，工作上又起到事半功倍的作用。

2.3 Less Fatty and Sweet Food

Mental workers consume much more mental power than physical strength, so balanced diet and nutrients are important. First, balanced diet means sufficient grains, vegetables, fruits, and meats. Second, some food like fish, particularly abyssopelagic fishes and nuts nourish brain.

Too little physical exercises or too much fatty and sweet food is the main reason for mental workers to develop obesity, diabetes, cardiovascular and cerebrovascular diseases. Therefore, they must control the diet in amounts and types, especially fatty

2.3 饮食合理，少食肥甘

脑力劳动者体力消耗较小，但脑力消耗较大，因此在饮食上要合理安排，保证充足的营养。首先要做到全面膳食，均衡营养，不偏嗜，不挑食，供给充足的谷蔬果肉。其次，要针对脑力消耗的情况，多选用益智健脑的食品，如鱼类（特别是深海鱼）、坚果类，以补脑健脑。

脑力劳动者运动量小，是肥胖症、糖尿病、心脑血管疾病的好发人群，过于肥甘的饮食也是主要病因之一。因此，该人群的饮食要注意

and sweet food, like fried food, fatty meat, animal organs, cream cake and ice cream, etc.

控制饮食总量,尤其注意少食肥甘之品,如油炸食品、肥肉、动物内脏、奶油蛋糕、冰淇淋等。

2.4 Appropriate Sports and Rest

Lack of sports may slow down the circulation of blood and qi, leaving the organs in need of nutrients, which finally lead to ailments for having lost functions to resist phlegm-rheum and blood stasis. Therefore, it is imperial for mental workers to do appropriate physical exercises including manual work to boost the circulation of qi, blood, and channels, improve the function of Zang Fu the competence of body systems, and work efficiency, and preserve exuberant energy and steady.

To associate activity and inertia for health as advocated by traditional Chinese medicine is quite helpful for mental workers. Based on personal interests, mental workers may do progressive, not exhausting sports, like walk, jogging, swimming, badminton, Taiji, Eight brocades, five animal exercises, etc, no less than half an hour each time and threes times every week. In office, some moderate sports, like bending and stretching limbs, neck, back and so on are applicable.

2.4 适度运动,动静结合

缺少运动,过于安逸,易导致气血运行不利,脏腑器官组织得不到气血的充分营养,功能减退,日久出现痰饮和瘀血等病理产物,变生他病。因此脑力劳动者在紧张的工作之余应进行适当的运动锻炼,包括参加力所能及的体力劳动,以促进气血顺畅运行,通畅经络,提高脏腑功能。同时运动可以提高机体的反应能力,有助于保持旺盛的精力和稳定的情绪,提高工作效率。

脑力劳动者的职业以静为主,辅之以适度运动,符合中医“动静结合”的养生要旨。具体运动方法,可根据个人的身体条件和喜好进行选择,以运动量适中,循序渐进,不引起疲劳为原则。如全身运动可选择步行、慢跑、游泳、羽毛球、乒乓球和传统健身术(太极拳、八段锦、五禽戏等)。保持每周 3 次以上的全身运动,每次不少于半小时。每天可在办公场所进行局部肢体运动,特别注意头颈和腰背运动,可利用工作间隙作若干次屈曲和伸展。

2.5 Massage for Flexible Channels

Massage on specific sinews and flesh or acupoints keep the vein open, boosts the circulation of blood and qi, dissipate fatigue, and prevent strain of muscle and lumbar. Massage can be applied by oneself or other people. The tips are as follows:

2.5 按摩保健,舒筋活络

为促进脑力劳动者经络气血的通畅,解除疲劳,可进行适当的保健按摩。保健按摩是通过对身体局部筋肉或穴位的刺激,以疏通经络,促进气血运行,可以达到舒筋活络、解除疲劳的作用,对于预防肌肉劳损及颈腰椎病也有一定的效果。保健按摩的实施可以由他人和本人来完成,以下为简易自我按摩的操作方法。

Head massage: ① Comb the hair with hands. Separate ten fingers and slightly bend them to comb hair from the root to end for 20 times; ②Smear the forehead. Bend the fingers like bows, press the inner side of the joints of the second finger against ophryon, and smear the forehead from middle to two sides for 20 times; ③Rub Greater yang points with finger pulps until soreness; ④ Knead the back of head. Rotate the finger pulps to knead the Feng Chi Point (GB 20) with strength, and then Nao Kong point(GB 19) until soreness.

头部按摩:①手梳头:两手十指分开,微曲,从前发际梳到后发际 20 次;②抹额:以两手食指屈成弓状,第二指节的内侧面紧贴印堂,由眉间向前额两侧抹 20 次;③揉太阳:以两手中指螺纹面按揉太阳穴,以酸胀为宜;④按揉脑后:以两手拇指螺纹面紧按风池穴,用力作旋转按揉,然后按揉脑空穴,以酸胀为宜。

Neck and shoulder massage: knead and grasp the muscles on each side of neck with finger pulps of thumbs up and down; knead and grasp muscles on shoulders with both hands; dab and swing arms for a couple of times.

颈、肩部按摩:用左右拇指指腹分别在颈项左、右侧,由上而下揉、拿颈部肌肉;左、右两手轮流揉、拿肩部肌肉;左右手分别拍打肩臂,并摆动数次。

Section 4 Health Preservation for Different Constitutions

第4节 辨体质施养

Under the guidance of TCM theory, to rectify the unbalanced constitution and expand life span, health preservation methods should be adopted correspondingly to constitution of the individuals.

辨体质施养,即在中医理论指导下,根据不同的体质,采用相应的养生方法和措施,纠正体质之偏,以达到却病延年的目的。

1 Basic Concepts of Constitution

Constitution refers to a special status that an individual develops during growing and aging. It, relatively stable in structure and function, is influenced by congenital and acquired factors and determines the specificity of the physiological reaction and the susceptibility to certain pathogenic factors and pathological changes. Learning from practice and experience, people have realized that constitution isn't unchangeable and can alter under the influence of external environment, development conditions and living conditions. Therefore, through positive health preserving measures, such as changing surrounding environment, improving working and living conditions and dietary nutrition, and strengthening the physical exercise, poor constitution can be improved, resistance to disease raised and unbalanced constitution rectified so as to prevent diseases and expand life expectancy.

1 体质的基本概念

体质是指人群及人群中个体禀赋于先天,受后天多种因素影响,在其生长发育和衰老过程中,所形成的结构上和功能上相对稳定的特殊状态,这种特殊状态往往决定其生理反应的特异性及对某些致病因素的易感性和病变过程的倾向性。人们在实践中认识到,体质不是固定不变的,外界环境和发育条件,生活条件的影响,都有可能使体质发生改变。因此,对于不良体质,可以通过有计划地改变周围环境,改善劳动、生活条件和饮食营养,以及加强体格锻炼等积极的养生措施,提高其对疾病的抵抗力,纠正其体质上的偏颇,从而达到防病延年之目的。

2 Causes of Different Constitutions

Congenital factors: Congenital factors, namely

2 体质差异形成的原因

先天因素:先天因素即

"endowment", include heredity and the nutritional status of fetus in wombs. On the one hand, constitution features of parents can pass on through inheritance to offspring, so descendants have similar individual characteristics; on the other hand, nutritional status during the development of the fetus also plays an important role in the formation of the characteristics of the constitution.

"禀赋",包括遗传和胎儿在母体里的发育营养状况。父母的体质特征通过遗传,使后代具有类似父母的个体特点,是先天因素的一个方面,而胎儿发育的营养状况,对体质特点的形成也起着重要的作用。

Gender: Gender not only forms different anatomical structures and constitution types, but also presents different physiological characteristics. In general, the male is muscular and fierce, while the female tends to be weak and tender. For male, qi is important; while for female, blood is essential.

性别因素:男女性别不仅形成各自不同的解剖结构和体质类型,而且在生理特性方面,也会显示出各自不同的特点。一般说,男子性多刚悍,女子性多柔弱,男子以气为重,女子以血为先。

Age: Age is related to the changes in the structure, function and metabolism of human body, which forms the differences of the constitution.

年龄因素:人体的结构、功能与代谢的变化同年龄有关,从而形成体质的差异。

Mental factors: Mental status, through influencing the functions of the viscera, qi and blood, can also change the constitution.

精神因素:人的精神状态,由于能影响脏腑气血的功能活动,所以也可以改变体质。

Geographical environment: In order to adapt to the objective environment, human beings, like other creatures, can gradually change their morphological structures and functions of qi transformation. Different geographical environments will give rise to different climates, products and dietary and living habits. Therefore, according to *Plain Questions* (Su Wen): different regions foster different constitutions. When treating different diseases with different therapeutic approaches, soil, climate, diet and living habits of different regions should be emphasized, for these factors affect the formation of

地理环境因素:人类和其他生物一样,其形态结构,气化功能在适应客观环境的过程中会逐渐发生变异。地理环境不同,则气候、物产,当地人的饮食、生活习惯等,与其他地区会有所不同,所以《素问》在论证不同区域有不同的体质,不同的多发病和不同的治疗方法的时候,特别强调了不同地区的水土、气候以及饮食、居住等生

constitution. It indicates that geographical environment is not only an important and but also an extremely complex factor in the variation of constitution.

活习惯，对体质形成的重大影响，说明地理环境对体质的变异，既是一个十分重要的因素，又是极其复杂的因素。

3 Classification of Constitutions

3 体质的分类

With the development of clinical medicine of TCM, to better the integrity of administration based on clinical pattern identification, modern TCM classifies the constitution into two groups—normal and poor—according to the deficiency, excess, exuberance and depletion of yin, yang, qi, blood and liquid. Those with strong body, luster complexion, fine sleep and appetite, smooth urination and bowel movements, normal pulse and no obvious exuberance and depletion of yin, yang, qi and blood are considered with normal constitution. On the contrary, those with obvious tendencies like deficiency of yin, yang, qi and blood, phlegm and dampness, exuberance of yang, blood stasis are regarded as individuals with poor constitutions. This taxonomy is called applied classification methods of constitution.

随着中医临床医学的发展，为了更好地与临床辨证相结合，现代中医常用的体质分类法着眼于阴阳气血津液的虚实盛衰，把人体分为正常体质和不良体质两大类。凡体力强壮、面色润泽、眠食均佳、二便通调，脉象正常、无明显阴阳气血偏盛偏衰倾向者，为正常体质。反之，有明显的阴虚、阳虚、气虚、血虚、痰湿、阳盛、血瘀等倾向（倾向与证候有微甚轻重之别）的属于不良体质，这种分类方法，可称之为实用体质分类法。

4 Essentials for Health Preservation Based on Different Constitutions

4 不同体质的养生要点

This section focuses on health preservation methods for poor constitutions like deficiencies of yin, yang, qi and blood, exuberance of yang, phlegm and dampness, blood stasis and qi depression. As for those with normal constitution characterized by balanced yin and yang, qi and blood, health preservation methods should be given based on age, gender and occupation and they are not discussed in this section.

此处着重介绍阴虚、阳虚、气虚、血虚、阳盛、痰湿、血瘀、气郁等不良体质的养生方法。至于阴阳气血平调的体质，应根据年龄、性别、职业等差异，采用不同的养生方法，不在此处讨论。

Latest research makes some rectifications on the types of poor constitutions. For example, yang exuberance is changed into dampness heat, blood deficiency is dropped and special inheritance is added. In the perspective of learning, previous classification is with more clarity and easier to master. Therefore, this section still introduces the previous one.

需要注意的是，中医界最新的研究中，将阳盛体质改为湿热质，并删去了血虚体质，增加了特禀质。但从学习的角度来看，旧的分类方法更加虚实分明、条理清楚，易于理解掌握，因此本教材沿用旧的体质分类法。

4.1 Yin Deficiency

4.1 阴虚体质

4.1.1 Characteristics

4.1.1 体质特点

Emaciation, postmeridian reddening of the face, scanty fluids of mouth and throat, occasional vexation, heat in the heart of the palms and soles, sleeplessness, dry stools and yellow urine, aversion to spring and summer, desire for cold drinks, fine rapid pulse with red tongue and scanty coating.

形体消瘦，午后面色潮红、口咽少津，心中时烦，手足心热，少眠，便干，尿黄，不耐春夏，多喜冷饮，脉细数，舌红少苔。

4.1.2 Essentials

4.1.2 养生要点

(1) Spirit adjustment: Yin deficiency leads to hyperactivity of fire, which often disrupts the mind. As a result, those with yin deficiency are often impatient, vexed and irritable. Therefore, individuals should strengthen self-improvement by reading books and developing habits of calmness. At work and in life avoid arguing with others and participating in competitive activities. Control desires to nourish mind.

(1) 精神调养：阴虚体质之人性情急躁、常常心烦易怒，这是阴虚火旺、火扰神明之故。平素应加强自我修养，常读提高涵养的书籍，自觉地养成冷静、沉着的习惯。在生活和工作中，对非原则性问题，少与人争，以减少激怒。要少参加争胜负的文娱活动，以免受到激惹。平常还要注意节制欲念，以保精养神。

(2) Environment: Those with yin deficiency often dislike heat and desires for cold. For them, winter is pleasant and summer is unbearable. Therefore, in summer, individuals should avoid the summer heat. If possible, they can go traveling to the

(2) 环境调摄：阴虚体质者，常畏热喜凉，冬寒易过，夏热难受。因此，每逢炎热的夏季，应注意避暑，有条件的应到海边、高山之地旅游。

seaside or in the mountains. It is important for those with yin deficiency to nourish yin in autumn and winter, especially in autumn when dry climate impairs yin. Therefore, it is appropriate to increase the humidity. It's better to live in a quiet house facing the south.

"秋冬养阴"对阴虚体质之人更为重要,特别是秋季气候干燥,更易伤阴,可适当增加环境的湿度。居室环境应安静,最好住坐北朝南的房子。

(3) Diet: The rule for diet is to preserve yin and subdue yang. It is better to have light food, such as Hei Zhi Ma(*Semen Sesami Nigrum*), glutinous rice, Feng Mi, diary products, sugarcane, vegetables, fruits, tofu and fish. Sha Shen (*Radix Glehniae*) Porridge, Bai He porridge, Gou Qi Zi porridge, Sang Shen(*Fructus Mori*)porridge, Shan Yao porridge are helpful. If possible, it's better to have swift's nest, tremella, trepang, mussel, tortoise meat, crab meat, Dong Chong Xia Cao (*Cordyceps*), and old duck. Keep away from spicy and stringent food like onion, ginger, garlic, chives and pepper.

(3) 饮食调养:饮食调理的原则是保阴潜阳,宜食芝麻、糯米、蜂蜜、乳品、甘蔗、蔬菜、水果、豆腐、鱼类等清淡食物,并着意食用沙参粥、百合粥、枸杞粥、桑椹粥、山药粥等。条件许可者,可食用燕窝、银耳、海参、淡菜、龟肉、蟹肉、冬虫夏草、老雄鸭等。对于葱、姜、蒜、韭、薤、椒等辛辣燥烈之品则应少吃。

(4) Exercise: Strenuous exercises are not available. Individuals should focus on regulating the functions of liver and kidney, therefore Tai Ji Quan and Eight Trigram Boxing (Ba Duan Jin) are suitable. Qi Gong, especially the essence-securing exercises, health preserving exercises and long life workouts are more suitable. Throat liquid exercise should be focused on.

(4) 体育锻炼:不宜剧烈活动,着重调养肝肾功能,以太极拳、八段锦等较为适合。气功宜固精功、保健功、长寿功等,着重咽津功法。

(5) Medication: Herbs that can enrich yin and clear heat, enrich and nourish liver and kidney can be selected, such as Nü Zhen Zi (*Fructus Ligustri Lucidi*), Wu Wei Zi (*Fructus Schisandrae Chinensis*), Han Lian Cao (*Herba Ecliptae*), Mai Dong (*Radix Ophiopogonis*), Tian Men Dong (*Radix Asparagi*), Huang Jing (*Rhizoma Polygonati*), Yu

(5) 药物养生:可选用滋阴清热、滋养肝肾之品,如女贞子、五味子、旱莲草、麦门冬、天门冬、黄精、玉竹、玄参、枸杞子、桑椹、龟板诸药,可依体质的偏颇程度选用。常用中药方剂有六味地黄

Zhu (*Rhizoma Polygonati Odorati*), Xuan Shen (*Radix Scrophulariae*), Gou Qi, Sang Shen and Gui Jia. These herbs can be chosen based on the degree of the constitutional unbalance. The common formulae are Liu Wei Di Huang Wan (*Rehmannia Pills with Six Ingredients*) and Da Bu Yin Wan (*Great Yin Supplementation Pills*). As yin deficiency can be classified into deficiency of lung yin, heart yin, stomach yin, kidney yin and liver yin, treatments should be differentiated. For deficiency of lung yin, Bai He Gu Jin Tang (*Lily Bulb Metal-Securing Decoction*) is helpful; for deficiency of heart yin, Tian Wang Bu Xin Wan (*Celestial Emperor Heart-Supplementing Pill*) is necessary; for deficiency of stomach yin, Shen Rou's Genuine yin -Nourishing Decoction (Shen Rou Yang Zhen Tang) is available; for deficiency of kidney yin, Liu Wei Di Huang Wan can be selected; for deficiency of liver yin, Yi Guan Jian (*All-the-Way-Through Brew*) can be chosen.

丸、大补阴丸等。由于阴虚体质又有肺阴虚、心阴虚、胃阴虚、肾阴虚、肝阴虚等不同，故应随其部位和程度而调补之，如肺阴虚，宜服百合固金汤；心阴虚，宜服天王补心丸；胃阴虚，宜服慎柔养真汤；肾阴虚，宜服六味地黄丸；肝阴虚，宜服一贯煎。

4.2 Yang Deficiency

4.2.1 Characteristics

Obesity or with white complexion, aversion to cold and desire for warmth, cold hands and feet, long voidings of clear urine, occasional lose stool, light-colored lips without taste of bitterness and thirst, frequent simultaneous sweating, deep and weak pulse with light-colored and enlarged tongue.

4.2.2 Essentials

(1) Spirit adjustment: Yang qi can warm the mind, so those with yang deficiency are often dispirited, depressed, absent-minded with lowered thinking capability. Therefore, various measures should be taken to regulate emotions. Take singing and dancing for example, they can manoeuvre vital-

4.2 阳虚体质

4.2.1 体质特点

形体白胖，或面色淡白，平素怕寒喜暖、手足欠温，小便清长，大便时稀，唇淡口和，常自汗出，脉沉乏力，舌淡胖。

4.2.2 养生要点

（1）精神调养：阳气对神具有温养作用，阳虚体质的人常有精神萎靡不振，情绪明显低落，注意力不集中，思考力下降等表现。因此，要善于运用多种方法，调节情

ity and keep up spirits.

绪，消除或减少不良情绪的影响。如采用歌舞的方法，结合肢体舞蹈和歌曲演唱调动活力，提振精神。

(2) Environment: Those with yang deficiency have poor adaptation to temperature changes, especially to cold weather. Therefore, they should avoid cold and keep warm in winter, cultivate and supplement yang in spring and summer. For example, taking sun bath for 20 to 30 times in summer with each time for 15 to 20 minutes can greatly improve the capability of adapting to cold weather in winter.

（2）环境调摄：此类人适应寒暑变化的能力差，尤其不耐寒冷。因此，在严寒的冬季，要“避寒就温”，注意保暖。在春夏之季，要注意培补阳气。在夏季进行20～30次日光浴，每次15～20分钟，可以大大提高适应冬季严寒气候的能力。

Nourishing yang in spring and summer emphasizes on keeping yang unharmed during these two seasons. In summer, yang tends to disperse in the exterior and pores and interstices are open. Therefore, those with yang deficiency mustn't sleep in the open or facing the fan directly. In air-conditioned rooms, temperature differences between the outside and the inside should be kept small. Don't stay in the shadow of trees, water pavilion and pathways where there are strong wind for a long time, otherwise it's easy to catch cold and wind will enter into the collaterals, leading to impediment pattern.

春夏养阳，强调春夏季节要保护阳气不受损害。由于夏季人体阳气趋向体表，毛孔、腠理开疏，阳虚体质之人切不可在室外露宿，睡眠时不要让电扇直吹；有空调设备的房间，要注意室内外的温差不要过大，同时避免在树阴下、水亭中及过堂风很大的过道久停，如果不注意夏季防寒，只图一时之快，更易着风受寒，甚至风邪入络而成痹症。

(3) Exercise: As motion generates yang, those with yang deficiency should do exercises once or twice a day persistently, such as walking, jogging, Tai Ji, Five-animal Boxing (Wu Qin Xi), Eight Trigram Boxing (Ba Duan Jin), Breathing Exercise, physical exercises during breaks, ball games and dancing. During exercises, sun bathe and air bathe can be combined to strengthen defensive yang. In

（3）体育锻炼：因“动则生阳”，故阳虚体质之人，要加强体育锻炼，春夏秋冬，坚持不懈，每日进行1～2次。具体项目可视体力强弱而定，如散步、慢跑、太极拳、五禽戏、八段锦、内养操、工间操、球类活动和各种舞蹈活

terms of qi gong, strengthening exercise, stake-standing, health-preserving exercise and long life workouts are helpful.

动等。在运动的同时可结合作日光浴、空气浴，强壮卫阳。气功方面，可坚持练强壮功、站桩功、保健功、长寿功等功法。

(4) Diet: Food with the function of warming can be helpful, such as mutton, dog meat and chicken. According to the rule of nourishing yang in spring and summer, during the dog days in summer, individuals can have Fu Zi (*Radix Aconiti Lateralis Preparata*) Porridge or Mutton and Fu Zi Porridge. Corresponding to the exuberant yang of the heaven and the earth, the porridge is effective in strengthening the yang of the body.

（4）饮食调养：应多食有温热作用的食品，如羊肉、狗肉、鸡肉等。根据“春夏养阳”的法则，夏日三伏，每伏可食附子粥或羊肉附子汤一次，配合天地阳旺之时，以壮人体之阳，颇为有效。

(5) Medication: Herbs that can supplement yang and disperse cold, warm and nourish liver and kidney can be selected, such as Lu Rong (*Cornu Cervi Pantotrichum*), Hai Gou Shen (*Callorhini Testes et Penis*), Ge Jie (*Gecko*), Dong Chong Xia Cao, Ba Ji Tian (*Radix Morindae Officinalis*), Yin Yang Huo, Xian Mao, Rou Cong Rong (*Herba Cistanches*), Bu Gu Zhi (*Fructus Psoraleae*), Hu Tao (*Juglandis Semen*), Du Zhong (*Cortex Eucommiae*), Xu Duan (*Radix Dipsaci*), Tu Si Zi. The common formulae include Jin Kui Shen Qi Wan (*Golden Chamber Kidney Qi Pills*), You Gui Wan (*Right-Restoring (Kidney Yang) Pill*) and Quan Lu Wan (*Whole Deer Pill*). Those with deficiency of heart yang can have Gui Zhi Gan Cao Tang (*Cinnamon and Liquorice Decoction*) combined with Rou Gui (*Cortex Cinnamomi*). If it is severe, add Ren Shen. For deficiency of spleen yang, Li Zhong Wan (*Center-Rectifying Pills*) or Fu Zi Li Zhong Wan (*Aconite Center-Rectifying Pills*) can be selected. Ji

（5）药物养生：可选用补阳祛寒、温养肝肾之品，常用药物有鹿茸、海狗肾、蛤蚧、冬虫夏草、巴戟天、淫羊藿、仙茅、肉苁蓉、补骨脂、胡桃、杜仲、续断、菟丝子等，成方可选用金匮肾气丸、右归丸、全鹿丸。若偏心阳虚者，宜桂枝甘草汤加肉桂常服，虚甚者可加人参；若偏脾阳虚者，选择理中丸，或附子理中丸；脾肾两虚者可用济生肾气丸。

Sheng Shen Qi Wan (*Life Saver Kidney Qi Pill*) is for deficiency of both spleen yang and kidney yang.

4.3 Qi Deficiency

4.3.1 Characteristics

Emaciation or overweight, fatigue and lassitude, low voice with timidity, frequent simultaneous sweating aggravated with motion, light-colored tongue with white coating and weak pulse.

4.3.2 Essentials

(1) Spirit adjustment: Those with qi deficiency are often dispirited, forgetful and absent-minded. To keep up spirit, individuals can listen to music, appreciate drama, cross talk or comedy when they feel depressed and upset.

(2) Exercise: Gentle exercises are necessary in rectifying constitutions and building up bodies, such as gymnastics, Tai Ji, walking, jogging, tuina for four limbs, chest and abdomen. Six-word Qi Gong (Liu Zi Jue), especially the blowing exercise, can be strengthened. Considering the weak constitution, exercises should be taken step by step to avoid overexertion.

(3) Diet: The following can be taken, such as non-glutinous rice, glutinous rice, millet, glutinous millet, barley, yam, indica rice, wheat, potato, Chinese-date, carrot, chicken, goose, rabbit, quail, pork, dog meat, black carp and chub. If with qi deficiency, herbal diet like Ginseng and Lotus Seed Soup is helpful.

(4) Medication: Those with qi deficiency can have herbs that can supplement qi, such as Ren

4.3 气虚体质

4.3.1 体质特点

形体消瘦或偏胖，神疲乏力，日常语声低怯，常自汗出，动则尤甚，舌淡苔白，脉虚弱。

4.3.2 养生要点

（1）精神调养：气虚的人，时常精神不振、健忘、注意力不集中，故应振奋精神。当烦闷不安，情绪不佳时，可以听一听音乐，欣赏一下戏剧，观赏一场幽默的相声或小品，以使精神振奋。

（2）体育锻炼：可选用较为柔缓的方式进行锻炼，如广播操、太极拳、散步、慢跑、按摩四肢及胸腹等，对纠正体质，增强身体素质有很好的帮助。气功可练六字诀中的“吹”字功。但由于体质虚弱不耐劳动，故应防止过度运动疲劳。

（3）饮食调养：可常食粳米、糯米、小米、黄米、大麦、山药、籼米、小麦、马铃薯、大枣、胡萝卜、鸡肉、鹅肉、兔肉、鹌鹑、牛肉、狗肉、青鱼、鲢鱼等。若气虚甚，可选用药膳人参莲肉汤补养。

（4）药物养生：平素常易气虚之人可选用人参、黄芪、

Shen, Huang Qi, Fu Ling (*Poria*), Bai Zhu, Da Zao and Shan Yao. If it is severe, formulae that can supplement qi can be used. For deficiency of spleen qi, Si Jun Zi Tang (*Four Nobles Decoction*), or Shen Ling Bai Zhu San (*Ginseng, Poria and Atractylodes Powder*) is necessary; for deficiency of lung qi, Bu Fei Tang (*Lung-supplementing Decoction*) can be selected; for deficiency of kidney qi, Shen Qi Wan (*Kidney Qi Pills*) is helpful.

茯苓、白术、大枣、山药等补气中药。气虚明显者加用补气的方剂，脾气虚，宜选四君子汤或参苓白术散；肺气虚，宜选补肺汤；肾气虚，可选肾气丸。

4.4 Blood Deficiency

4.4 血虚体质

4.4.1 Characteristics

4.4.1 体质特点

Pale and lusterless or yellowish complexion, light white lips, dizziness and blurred eyes, easy to be tired, sleeplessness, light-colored tongue with fine weak pulse.

面色苍白无华或萎黄，唇色淡白，头晕目眩，不耐劳作，易失眠，舌质淡，脉细无力。

4.4.2 Essentials

4.4.2 养生要点

(1) Spirit adjustment: Maintain inner peace and stable emotion. Listen to lyric music or appreciate drama when feel vexed and depressed.

（1）精神调养：保持内心平静和情绪稳定。心烦郁闷时，可听柔和抒情的音乐和戏曲来帮助舒缓情绪。

(2) Daily life: Have adequate rest and enough sleep. Avoid long-time reading and writing, for it will impair blood. Keep away from worries, in case heart blood is consumed.

（2）起居调摄：注意休息，保证睡眠时间；看书写作要适量，谨防“久视伤血”；不可劳心过度，避免心血暗耗。

(3) Diet: The following food that can supplement and nourish blood is helpful, such as Chinese-date, black fungus, spinach, carrots, beef, pork, mutton, beef liver, lamb liver, turtles, sea cucumber and milk.

（3）饮食调养：可选用红枣、黑木耳、菠菜、胡萝卜、牛肉、猪肉、羊肉、牛肝、羊肝、甲鱼、海参、牛奶等有补血养血作用食物。

(4) Medication: Herbs like Dang Gui, He Shou Wu (*Radix Polygoni Multiflori*), E Jiao can be selected. If blood deficiency is severe, the following formulae are necessary: Dang Gui Bu Xue Tang

（4）药物养生：可选用当归、何首乌、阿胶等药物，血虚明显者，可选择当归补血汤、四物汤、归脾汤、八珍汤、

(*Angelica Blood-Supplementing Decoction*), Si Wu Tang (*Four Agents Decoction*), Gui Pi Tang (*Spleen-Returning Decoction*), Ba Zhen Tang (*Eight Jewel Decoction*), Shi Quan Da Bu Tang (*Perfect Major Supplementation Decoction*) and Ren Shen Yang Rong Tang or Wan (*Ginseng Construction-Nourishing Decoction (Pill)*).

十全大补汤、人参养荣汤(丸)等。

4.5 Yang Exuberance

4.5.1 Characteristics

Strong body with red complexion, high voice and gruff breathing, aversion to heat and desire for cold and cold drinks, heat and red urine, smelly stools, red tongue with yellow coating and large pulse.

4.5.2 Essentials

(1) Spirit adjustment: People with yang exuberance are irritable. Therefore, moral cultivation and the will power must be strengthened. Control the temper consciously when feeling angry.

(2) Exercise: Take an active part in sports activities to disperse the extra yang. Swimming is preferred. In addition, running, martial arts and ball games can also be chosen according to the hobbies.

(3) Diet: Avoid spicy and dry foods, such as pepper, garlic, ginger, spring onion. Eat more fruits and vegetables, such as bananas, watermelon, persimmon, balsam pear, cucumber, tomato and lotus root, instead of those warm in nature, such as beef, dog meat, chicken and venison. As wine is stringent and heat in feature and upward in motion, those with yang exuberance should strictly avoid

4.5 阳盛体质

4.5.1 体质特点

形体壮实，面赤，声高气粗、喜凉怕热，喜冷饮，小便热赤，大便熏臭，舌红苔黄，脉大。

4.5.2 养生要点

(1) 精神调养：阳盛之人好动易发怒，故平日要加强道德修养和意志锻炼，培养良好的性格，有意识控制自己，遇到可怒之事，用理性克服情感上的冲动。

(2) 体育锻炼：积极参加体育活动，让多余阳气散发出来。游泳锻炼是首选项目。此外，跑步、武术、球类等，也可根据爱好进行选择。

(3) 饮食调理：忌辛辣燥烈食物，如辣椒、蒜、姜、葱等，对于牛肉、狗肉、鸡肉、鹿肉等温性食物宜少食用。可多食水果、蔬菜，如香蕉、西瓜、柿子、苦瓜、黄瓜、番茄、莲藕等。酒性辛热上行，阳盛之人力戒酗酒。

drinking alcohol.

(4) Medication: Herbal tea with Ju Hua (*Flos Chrysanthemi*), Jue Ming Zi (*Semen Cassiae*), Ku Ding Cha (*Folium llicis Latifoliae*) is necessary. With dry stool, Ma Zi Ren Wan (*Hemp Seed Pills*) or Run Chang Wan (*Intestine-Moisturizing Pills*) is helpful; for dry mouth and tongue, Mai Men Dong Tang (*Ophiopogon Decoction*) is available; for vexation and irritability, Dan Zhi Xiao Yao San (*Cortex Moutan, Fructus Gardeniae and Free Wanderer Powder*) is necessary.

（4）药物调养：可以常用菊花、决明子、苦丁茶沸水泡服。大便干燥者，用麻子仁丸或润肠丸；口干舌燥者，用麦门冬汤；心烦易怒者，宜服丹栀逍遥散。

4.6 Blood Stasis

4.6 血瘀体质

4.6.1 Characteristics

Dark complexion, purple mouth and lips, black eye socket, scaly dry skin, purple dark tongue with stasis spots, fine rough pulse.

4.6.1 体质特点

面色晦滞，口唇色暗，眼眶黯黑，肌肤甲错，舌紫暗或有瘀点，脉细涩。

4.6.2 Essentials

(1) Spirit adjustment: For those with blood stasis, optimism should be cultivated. Happiness can promote the harmony and free flow of qi and blood, and smooth circulation of nutrition qi and defensive qi. As a result, blood stasis can be relieved. Vice versa, depression will aggravate the blood stasis.

(2) Exercise: Exercises that are good for the heart and blood vessels can be taken, such as dancing, Tai Ji, Eight Trigram Boxing (Ba Duan Jin), long life workouts, breathing exercise, health-preserving tuina. Exercises that can activate various parts of the body and promote circulation of qi and blood can be implemented.

(3) Diet: Foods that can quicken the blood and eliminate stasis are available, such as peach kernel, rape, arrowhead, black soya bean and Shan Zha. Small-amount low alcoholic drink like rice wine,

4.6.2 养生要点

（1）精神调养：血瘀体质在精神调养上，要培养乐观的情绪。精神愉快则气血和畅，营卫流通，有利于血瘀体质的改善。反之，苦闷、忧郁则可加重血瘀倾向。

（2）体育锻炼：多做有益于心运血脉的活动，如各种舞蹈、太极拳、八段锦、长寿功、内养功、保健按摩术，均可实施，总以全身各部都能活动，以助气血运行为原则。

（3）饮食调理：可常食桃仁、油菜、慈菇、黑大豆、山楂等具有活血祛瘀作用的食物，米酒、黄酒和红酒等低度

yellow rice wine and red wine can be regularly taken.

酒可少量常饮。

(4) Medication: Herbs with the function of quickening and nourishing the blood can be chosen, such as Hong Hua (*Flos Carthami*), Sheng Di Huang (*Radix Rehmanniae*), Dan Shen (*salvia miltiorrhiza*), Chuan Xiong (*Rhizoma Chuanxiong*), Dang Gui, San Qi (*Radix Notoginseng*), Xu Duan (*Radix Dipsaci*), Chong Wei Zi (*Fructus Leonuri*). If blood stasis is severe, formulae that can quicken the blood and transform blood stasis are helpful, such as Si Wu Tang (*Four Agents Decoction*), and Tao Hong Si Wu Tang (*Peach Pit, Safflower and Four Agents Decoction*).

(4) 药物养生：可选用活血养血之品，如红花、生地黄、丹参、川芎、当归、三七、续断、茺蔚子等。瘀血明显者，可选用四物汤、桃红四物汤等活血化瘀的方剂。

4.7 Phlegm-dampness

4.7 痰湿体质

4.7.1 Characteristics

Overweight with loose muscles, desire for greasy and sweet food, fatigue and heaviness in the body, laziness and somnolence, sticky taste, or loose stool, enlarged tongue with slippery and greasy coating, soggy and slippery pulse.

4.7.1 体质特点

形体肥胖，肌肉松弛，嗜食肥甘，神倦身重，懒动嗜睡，口中黏腻，或便溏，舌体胖，苔滑腻，脉濡而滑。

4.7.2 Essentials

(1) Spirit adjustment: Phlegm-dampness easily obstructs qi movements, causing poor circulation of qi. Therefore, those with this constitution are often depressed. So they should adjust the state of mind, face the life and work positively, frequently communicate with family and friends, regularly listen to lively and cheerful music and watch comedies and inspirational films.

(2) Environment: Avoid living in damp environment. Be careful for the dampness attack during the rainy season.

(3) Exercise: Those with phlegm-dampness are

4.7.2 养生要点

(1) 精神调养：痰湿体质者气机容易受阻，气机失于条畅，可见精神抑郁，情绪低落，故要调节心境，以主动积极的心态来面对生活和工作，多与家人和朋友沟通，多听欢快令人愉悦的音乐，观看喜剧和励志的电影。

(2) 环境调摄：不宜居住在潮湿的环境里；在阴雨季节，要注意慎防湿邪的侵袭。

(3) 体育锻炼：痰湿之体

often overweight, flaccid and usually feel heaviness. Therefore, they should do exercises persistently, such as walking, jogging, ball games, martial arts, Eight Trigram Boxing (Ba Duan Jin), Five-animal Boxing (Wu Qin Xi) as well as a variety of dances. These exercises should be gradually strengthened so that the loose muscles can gradually turn into strong and tight ones. In terms of Qi Gong, stake-standing, health-preserving exercise, long life workouts are necessary. Breathing exercise can also be strengthened.

质，多形体肥胖，身重易倦，故应长期坚持体育锻炼，散步、慢跑、球类、武术、八段锦、五禽戏，以及各种舞蹈，均可选择。活动量应逐渐增强，让疏松的皮肉逐渐转变成结实、致密之肌肉。气功方面，以站桩功、保健功、长寿功为宜，加强运气功法。

(4) Diet: Eat less greasy and sweet food, and drink less alcohol. Don't eat too much. Have more foods that have the function of fortifying spleen and removing dampness, transforming phlegm and eliminating dampness, such as radish, water chestnut, laver, jellyfish, onion, loquat, Bai Guo (*Semen Ginkgo*), Da Zao(*Fructus Jujubae*), Bai Bian Dou(*Semen Lablab Album*), Yi Yi Ren (*Semen Coicis*), Chi Xiao Dou (*Semen Vignae*), broad beans, etc.

(4) 饮食调理：少食肥甘厚味、酒类也不宜多饮，切勿过饱。一些具有健脾利湿，化痰祛湿的食物，应多食之，如白萝卜、荸荠、紫菜、海蜇、洋葱、枇杷、白果、大枣、扁豆、薏苡仁、红小豆、蚕豆等。

(5) Medication: The generation of phlegm and dampness is closely related with lung, spleen and kidney. Therefore, the focus is on regulating and supplementing these three zang-organs. When lung fails to diffuse and descend, liquids are not regulated and fluids are accumulated into phlegm. Er Chen Tang (*Double Vintage Decoction*) is used to disperse lung and transform phlegm. When spleen fails to transform, dampness coagulates into phlegm. Liu Jun Zi Tang (*Six Nobles Decoction*) or Xiang Sha Liu Jun Zi Tang (*Costus Root and Amomum with Six Nobles Decoction*) is necessary in fortifying spleen and transforming phlegm. If the kid-

(5) 药物养生：痰湿之生与肺脾肾三脏关系最为密切，故养生重点在于调补肺脾肾三脏。若因肺失宣降，津失通调，液聚生痰者，当宣肺化痰，方选二陈汤；若因脾不健运，湿聚成痰者，当健脾化痰，方选六君子汤，或香砂六君子汤；若肾虚不能制水，水泛为痰者，当温阳化痰，方选苓桂术甘汤。

ney fails to manage water due to deficiency and water transforms into phlegm, Ling Gui Zhu Gan Tang (*Poria, Cinnamon, Atractylodes and Liquorice Decoction*) is helpful in warming yang and transforming phlegm.

4.8 Qi Depression

4.8.1 Characteristics

Emaciation or overweight, pale dark or yellowish complexion, sometimes impatient and irritable, sometimes depressed, chest stuffiness with desire to heave a deep sigh, light-red tongue with white coating and string-like pulse.

4.8.2 Essentials

(1) Spirit adjustment: People with such constitution are introverted and easily depressed. So they should take the initiative to seek happiness by frequently participating in social activities and entertainment activities, such as watching comedy and burlesque, appreciating the cross talk and inspirational films instead of tragedy, listening to light, cheerful and exciting music to keep up the spirits and reading more books that are positive, encouraging, funny and prospective to foster a bright and cheerful character. Don't care too much about gain and loss on the fame and fortune. Be content about what you have now.

(2) Exercise and tourism activities: Sports and tourism activities can build up the body and promote the circulation of qi and blood. Through these activities, individuals not only appreciate the natural beauty, adjust the spirit and breathe the fresh air, but also bathe in the sunshine and build up the body. In terms of Qi Gong, strengthening exercise, health-preserving exercise, stake standing are help-

4.8 气郁体质

4.8.1 体质特点

形体消瘦或偏胖，面色苍暗或萎黄，时或性情急躁易怒，易于激动，时或忧郁寡欢，胸闷不舒，时欲太息，舌淡红、苔白，脉弦。

4.8.2 养生要点

（1）精神调摄：此种人性格内向，容易处于抑郁状态，应主动寻求快乐，多参加社会活动、集体文娱活动，常看喜剧、滑稽剧，听相声，以及富有鼓励、激励的影视作品，勿看悲剧、苦剧。多听轻松、开朗、激动的音乐，以提高情志。多读积极的、鼓励的、富有乐趣的、展现美好生活前景的书籍，以培养开朗、豁达的性格。注意在名利上不计较得失，知足常乐。

（2）多参加体育锻炼及旅游活动：因体育和旅游活动均能运动身体，流通气血。既欣赏了自然美景，调节了精神，呼吸了新鲜空气，又能沐浴阳光，增强身体素质。气功方面，以强壮功、保健功、站桩功为主，着意锻炼呼

ful. Breathing exercise can be strengthened to conduct the depression.

吸吐纳功法，以开导郁滞。

(3) Diet: Small-amount alcohol can be taken to quicken the blood, free the network vessels and keep up the spirits. Eat more foods that can promote the circulation of qi, such as bergamot, orange, orange peel, buckwheat, leek, fennel, garlic, ham, sorghum, Dao Dou (*Semen Canavaliae*), Xiang Yuan (*Fructus Citri*), etc.

（3）饮食调养：可少量饮酒，以活血通脉，提高情绪。多食一些行气的食物，如佛手、橙子、柑皮、荞麦、韭菜、茴香菜、大蒜、火腿、高粱、刀豆、香橼等。

(4) Medication: Scented tea that can relieve the depression is helpful, such as rose tea and bergamot flower tea. Formulae, which are made up of herbs with the function of soothing liver, regulating qi and relieving depression like Xiang Fu (*Rhizoma Cyperi*), Wu Yao (*Radix Linderae*), Chuan Lian Zi (*Fructus Toosendan*), Xiao Hui Xiang, Qing Pi (*Pericarpium Citri Reticulatae Viride*) and Yu Jin (*Radix Curcumae*), can be selected, such as Stagnancy-Relieving Pills (Yue Ju Wan). If qi depression leads to blood stasis, herbs that can quicken the blood and transform stasis may be added.

（4）药物养生：可常以玫瑰花、佛手花等具有解郁作用的花类泡茶。选用香附、乌药、川楝子、小茴香、青皮、郁金等善于疏肝理气解郁的药为主组成方剂调理，如越鞠丸等。若气郁引起血瘀，当配伍活血化瘀药。

Chapter 11 Health Preservation for Five Viscera

第 11 章 五脏保养

Centered on the five viscera, human body is an organic whole with six bowels, five constituents, nine orifices, four limbs and skeleton connected through the meridian system. Physiologically, the five systems are not only connected with each other, but also function independently to complete the physiological activities of the body. Pathologically, the lesions of one viscus can influence and even transmit to other viscera. The physiological functions of viscera and bowels and the balance between them are important factors to maintain relative stability of the internal and external environment. Therefore, five viscera are the core to the health preservation.

人体以五脏为中心，通过经络系统，把六腑、五体、九窍、四肢百骸等全身组织器官联系成为一个有机整体。在生理状态下，五大系统既相互联系，又分工合作，共同完成人体的生理活动；病理状态时，内在脏腑的病变可以相互影响，相互传变。脏腑生理功能和相互之间的平衡协调是维持机体内外环境相对恒定的重要条件，因此，养生保健的核心内容之一就是五脏保养。

Section 1 Heart

第 1 节 心脏保养

According to the TCM theory of visceral manifestation, heart not only governs the complete circulation system including blood and veins, but also manages spirit, consciousness and thinking activity. In addition, heart is regarded as the "big master" of the five viscera and six bowels and as the monarch,

在中医藏象学说中，心的生理功能，不仅包括主宰血、脉在内的完整循环系统，而且还包括主宰精神、意识、思维活动。同时，中医强调心为五脏六腑之“大主”、为

which indicates the important position of heart in the viscera and in life activities. Therefore, to preserve health, it is necessary to keep heart in good condition.

“君主之官”，说明了心在脏腑中的重要地位和在人体生命活动中的重要性。因此，养生首先要做好心的保健。

1 Care in Pregnancy

Due to contraction of external pathogenic factors, over age pregnancy, inappropriate medications, exposure to harmful materials such as radiation, fright, unstable life and even poor rest, fetus may develop congenital heart diseases in pregnancy within three months. As a result, to prevent them, mother should be careful during pregnancy. For example, adjust to temperature changes to avoid contraction of external pathogenic factors; take medicines under the guidance of doctors; have balanced diet to prevent nutrients deficiency; keep stable moods and avoid emotional stimulus; have enough rest and so on.

1 重视养胎

母亲怀孕 3 个月内，因感受外邪，或母亲年龄过大，或服用不当的药物，或接受放射等有害物质，或受过惊吓、生活不安定、休息不佳等因素，可能使胎儿罹患先天性心脏病。因此，母亲在怀孕期间，要重视养胎。养胎着重要调适寒温，避免感受外邪；要在医生的指导下服用药物；注意膳食合理，避免营养缺乏；保持情绪稳定，避免接触容易引起情绪大起大落的事物；注意劳逸结合，从而预防先天性心脏病的发生。

2 Proper Diet

First of all, diet should be light. According to *The Yellow Emperor's Inner Canon* (Huang Di Nei Jing), salty diet does harms to the heart and blood vessels. Modern medicine has also confirmed that excessive intake of salt can cause or aggravate high blood pressure, and even give rise to heart disease. Therefore, in order to preserve heart, it is advisable not to take salty food and the daily intake of salt should be controlled below 6 g.

Secondly, eat less greasy and sweet food. Long-term intake of greasy and sweet food will cause poor circulation of qi and blood, leaving phlegm and sta-

2 合理饮食

首先应注意饮食宜淡。《黄帝内经》中就已经认为，饮食过咸对心脏及其所主血脉会造成危害。现代医学也证实，过多摄入食盐，易导致或加重高血压，容易引起心脏病。故为了保养心脏，饮食不可过咸，每天食盐摄入量小于 6 克为宜。

其次要少食肥甘。长期过食肥甘之品，容易导致气血运行不畅，痰瘀留结于血

sis blocking the vessels and heart deprived of nourishment. Subsequently, heart disease is developed. Therefore, for the middle-aged and even older people, to protect the heart, it is necessary to eat less greasy and sweet food. Vegetables and fruits are advised, such as radish, cucumber, wax gourd, corn, millet, celery, leek, agaric, day-lily flower, apples, pears, He Tao Ren(*Semen Juglandis*), Shan Zha (*Fructus Crataegi*), etc.

脉,心失所养,导致心脏病发生。所以,对于中年以后的人群,为保护心脏,应少食肥甘,多食谷蔬与水果,谷蔬如萝卜、黄瓜、冬瓜、玉米、小米、芹菜、韭菜、木耳、黄花菜等;水果如苹果、生梨、核桃、山楂等。

3 Moderate Exercise

According to TCM, smooth flow of qi and blood is the basic condition to stay healthy. Moderate exercise is good for heart cultivation by promoting circulation of qi and blood and maintaining smooth blood flow. Of course, the intensity, frequency, time and the way of exercise vary from person to person. Few exercise is not enough to build up the body, while much exercise will consume qi and injure the body. Therefore, individuals, especially the elderly, should choose the proper exercise according to their own conditions.

3 适度运动

中医强调经络气血通畅是保持健康的基本条件。适度的运动,可以促进气血运行,保持血脉通畅,对心脏具有保养作用。当然,运动的强度、频度、时间和方式要因人而异。运动量过小,达不到锻炼效果;运动量过大,则耗气伤形,尤其老年人,更应根据自身情况,量力而行,不可过于疲劳。

4 Mind Cultivation

Heart governs mind. If a person feels nervous, depressed, frightened and sad for a long time, the mind will be damaged, leading to depression, vexation, palpitations, insomnia, dizziness, headache, etc.

Heart is related to joy. In general, joy is advantageous and is good for the role of heart in governing blood vessels. But excessive joy can dissipate heart qi and damage mind. Therefore, there is a saying in TCM that joy impairs heart.

Therefore, to cultivate mind, it is a key to keep

4 保养心神

心主神明,如果长期情志过极,处于紧张、郁怒、恐惧、悲伤等负面情绪中,可损伤心神,导致抑郁、心烦、心悸、失眠、头晕头痛等。

心在志为“喜”,一般来说,喜属良性刺激,有益于心主血脉的功能。但是喜乐过度,可使心气涣散,心神受伤,故中医学素有“喜伤心”之说。

因此,保持一种恒定淡

a constant cool attitude and be open-minded. Don't be pleased by external gains and saddened by personal losses.

然的心态，不以物喜，不以己悲，使心神安定，心态豁达，为保养心神的要点。

5 Nourishing Heart in Summer

According to the theory of five elements, heart pertains to fire and interlinked to summer. The warmth in summer is beneficial to the role of heart in governing blood vessels. If coupled with appropriate exercise and proper diet, the heart function will be better strengthened. According to *Plain Questions* (Su Wen), it is important for heart nourishing to nourish yang-qi in spring and summer when yang is exuberant. For example, don't stay outside for coolness or in air-conditioned rooms for a long time and avoid excessive intake of cold food. If possible, take a sun bath.

5 夏季养心

心在五行属火，与夏季相通，夏季的温热气候本身有利于心主血脉的功能，如果再加上合适的运动锻炼和饮食调养，就会收到更好的强心健心功效。《素问》提倡在春夏阳盛之时，保养阳气，这对于心脏保养尤其重要。所以，夏季不要过度在室外纳凉，或长期在室内吹空调，不要过多食用生冷食品，应适当接受阳光浴等，都是夏季养心的要点。

Section 2 Lungs

第2节 肺脏保养

Lungs play a very important role in life activities, for they aid heart to govern blood and vessels. The main physiological functions of lung are: it governs qi and respiration and controls diffusing and descending of qi and body fluids. According to TCM, lung, also called delicate viscus, is the canopy of five viscera. Through respiration, lung is directly linked to the outside world. It follows that the temperature changes of the outside world and a variety of pathogenic factors like microorganism and dirt always affects the lungs. If the morphologi-

肺具有帮助心治理血脉的功能，对人体的生命活动过程起着非常重要的作用。肺的主要生理功能是主气、司呼吸、主宣发和肃降，通调水道。中医认为，肺为五脏之华盖，称为“娇脏”，是非常娇弱的脏器。肺在呼吸过程中，与外界直接相通，外界的冷暖变化和各种致病微生物、灰尘等有害因素，都时刻影响

cal structure and function of lungs are degraded, the body is more susceptible to harmful factors. Therefore, lungs cultivation is an important part of diseases prevention, health improvement, aging delaying.

着肺脏。若肺脏的形态结构和功能退化,人体更易受外界有害因素的侵袭。因此,肺脏保养是预防疾病、增进健康、抗衰防老的重要环节。

1 Breathing Fresh Air

Lungs governs air and qi, and regulates the ascending, descending, entering and exiting of qi. They ensure normal metabolism of human body by inhaling the clear and exhaling the turbid. To protect the lungs, first of all, the quality of air should be improved so that the impurities in the air and toxic gases, such as carbon dioxide, carbon monoxide, sulfur dioxide, chlorine, formaldehyde, organophosphorus pesticide, and inhalable particles, won't be inhaled. Excessive inhalation of poisonous and harmful materials can lead to pulmonary lesions and even systemic diseases.

Therefore, air pollution should be actively prevented and controlled by improving the environment of the workplace and residences, such as purifying the dusty environment. Preventive measures may be taken in poor environment, such as implementing dust-preventing equipment, ventilation equipment and air purification equipment, and wearing dust-preventing masks, etc.

1 呼吸清洁空气

肺主呼吸之气和一身之气,调节气的升降出入运动,吸清呼浊,吐故纳新,从而保证人体新陈代谢的正常进行。保护肺脏健康,首先应提高空气质量,尽量避免吸入空气中的杂质和有毒气体。如:二氧化碳、一氧化碳、二氧化硫、氯气、甲醛、有机磷农药,还有空气中的可吸入颗粒物。有毒有害物质吸入过多,可引起肺部病变和全身病变。

因此,要积极预防和控制空气污染,改善劳动环境、居住环境、居室环境,对灰尘多的环境进行“净化”处理,搞好环境卫生。在空气不尽如人意的环境中,要主动采取预防措施,如添置防尘器具、通风设备、空气净化设备,佩戴防尘口罩等。

2 Developing Good Lifestyle

Good lifestyle is conducive to lung cultivation. When compared with non-smokers, long-term smokers have a 10-20 times higher incidence of lung cancer. Therefore, don't smoke or smoke less. Be careful for the diet. As lung is delicate, food

2 培养良好生活习惯

良好的生活习惯有助于对肺脏的保养,尤其要不吸烟或少吸烟,长期吸烟者的肺癌发病率比不吸烟者高10～20倍。注意饮食宜忌,

shouldn't be spicy and greasy. Overheat or over-cold diets, especially the cold drinks, easily do harms to lungs.

肺为"娇脏",饮食宜少吃辛辣厚味,切勿过寒过热,尤其是寒凉冷饮,否则易伤肺。

3 Moderate Exercise

It is necessary to do morning and evening exercises in a place with fresh air, such as walking, gymnastics, taiji quan, and qigong. Exercises can effectively build up the body and improve cardiopulmonary function. Abdominal breathing can be trained on a regular basis for 5 - 10 minutes each time to replace pectoral breathing, for abdominal breathing can improve lung function by strengthening the activities of the diaphragm and abdominal muscles, deepening breathing extent, increasing ventilation and reducing the residual capacity.

3 适度运动锻炼

早晚到空气新鲜的地方活动肢体,散步、做广播体操、打太极拳、练气功等,可有效地增强体质,改善心肺功能;经常训练腹式呼吸以代替胸式呼吸,每次持续 5~10 分钟,通过腹式呼吸,可以增强膈肌、腹肌等的活动,加深呼吸幅度,增大通气量,减少残气量,从而改善肺功能等。

4 Preventing Cold and Keeping Warm

It is easy to catch cold and trigger bronchitis in cold seasons or during temperature changes. Therefore, individuals may adapt to the climate change of the outside world. Take off or put on clothes according to the temperature. Avoid wind when sweating. Rooms can be keep in an appropriate temperature and humidity with good ventilation. Don't face the wind directly. Chest should always be protected while the back warmed. If warmed, lung qi won't be impaired.

4 注重防寒保暖

寒冷季节或气温突变时,最易患感冒,诱发支气管炎。因此,要适应外界自然气候变化,注意防寒保暖。随气温变化而随时增减衣服,汗出之时要避风。室内温湿度要适宜,通风良好,但不宜直接吹风。胸宜常护,背宜常暖,暖则肺气不伤。

To enhance the capacity of resisting cold and prevent common cold, it is advisable to strengthen cold-resistant exercise from autumn, such as washing face with cold water, taking air bath and massaging noses.

加强耐寒锻炼。可从秋季开始,施行冷水洗面、空气浴、按摩健鼻等方法,增强机体耐寒能力,预防感冒。

In addition, the method of treating winter diseases in summer is also necessary. In summer when

此外,可用"冬病夏治"之法,在夏季未发病之时,采

the disease doesn't occur, medications or acupuncture may be applied to secure the root, strengthen the healthy qi and enhance the resistance. When autumn or winter comes, diseases will develop less frequently or even won't occur.

用方药或针灸固本扶正之法，增强抵抗力，到了秋冬季就可少发病或不发病。

5 Nourishing Lungs in Autumn

According to TCM, lung is related to autumn. In autumn, due to less raining and dry weather, the body is vulnerable to dryness and lungs easily get impaired, causing chapped skin, dry mouth and throat, cough with scanty sputum. Common cold, fever, asthma and other diseases are gradually intensified. So the key of health preservation in autumn is to astringe healthy qi, protect fluids and nourish lung qi. Based on the principle of less pungent and more acid, acid foods like orange and Shan Zha instead of pungent ones like ginger, onions, garlic and chili can be frequently taken. It is better for the elderly patients with upper respiratory tract infection to have porridge for breakfast. In autumn, drink water more frequently and slowly but with less quantity at each time. To moisten lungs, it is advisable to drink 200 ml water before morning exercise and bedtime respectively and 800 ml between two meals during the day.

5 秋季养肺

中医认为，肺“通于秋气”。秋季雨水渐少，天气干燥，人体易受燥邪侵袭损伤肺，出现皮肤干裂、口干咽燥、咳嗽少痰等秋燥病证，感冒、发烧、哮喘等疾病也渐进入高发期。故秋季养生应注重收敛正气，保护津液，以养肺气。饮食以“少辛增酸”为原则，即少吃姜、葱、蒜、辣椒等，而多吃一些酸性食品如柑橙、山楂等。有上呼吸道感染的老年患者早晨饮食以粥为主。秋季养肺还应主动喝水，喝水时一次不宜大量、快速地喝，要多次少喝。最好是在清晨锻炼前和晚上睡觉前各喝水 200 毫升，白天的两餐之间可喝水 800 毫升左右，这样可使肺脏滋润。

Section 3 Spleen and Stomach

第 3 节 脾胃保养

Spleen and stomach are the sources of qi and blood. All nutrients for growing and life sustaining

脾胃是气血生化之源。出生以后人体生长发育、维

after birth are largely depended on the transportation and transformation of spleen and stomach. If the functions of spleen and stomach are declined, the growth, development and metabolism of the body will be severely affected. Therefore, much importance is attached to the spleen and stomach by generations of experts in health preservation. They all hold that it is a must to protect the qi of spleen and stomach.

持生命的一切营养物质，主要靠脾胃运化水谷以供给。若脾胃功能减弱，则人体的生长发育、新陈代谢就会受到严重影响。所以历代养生家特别强调“脾胃”的重要性，认为养生必须要保养脾胃之气。

1 Proper Diet

First of all, have regular meals with fixed amount of food. According to Su Wen, overeating will damage the function of spleen and stomach. It is suggested that individuals should be 80% full for every meal so that they will be moderately hungry before the next meal. In this case, they will always have a good appetite and well-functioned digestion and absorption. The elderly, in particular, should eat less but more frequently, which not only ensures nutrition, but protect the spleen and stomach.

Secondly, the diet should be light, properly mixed with refined and coarse grains, and rich in vegetables and fruits. Such meal can not only guarantee balanced nutrition and necessary dietary fibers, but also promote peristalsis of guts with a certain amount of water. Furthermore, it can help digestion and prevent constipation. The elderly, in particular, may have less fatty, fried and salty food, limit the intake of animal fat, drink less alcohol, and quit smoking and alcohol.

In addition, warm, cooked and soft diets are advised. Eat less or even don't eat raw and cold

1 饮食有节

首先要定时定量。《素问》指出饮食过饱，会损伤脾胃功能。建议每餐只吃八分饱，在吃下一顿饭前保持适度的饥饿感，可始终保有旺盛的食欲和良好的消化吸收功能。对于老年人来说，更应少食多餐，既保证营养供应，又不伤脾胃。

其次，饮食宜清淡。每餐粗细粮搭配合理，多吃蔬菜、水果，既可均衡营养，又能保证每天摄入必要的纤维素，促进食物在肠道中的移动，保持肠道中含有一定量的水分，帮助消化，防止便秘。特别是中老年人，不宜多吃肥腻、油煎、过咸的食物，要限制动物脂肪的摄入，戒烟、酒或少量饮酒。

此外，饮食宜温、熟、软，勿食或少食生冷。老年人由

food. The elderly, due to loose teeth, must have soft diet and keep away from those sticky, hard and indigestible foods.

于牙齿松动,一定要食用软食,忌食黏硬不易消化的食物。

Proper diet also includes other aspects such as food hygiene, feeding methods and balanced nutrition, and they can be referred to relevant chapters.

其他诸如饮食卫生、进食方法、营养全面都属饮食有节的具体内容,可参照相关章节内容。

2 Keeping Good Mood

2 舒畅情志

Depression leads to stagnation of liver qi. Due to the fact that the wood can't sooth the earth, it will further affect the rotting and ripening of stomach and transporting and transforming of spleen, causing poor appetite, distention and fullness of stomach and epigastric region, and thin loose stools. Essence of water and grains are not well distributed to nourish the body, resulting in heaviness of the body and lassitude. Good state of mind can improve digestion and enhance appetite. Therefore, mind adjusting and a good mood are important factors to ensure normal function of spleen and stomach.

情志抑郁导致肝气郁结,木不疏土,会影响脾胃腐熟和运化水谷的功能。导致纳谷不香,胃脘胀满,大便溏薄等症状;水谷精微得不到转输,不能灌溉四傍,则会有身体滞重、倦怠等表现。良好的精神状态可以提高人的消化能力,增强食欲,因此调节心理状态,保持情志舒畅,是保证脾胃功能正常发挥作用的重要方面。

3 Teeth Knocking and Saliva Swallowing

3 叩齿咽唾

Teeth and saliva play an important role in digestion and absorption. With poor teeth and lack of saliva, the functions of spleen and stomach are bound to be impaired. Therefore, to preserve spleen and stomach, it is necessary to maintain the normal function of teeth and adequacy of saliva. To knock teeth, individuals should be fully relaxed with distractions eliminated and mouth shut, and then the upper teeth rhythmically and gently knock the lower ones for 36 times.

牙齿和唾液对人体的消化吸收功能有重要作用,牙齿不好,缺乏唾液的人,脾胃功能必然受损。因此,保健脾胃应保持牙齿功能正常和唾液充足。叩齿的具体做法是:摒除杂念,全身放松,口唇轻闭,然后上下牙齿有节律地互相轻轻叩击36次。

Saliva is considered as golden liquid and jade

唾液,古称为"金津玉

fluids in ancient times. The experts in health preservation in ancient China held that adequate saliva is the guarantee of health and longevity. To swallow saliva, after rinsing in the morning, individuals may close the mouth calmly, and then knock teeth for 36 times. Afterwards, clench teeth and stir the tongue around in the mouth for several times until the mouth is filled with saliva. Finally slowly swallow the saliva for three times.

液”，中国古代养生家认为口中津液充盈，是健康长寿的保证。咽唾的方法是：晨起漱口之后，宁神闭口，先叩齿36次，然后咬紧牙齿，用舌在口腔中四下搅动，不拘次数，以津液满口为度，再分三次缓缓咽下。

4 Abdominal Rubbing and Walking after Meals

Don't lie on the bed immediately after a meal. Instead, individuals should walk slowly and rub hands until they are warmed and then gently rub the abdomen around navel. Long-time abdominal rubbing is conducive to adjusting gastrointestinal functions, promoting digestion and absorption, preventing and treating indigestion and chronic gastrointestinal tract diseases.

After-meal walking is suitable for those who seldom exercise, work at desks for long time, and are overweight. Such person could start walking 20 to 30 minutes after meals, which helps to reduce fat accumulation and over-secretion of gastric acid. But for those who are weak and sick, especially those with gastroptosis, after-meal walking is prohibited. Instead, they should lie down for 10 minutes. If with cardiovascular diseases such as hypertension and coronary heart disease, individuals may begin walking two hours after dinner. Walking may be reduced to the point where individuals slightly perspire without shortness of breath. Each time walk for 15 to 20 minutes and take a break according to the condition. In summary, after-meal walking va-

4 饭后摩腹散步

饭后切忌立即躺在床上，应当缓慢散步，并将手搓热，轻轻绕脐揉摩腹部。长期坚持，对调整胃肠功能，促进食物的消化及吸收，防治消化不良和胃肠道慢性疾病大有益处。

饭后散步适合平时活动较少、长时间伏案工作、形体较胖的人。这类人可在饭后20～30分钟之后开始散步，有助于减少脂肪堆积和胃酸分泌过盛。而体质较差、体弱多病者，尤其是患有胃下垂等疾病的人，饭后非但不能散步，还应平卧10分钟；若患有心脑血管疾病如高血压、冠心病等，步行锻炼最好在晚餐后两小时，以没有气急、气短，身体微出汗为限度，每次可行走15至20分钟，中途还可依据自身情况

ries from person to person.

Abdominal rubbing after meals also needs timing and skills. There are many important organs in the abdomen, where various vessels are connected. Therefore, rubbing abdomen frequently can build up bodies and expand life span by freeing meridians and network vessels, and accelerating circulation of qi and blood. But rubbing abdomen immediately after meals can accelerate the peristalsis of the stomach and push those partially digested food into the small intestine prematurely, which subsequently not only increases the burden of the small intestine, but also leads to the fact that the nutrients in food are not fully digested and absorbed. Therefore, it is better to rub abdomen after dinner and before bedtime. And it is better to rub abdomen gently after dinner Shen Que (CV 8), in the middle of the umbilicus, has the function of tonifying deficiency, securing the root and quieting the spirit. The abdomen is divided into the upper and lower parts by Shen Que (CV 8). Rub Shen Que (CV 8), then the upper abdomen and finally the lower abdomen counterclockwise and clockwise for 108 times respectively with one hand placed on the other. This way can not only treat many diseases, but also lose weight and enhance sleep.

5 Preventing Dampness in Late Summer

Late summer refers to the period between late summer and early autumn. It is characterized by high humidity, so health preservation in this period may focus on dampness prevention. In late summer, it rains frequently and the evaporation of rains in-

休息。所以,饭后散步应该因人而异,不可拘泥。

饭后摩腹也应注意时间和技巧。人体腹腔内有重要的脏器,是诸多脉络的起止联络处,经常按摩腹部,可疏通经络,加速气血运行,起到强身健体,延年益寿的作用。但是如果饭后即刻大力按摩腹部,会加快胃的蠕动,令那些还未消化完的食物过早地被推入小肠,不仅增加了小肠的负担,而且也会使食物的营养素得不到充分的消化和吸收。揉腹最佳时间应在晚饭后、临睡前,食后若行摩腹,则手法宜轻柔。脐窝正中的神阙穴具有补虚、固本、安神的作用。以此为中心,分上、下腹。先按神阙,再按上腹和下腹。具体方法:双手重叠先逆时针后顺时针方向略用力搓摩腹部各 108 次,这样,不仅可以调理许多疾病,还能减肥,调节睡眠。

5 长夏防湿邪

长夏指夏末秋初时期,其气候特点是多湿,所以养生应防湿邪伤人。长夏多雨潮湿,水气上升,空气中湿度最大,加之或因外伤雾露,或

creases the humidity in the air. If a person is attacked by fog, wet with sweat or caught by rains, or lives in a damp place, he will contract dampness and develop diseases. Modern scientific researches have also confirmed that relatively high humidity in the air hinders the cooling of the body in an evaporative way. Evaporation is recognized as the main way to dissipate heat in heated condition. Large amount of moisture in the air makes it difficult to balance the heat by evaporation, which leads to obstacles in body temperature regulation, presenting chest tightness, palpitation, depression and fatigue.

因汗出沾衣,或因涉水淋雨,或因居处潮湿,以至感受湿邪而发病者多。现代研究表明,当环境中空气湿度相对大时,有碍于机体蒸发散热,而高温条件下蒸发是人体的主要散热形式。空气中大量水分使机体难以通过水分蒸发而保持产热和散热的平衡,出现体温调节障碍,常常表现出胸闷、心悸、精神萎靡、全身乏力。

In late summer, it is better to eat more light and digestive foods instead of greasy ones. Despite the humid weather, diet should not be too cold, because cold food easily hurts the spleen yang, which may cause devitalized spleen yang. In addition, due to the saying that diseases originate from food, keep away from rotten and spoiled food and unboiled water. Raw fruits and vegetables must be cleaned. To discharge dampness and heat through urine, it is necessary to eat more foods with the function of clearing heat and disinhibiting dampness, such as mung bean porridge, lotus leaf porridge and red bean porridge.

长夏季节最好少吃油腻食物,多吃清淡易于消化的食物。天气虽然潮湿闷热,但饮食也不应过凉,因为寒凉饮食最易伤脾的阳气,造成脾阳不振。此外,一定要把好"病从口入"这一关,不吃腐烂变质食物,不喝生水,生吃瓜果蔬菜一定要洗净,并应多食清热利湿的食物,使体内湿热之邪从小便排出。常用清热利湿食物,以绿豆粥、荷叶粥、红小豆粥较为理想。

Section 4 Liver

第4节 肝脏保养

Liver, as the hub of ascending, descending, entering and exiting of qi, governs free coursing and regulates qi activity. It governs blood storage and

肝主疏泄,调理全身气机,是气机升降出入的枢纽;肝主藏血,是贮藏血液、调节

adjusts the blood volume. The two functions of liver-free coursing and blood storing-are mutually connected and balanced. If liver fails to course freely, liver qi will be depressed, inducing qi stagnation and blood stasis; if liver over-courses, the function of storing blood will be affected, leading to bleeding. Therefore, liver cultivation should be centered on these two aspects.

血量的重要器官。肝主疏泄与主藏血功能相互联系、协调平衡。如果疏泄不及，肝气郁结，可致各种气滞血瘀的病理变化；如果疏泄太过，影响藏血功能，又可导致各种出血之症。所以肝脏保健应以二者为中心。

1 Proper Diet

Free coursing is an important factor to promote the transportation and transformation of spleen and stomach. Protein and sugar that liver needs can be obtained from diet. So it is necessary to keep a balanced diet. Protein, carbohydrate, fat, vitamins and minerals in foods should be kept in corresponding proportions. Eat more fresh vegetables and fruits instead of spicy foods. Foods rich in fiber are advised, for they can prevent constipation and promote bile secretion and excretion. Therefore it is an important approach to improve free coursing. Don't overeat or starve yourself, for irregular eating habits can cause abnormal secretion of digestive juices and disorders of liver function.

1 合理饮食

肝的疏泄功能是促进脾胃运化功能的一个重要环节。肝脏本身必需的蛋白质和糖类等，要从饮食中获得。所以饮食要保持均衡，食物中的蛋白质、碳水化合物、脂肪、维生素、矿物质等要保持相应的比例；尽量少吃辛辣食品，多吃新鲜蔬菜、水果等。同时，还宜适当食用含纤维素多的食物，高纤维食物有助于保持大便通畅，有利于胆汁的分泌和排泄，这是促进肝脏疏泄功能的一项重要措施。不要暴饮暴食或常忍饥不食，饥、饱不匀的饮食习惯，会引起消化液分泌异常，导致肝脏功能的失调。

To protect liver, it is unfavorable to eat too much fat. Avoid alcoholism, for liver has a limit role in alcohol metabolism. Excessive alcohol drinking can cause loss of appetite, deficiency of protein and B vitamins, and even alcoholic intoxication. Long-term alcohol abuse can also lead to fatty liver

为保护肝脏，不宜进食太多的脂肪。切忌嗜酒，肝脏代谢酒精的能力是有限的，过量饮酒可引起食欲减退，造成蛋白质及 B 族维生素缺乏，甚则发生酒精中毒，

and hepatic cirrhosis. Healthy people weighed below 60 kilograms can only metabolize 60 grams of alcohol per day. If more alcohol is drunk, the health of liver will be affected. What's worse is that the life will be threatened. Therefore, to protect liver in daily life, excessive alcohol drinking should be avoided.

长期酗酒还可导致脂肪肝、肝硬化。体重60千克的健康人,每天只能代谢60克酒精,若超过限量,就会影响肝脏健康,甚至危及生命。因此,日常生活中切忌过量饮酒,以免损伤肝脏。

2 Avoiding Anger and Preventing Depression

2 戒怒防郁

Moods are closely related to the role of liver in free coursing. Repeat, persistent or radical moods will directly affect the free coursing of liver. Liver likes orderly reaching and is related to anger, so depression and rage will impair liver, resulting in depressed liver qi or hyperactivity of liver fire. Therefore, it is necessary to gradually cultivate the capability of controlling extreme emotions and eliminating bad moods. Try to be calm, optimistic and cheerful so that liver fire can be calmed and liver qi can be flowed smoothly.

人的情志调畅与肝的疏泄功能密切相关。反复、持久或过激的情志,都会直接影响肝的疏泄功能。肝喜条达,在志为怒,抑郁、暴怒最易伤肝,导致肝气郁结或肝火亢盛的病理变化。因此,要逐渐培养控制自己的过激情绪和疏导不良情绪的能力,要尽力做到心平气和、乐观开朗、无忧无虑,从而使肝火平息,肝气得顺。

3 Preventing Disease and Nourishing Liver

3 防病健肝

Preventive care should be focused on two aspects: on the one hand, to prevent the invasion of pathogenic factors, especially the infectious hepatitis in China; on the other hand, exercise for health preservation may be strengthened to improve liver function and enhance disease resistance.

预防保健的要求应着眼于两个方面:一方面是预防病邪入侵,在我国应特别注意预防传染性肝炎;另一方面是经常进行保健锻炼,增强肝脏功能,提高抗病能力。

3.1 Preventing Infectious Hepatitis

3.1 预防传染性肝炎

Prevention of hepatitis is a positive and active measure to protect liver. The effective ways are: to decrease sources by census and vaccination, to block transmission through improving food hygiene and good management of blood products. In addition,

预防肝炎是保护肝脏的一项积极、主动措施。其有效的方法是:做好普查和预防接种工作,减少传染源;搞好饮食卫生,阻断饮食传染

medications are necessary. For example, Yin Chen (*Herba Artemisiae Scopariae*), Ban Lan Gen (*Radix Isatidis*), Jin Qian Cao (*Herba Lysimachiae*), Shan Zha, Mai Ya (*Fructus Hordei Germinatus*, Stir-fried), Shen Qu (*Medicated Leaven*, Stir-fried) are effective in preventing Hepatitis A.

途径;管理好血液制品,阻断输血传染途径;同时可配合药物,如服用茵陈、板蓝根、金钱草、焦三仙(焦山楂、炒麦芽、炒神曲)等药物对预防甲肝有一定效果。

Additionally, it is forbidden to take large dose of drugs that do harms to liver for a long time, such as chlorpromazine sulfanilamide, isoniazide and phenobarbital preparations. If necessary, liver-protecting drugs and other comprehensive measures can be used to protect liver functions. Besides, drink more water to supplement the body fluid, enhance the blood circulation, promote metabolism and glands secretion, improve digestion, absorption and waste elimination, and lower the damage of metabolites and toxins to the liver.

另外,应避免长期大量服用损害肝脏的药物。如氯丙嗪磺胺、异烟肼、苯巴比妥制剂等,如因治疗需要,则应配合一些保肝药物及其他综合性保肝措施,以免损伤肝脏功能。同时,多喝水以补充体液,增强血液循环,促进新陈代谢,促进腺体分泌,以利消化、吸收和废物的排除,减少代谢产物和毒素对肝脏的损害。

3.2 Exercise for Liver Nourish

The principles of liver-preserving exercise is to stretch smoothly and slowly, which conforms to the features of upbearing, effusing and orderly reaching of liver. Therefore, walking, outing in spring, ball games and those traditional workouts, such as taiji quan, Eight Trigram Boxing (Ba Duan Jin), Sinew-transformation exercise (Yi Jin Jing) can not only promote smooth flow of qi and blood, exhalation of the old and inhalation of the new, but also keep body strong, nourish the liver and cultivate the mind. Subsequently the liver is preserved.

3.2 健肝锻炼

保健肝脏的运动锻炼的原则是动作舒展、畅达、缓慢,符合肝气升发、畅达的特点。散步、踏青、打球,及传统的健身术诸如太极拳、八段锦、易筋经等,既能使人气血通畅,促进吐故纳新,强健身体,又可以怡情养肝,达到护肝保健之目的。

4 Nourishing Liver in Spring

Liver is related to spring. In warm spring, human activity is gradually increased and metabolism

4 春季养肝

肝主春,肝气与春季相通应。春天温暖的气候里,

is increasingly vigorous. Therefore, blood circulation should be sped up and nutrition supply should be increased so as to meet the needs of human life activities. The speeding up of blood circulation mainly lies in the regulation of blood, while the increase of nutrition supply largely depends on digestion and absorption. Both of them are associated with the physiological functions of liver. If liver functions abnormally and can not adapt to the physiological changes in spring, a series of diseases will be presented. Mental diseases and liver diseases, in particular, are easily developed in the spring. According to the statistics, the incidence of mental diseases is the highest in March and April, which indicates a response to the season. Therefore, don't work too hard, otherwise it will increase the burden of liver. Apart from taking liver-protecting and hypotensive drugs, patients with liver disease and hypertension should closely monitor liver function, blood lipid and blood pressure in spring. To prevent worsening, those with mental disorders should stay away from mental stimulation.

人的活动量日渐增加,新陈代谢亦将日趋旺盛。因而,在人体内,无论是血液循环,还是营养供给,都要相应加快、增多,以适应人体各种生命活动的需要。血液循环的加快主要在于血量的调节;营养供给的增加则重在消化、吸收。这些均与肝脏的生理功能有关。若肝脏功能失常,不能适应春季的生理变化,则出现一系列病证。特别是精神病及肝病患者,易在春季发病。据统计,精神病发病率以三四月份最高,这是季节对机体影响的一种反应。所以,春天不要过分劳累,以免加重肝脏的负担。素有肝病及高血压病的患者,在春季,除按医嘱服用养肝、降压的药物外,应特别注意监测肝功能、血脂和血压。有精神疾患者在春天要注意避免精神刺激,以免加重病情。

Section 5 Kidney

第5节 肾脏保养

According to TCM, the growth, development and aging are closely related to kidneys. To be more specific, the speed of aging and the extent of lifespan largely depend on kidney essence. Rich kidney

中医学认为,人体生长发育、衰老与肾关系密切。可以说衰老与否、衰老速度、寿命长短,在很大程度上决

essence can slow the aging process and prolong lifespan. On the contrary, deficient kidney essence will lead to early aging, rapid aging speed, and short life expectancy. Therefore, kidney cultivation should mainly focus on the maintenance of kidney essence.

1 Proper Diet

Kidneys itself need plenty of protein and carbohydrate, so foods rich in protein and vitamin, low in fat, cholesterol and salt are conducive to kidney, such as lean meat, fish, bean products, mushrooms, fruits, vegetables, winter melon, watermelon, green beans, red beans, etc.

1.1 Moderate Intake of Protein

High-protein diet will produce more metabolites that must be discharged from kidneys, such as ketone body and non-essential amino acids, which will increase the burden of kidney and do harms to kidney. On the contrary, small intake of protein can affect re-synthesis of tissues. Therefore, protein intake should be moderate.

1.2 Avoid High-fat, High-sugar and High-salt Foods

Starchy foods are rich in sugar. Excessive intake of sugar and fat will lead to the accumulation of glycogen and lipid in the body, which results in increased weight and blood fat, causing atherosclerosis, thrombosis and hypertension. Subsequently, kidneys are atrophied and degenerated. High-salt

定于肾中精气的强弱。肾气旺盛，人就不易衰老，衰老速度也缓慢，寿命长；反之，肾气衰，衰老就提前，衰老的速度也快，寿命会相应缩短。所以中医养生，尤重养肾。肾脏保养主要着眼于保养肾中精气。

1 饮食保肾

肾脏本身需要较大量的蛋白质和糖类，故有利于肾脏的饮食宜适当选择高蛋白、高维生素、低脂肪、低胆固醇、低盐的食物。常选用的食品有瘦肉、鱼类、豆制品、蘑菇、水果、蔬菜、冬瓜、西瓜、绿豆、赤小豆等。

1.1 摄入蛋白质应适量

过高的蛋白饮食会产生较多的代谢产物从肾排出，如酮体和非必需氨基酸都必须从肾排出，加重肾脏负担而不利肾脏健康；但蛋白质过少会影响组织重新合成。因此要注意摄入蛋白质应适量。

1.2 避免高脂、高糖、高盐食物

淀粉类食物主要含糖类，糖和脂肪摄入过多，则体内糖原和脂质沉积，使人肥胖，血脂增高，易致动脉粥样硬化、血栓形成、高血压等，使肾脏萎缩变性，严重危害

diet affects water metabolism and increases burdens on kidneys. It is advisable to keep the daily intake of salt below 6 g.

肾脏。高盐饮食影响水液代谢,加重肾脏负担。每日用盐以少于6克为好。

1.3 Moderate Water Drinking

Individuals should drink water based on their own needs. It is unnecessary to drink too much water, or to control the water drinking. Either extremity of water drinking can impair kidneys: drinking too much will increase burdens on kidneys; drinking too little will lead to the deposition of uric acid salt in kidneys. Therefore, the daily consumption of water should be kept above 1 200 ml, which means 2-3 bottles of mineral water.

1.3 适量饮水

饮水的多少,应根据需要,不必过多饮用,更无必要自己控制,应以自觉舒适为度,过多过少都可伤肾,过多则加重肾脏负担,过少则易引起肾中尿酸盐沉着。一般每日饮水量不能少于1 200毫升,即普通矿泉水瓶2～3瓶。

1.4 Be Cautious with Drugs

Some drugs are harmful to kidneys, such as mercury chloride, carbon tetrachloride, barbitone kind, sulfanilamide preparations, polymyxin, cephalothin, kanamycin and neomycin, griseofulvin, streptomycin and so on. These drugs should be used carefully. If necessary, take small dose of these drugs or add other drugs so as to avoid damage to kidney functions.

1.4 慎用药物

有些药物对肾脏有损害,如二氯化汞、四氯化碳、巴比妥类、磺胺制剂、多黏菌素、先锋霉素、卡那霉素、新霉素、灰黄霉素、链霉素等等,这些药宜慎用。非用不可时,应采取短期少量或适当配伍,以免损伤肾功能。

2 Preserving Essence through Continence

Essence is regarded as one of three treasures of the human body. Therefore, essence cultivation is an important part of body building up. Individuals should prevent masturbation before getting married and avoid sexual indulgence during married life. Kidney damage is caused by loss of essence. Therefore, to preserve essence through continence is an important method to strengthen kidneys. According to modern immunology, long-term sexual indulgence can decline the regulating function of the immune

2 节欲保精

精为人身三宝之一,保精是强身的重要环节。在未婚之前要防止"手淫",既婚则需节欲,绝不可放纵性欲。所谓"伤肾"实由失精过多引起,因此,节欲保精,是强肾的重要方法之一。现代免疫学亦认为,长期的性生活过度,会使人体的免疫系统的调节功能减退,因为性交频

system, as frequent intercourse can cause intense excitement systemically in a short time, consume enormous energy and weaken the adaptability of organ functions.

繁,在短时间内多次引起高度的全身性兴奋,可使人体能量大量消耗,器官功能的适应性减弱。

3 Supplementing Kidney through Medication

3 药物补肾

After the age of 35 for a female and 40 for a male, the essence in kidney becomes deficient, which results in the recession of qi and blood in yangming meridians, presenting gradually wilted complexion and hair loss. Therefore, to preserve kidney essence, herbs that can enrich and nourish kidney yin and warm and supplement kidney qi are necessary for women aged above 35 and men above 40. The common medications are:

女性35岁、男子40岁以后,肾中精气不足,导致阳明经脉中的气血衰退,表现为面部开始憔悴,头发逐渐脱落。因此,妇女在35岁、男子40岁后宜服用滋养肾阴、温补肾气药物以养肾之精气。常用方药如:

Qing Gong Shou Tao Wan (*Peach Pills in Qing Court*): It, previous called Flat Peach Pill, is a widely used patent drug to supplement yin and assist yang in the court of Qing dynasty palace. It consists of more than ten kidney-supplementing herbs, such as Yi Zhi Ren (*Fructus Alpiniae Oxyphyllae*), Sheng Di (*Radix Rehmanniae*), Gou Qi Zi (*Fructus Lycii*) and Hu Tao (*Semen Juglandis*). Based on supplementing kidney and nourishing yang, securing root and cultivating the origin, this drug can effectively supply the congenital and acquired essence, supplement and regulate qi and blood, free network vessels and collaterals, and as well as eliminate stasis and dispel stagnation. In this way, viscera are nourished; illnesses, prevented and treated; aging, prevented; lifespan, prolonged.

清宫寿桃丸:原名蟠桃丸,系清代宫廷中广为应用的补阴助阳的中成药。该方由益智仁、生地、枸杞子、胡桃等十余种补肾中药组成,以补肾养阳、固本培元为根本,能够有效补充人体先天及后天之精气,调补气血,通经活络,消瘀祛滞,滋养脏腑,祛病防病,延缓衰老,延年益寿。

Gui Ling Ji (*Longevity set*): This drug was offered to Emperor Jiajing by Shao Zhijie, a noble in Ming dynasty. It was advocated by many emperors

龟龄集:此药为明代乡士邵之节献给嘉靖皇帝的宝药,历代皇帝大多对此十分

and then introduced to the folk. The drug is made up of 33 herbs, such as Lu Rong (*Cornu Cervi Pantotrichum*), Ren Shen (*Radix Ginseng*), Shu Di Huang (*Radix Rehmanniae Preparata*), Hai Ma (*hippocampus*), Du Zhong (*Cortex Eucommiae*), Rou Cong Rong (*Herba Cistanches*), Bu Gu Zhi (*Fructus Psoraleae*), Tu Si Zi (*Semen Cuscutae*), Gou Qi Zi (*Fructus Lycii*), Yin Yang Huo (*Herba Epimedii*), Ding Xiang (*Flos Caryophylli*), Da Qing Ye (*Folium Isatidis*), Sha Ren (*Fructus Amomi*), Fu Ling (*Poria*), silkworm moth, Tian Dong (*Radix Asparagi*) and Dang Gui (*Radix Angelicae Sinensis*). It has the function of warming kidney, assisting yang and boosting qi and blood. Studies have demonstrated that this drug can improve the adaptation, enhance non-specific and specific immune function, stimulate and inhibit the central nervous system, and directly stimulate cardiac muscles. Taking the drug regularly can delay the aging by promoting the metabolism of declining protein and the important nucleic acid in the cells.

推崇，后传入民间。此药由鹿茸、人参、熟地黄、海马、杜仲、肉苁蓉、补骨脂、菟丝子、枸杞子、淫羊藿、丁香、大青叶、砂仁、茯苓、蚕蛾、天冬、当归等 33 种药物组成。功能温肾助阳、补益气血。实验表明它可提高机体适应能力，增强免疫功能；增强调节中枢神经系统能力，有兴奋和抑制中枢双向作用；有强心作用，并以直接兴奋心肌为主。老年人常服本品，可促进老年人日已衰退的蛋白质及细胞内重要物质核酸的代谢，从而延缓衰老。

4 Strengthening Kidney through Exercises

4 练功强肾

4.1 Lifting with Elbow Flexed

4.1 屈肘上举

Sit straight with one leg shoulder-width apart from the other, and then lift two hands laterally to reach the horizon of ears with elbow flexed and fingers extended. Finally, further elevate hands to the point where ribs are stretched and then withdraw the hands. This exercise should be done for 3 to 5 times a day with 3 to 5 elevations every time.

端坐，两腿自然分开，与肩同宽，双手屈肘侧举，手指伸直向上，与两耳平。然后，双手上举，以两胁部感觉有所牵动为度，随即复原，连续做 3～5 次为一遍，每日做 3～5 遍。

4.2 Casting

4.2 抛空

Sit with left palm rested on the left leg, and then flex right elbow and do casting for 3 to 5 times

端坐，左臂自然屈肘，掌朝下放于左腿上；右臂屈肘，

with the palm facing upside. Switch to the left elbow and do the same movements. This exercise can be done for 3 to 5 times a day. Attention should be paid to the breathing: inhale while casting and exhale while withdrawing.

手掌向上，做抛物动作 3～5 次，然后，右臂放于右腿上，左手做抛空动作，与右手动作相同，每日可做 3～5 遍。在做抛物动作时，要注意与呼吸配合：手上抛时吸气，复原时呼气。

4.3 Swinging Legs

Whiling sitting with legs naturally placed, individuals first slowly turn the body around for 3-5 times, and then dangle two feet and sway them back and forth for more than 10 times. This set of movements can exercise waist and knees, and boost kidneys and strengthen waist.

4.3 荡腿

端坐，两腿自然下垂，先缓慢左右转动身体 3～5 次，然后两脚悬空，前后摆动十余次。此动作可活动腰、膝，有益肾强腰之功效。

4.4 Rubbing Waist

While sitting with clothes and belt loosened, individuals are instructed to rub hands until they are warmed and then place hands on the waist and rub it from the superior to the inferior until the waist is warmed. To rub waist is actually to tuina acupoints on the waist, such as Ming Men (GV 4), Shen Shu (BL 23), Qihai Shu (BL 24) and Dachang Shu (BL 25). Most of these acupoints are related to kidneys. When waist is rubbed warm, it can dredge meridian and network vessels, move qi and quicken the blood and warm kidneys and strengthen waist.

4.4 摩腰

端坐，宽衣，将腰带松开，双手相搓，以略觉发热为度；再将双手置于腰间，上下搓摩腰部，直至腰部感觉发热为止。搓摩腰部，实际是对腰部命门、肾俞、气海俞、大肠俞等穴的自我按摩，而这些穴位大多与肾脏有关。待搓至发热时，可起到疏通经络，行气活血、温肾壮腰的作用。

4.5 Pronouncing Chui Sound

Stand straight with two feet placed together. First lift crossed hands to the ceiling and bend down with hands touching the ground, and then squat with hands placed on knees and pronounce the Chinese character Chui silently. It could be done for more than ten times in succession. This exercise is one part of Six-word Qi Gong and can secure kidney

4.5 "吹"字功

直立，双脚并拢，两手交叉上举过头，然后弯腰，双手触地，继而下蹲，双手抱膝，心中默念"吹"字音，可连续做十余次。本功属于"六字诀"中的"吹"字功，常做可固肾气。

qi.

5 Nourishing kidney in winter

Kidney is related to winter. In winter, yang stores inside the body and the physiological activities are also slowed. At this point, kidneys need to prepare enough energy for the winter and stores a certain amount of energy for the coming year, so it is very important to preserve kidneys. To preserve kidneys, we should be careful with the diet. Energy, vitamins and inorganic salt should be supplied. Animal-based foods and beans are advised. Foods like, mutton, goose and duck meat, beans, walnuts, chestnuts, black fungus, sesame seed, yams and carrots are necessary in winter.

5 冬季养肾

肾通于冬气。冬季，人体阳气内敛，人体的生理活动也有所收敛。此时，肾既要为维持冬季热量支出准备足够的能量，又要为来年贮存一定的能量，所以此时养肾至关重要。饮食上就要时刻关注肾的调养，注意热量的补充，要多吃些动物性食品和豆类，补充维生素和无机盐。羊肉、鹅肉、鸭肉、大豆、核桃、栗子、木耳、芝麻、红薯、萝卜等均是冬季适宜食物。

Part Two
Rehabilitation of Traditional Chinese Medicine

下篇
中医康复学

Introduction

概　论

Rehabilitation (Kang Fu) of traditional Chinese medicine has a long history. Both characters of "Kang" and "Fu" were explained in *Explanation to Semantics* (Er Ya). In The Old *Book of Tang Dynasty* (Jiu Tang Shu), the phrase "Kang Fu" was appeared in a sentence describing Wu Zetian, a female emperor in Tang dynasty. In *Recovery of All Diseases* (Wan Bing Hui Chun) by GONG Tingxian in Ming dynasty, the phrase "Kang Fu" was officially included in TCM literature as a medical word. Actually, many words such as Pin Fu, Kang Jian, Zai Zao, Fu Jiu and Fu Kang are similar to Kang Fu in meanings. Over the past thousands years, with the efforts made by medical experts of dynasties, rehabilitation of TCM has been constantly supplemented and gradually developed into a comprehensive discipline as an important part of TCM. With the deepening of the clinical practice of TCM rehabilitation, more and more importance is attached to the research and conclusion of the theories and methods of TCM rehabilitation.

中医康复具有悠久的历史。早在《尔雅》中就有对"康"和"复"的解释。在《旧唐书》中记载武则天的内容里有"上以所疾康复",已经出现"康复"一词,到明代龚廷贤的《万病回春》,明确将"康复"一词引入了中医学典籍。历代中医古籍文献中,"平复""康健""再造""复旧""福康"等常用语中,也都蕴含"康复"的意思。数千年来,在历代医家的努力下,中医康复学术内容不断得到补充与发展,渐形成的一门综合性学科,成为中医学的重要组成部分。随着中医康复临床实践的深入开展,对中医康复学理论和方法的研究和总结,越来越引起人们的重视。

1 Definition of TCM Rehabilitation

1 中医康复学的学科定义

Under the guidance of TCM theory, TCM rehabilitation refers to a discipline that researches on

中医康复学是在中医学理论指导下,研究中医康复

the basic theory, methods and application of rehabilitation with TCM. To cure physical impairments and disabilities caused by internal or surgical, chronic or acute diseases and aging, TCM rehabilitation, under the guidance of TCM basic theories, focuses on how to apply methods such as acupuncture, Chinese herbs, tuina, lifestyle regulation, diet, entertainment, natural factors, exercises and daoyin to improve and restore the body functions in physiological, psychological and social statuses.

学基本理论、方法及其应用的一门学科。是针对各种内外科急慢性病症,以及年迈体衰等,导致机体的病损伤残诸症,以中医基础理论为指导,研究如何辨证综合地运用针药按摩、起居作息、饮食娱乐、自然因子、功法导引等多种方法,使受损机体在生理机能、心理道德、社会适应诸方面得以改善或恢复正常的中医分支学科。

1.1 Research Subjects and Scope

The academic research focuses on disorders. TCM rehabilitation aims at improving and restoring body functions. Centering on this focus, the subjects mainly are patients with disabilities, chronic diseases, aging problems, malignant tumors and acute febrile diseases. As a applied discipline, TCM rehabilitation can be divided into three parts, namely basic theory, basic method and clinical practice. Extended from its academic core, the contents include basic theory, fundamental concept and principle of TCM rehabilitation, diagnosis, treatment and assessment of rehabilitation and as well as diagnosis and treatment for specific diseases.

1.1 学科研究对象与范畴

中医康复学的学术研究的核心着眼点是“障碍”,目标是出现障碍后机体的“恢复”和“改善”。围绕这一核心,其学科研究的人群对象主要是伤残疾患、慢性病、老年病、恶性肿瘤及急性热病后等存在功能障碍的患者。作为一门应用学科,其学科性质决定其研究范畴划分为:学科基础理论、基本方法和临床应用三大版块体系;并由其学术核心具体延伸展开其内容,包括中医康复学的理论基础、基本观念和原则、康复诊断、康复疗法、康复评价,以及针对具体病证的康复诊疗等。

1.2 Discipline Orientation

Pertaining to TCM, TCM rehabilitation is a branch discipline with independent content and

1.2 学科定位

中医康复学是隶属于中医学,具有自己相对独立内

tasks and close relations with other TCM disciplines. The basic theory, fundamental concept and rudimentary methods of TCM are all deepened and applied in TCM rehabilitation. Therefore, this discipline is interrelated with TCM basic theory, TCM diagnostics, science of Chinese materia medica, science of formulas, acupuncture and moxibustion, tuina and as well as herbal diet. As a science on lives, the scope of TCM rehabilitation can be divided based on the statuses of life existences. It is closely related with the following branches of TCM.

容与任务的中医分支学科，并与中医学其他学科存在紧密的联系。中医康复学作为中医学的重要组成部分，中医学的基础理论、基本观念、基本方法等同样在本学科渗透并得以深化运用。因此，本学科与中医基础理论、中医诊断学、中药学、方剂学、针灸学、推拿学、药膳食疗学等存在错综交叉的关系。中医学是一门生命科学，以生命存在的状态为依据分化其学科范畴，中医康复学与下列几大中医分支学科关系密切。

First, TCM rehabilitation is independently equal to TCM preventive medicine and TCM clinical medicine. Due to the consistency of life, these disciplines are interrelated with each other and form into a unity.

首先，中医康复学与中医预防医学、中医临床医学是相对独立的平级学科关系。但由于生命状态的连续性，病前、病中、病后实无泾渭分明的界限，因此这几门学科是相互渗透、紧密联系的关系，共同形成一个统一体。

Secondly, the relations between TCM rehabilitation and TCM health preservation is close and complicated. Health preservation is to nurture life, and it involves all statuses from the birth to death. The science of TCM health preservation is a comprehensive integrity involving prevention, health care, treatment, rehabilitation, psychology, behavior and society. In terms of the scope, TCM rehabilitation is a part of health preservation. As for the

其次，中医康复学与中医养生学关系更为紧密而复杂。养生就是“养护生命”，涵盖了生命从孕育到消亡的全部状态，中医养生学实质是涉及预防、保健、治疗、康复、心理、行为、社会等领域的一个多学科群综合体。从研究对象范畴上看，中医康

task or target, health preservation aims at longevity, while rehabilitation targets at improving and restoring body functions. From this point, two disciplines are relatively independent. Meanwhile, how to restore health and reduce the consumption is also the way to reach longevity, which is also an important part of health preservation. Therefore, the science of TCM rehabilitation has absorbed a great amount of achievements from the science of TCM health preservation, enriched its content and formed into a unique system with the theories and methods of preventive rehabilitation, health-preserving rehabilitation and therapeutic rehabilitation. As a matter of fact, TCM rehabilitation and TCM health preservation share many approaches, such as acupuncture, tuina, qi gong, diet, entertainment and medication. These methods are characterized by preserving and treating. The science of health preservation focuses on preserving, while rehabilitation on preserving or treating or even the combination of both on the basis of the specific condition.

复学可视为中医养生学的一部分。同时，从一门学科的任务或者目标来看，中医养生学是以“健康长寿”为其最高学术目标，中医康复学的学术目标则是障碍后机体的“恢复”和“改善”，由此可见两者又是相对独立的。应该看到：病后如何恢复健康、减少生命耗损，从而达到相对长寿的目的，也是中医养生学研究的重要内容。正因如此，中医康复学在其学科的发展过程中，吸取大量中医养生学的成就，丰富其专业内容，形成了独具特色的预防康复、养生康复和疗养保健等中医康复学的理论与方法体系；中医康复学与中医养生学所采用的方法，有许多相同，如针灸、按摩、气功、饮食、娱乐、药物调养等，这些方法具有“养”和“治”兼备的特点，养生学侧重于利用其“养”，中医康复学则针对患者不同的康复阶段而选择其“养”或“治”或“养治结合”。

1.3 Academic Characteristics

Under the guidance of basic thoughts and theory of TCM, the science of TCM rehabilitation has evolved along the path of "theory-practice-theory-practice". Over the past thousands years, unique academic characteristics have been formed.

1.3 学术特点

中医康复学在历经数千年的发展过程中，在中医学的基本思想和理论对其学术起着根本性的指导作用下，在从“理论-实践-理论-实践”

循环往复的发展前进中，形成了其颇具特色的学术特点。

First, the integrity of prevention, treatment, health preservation and rehabilitation. Sticking to practice these four parts, the approaches adopted have multiple functions. For example, qi gong and daoyin, diet, medication, bathing, sun bathe and emotion regulation can not only prevent diseases, but also treat diseases.

其一，是“预防-治疗-养生-康复”一体的特点。中医康复学始终坚持四位一体的实践。所采用的方法往往同时具有预防保健、祛病延年等多重作用，如气功导引、食物调养、药物调摄、泉水饮浴、日光沐浴、情志调适等方法，既能施于未病之先又能用于既病之后，既可用于养生防病又可用于医疗康复。

Secondly, holism outweighs function recovery. Rehabilitation aims at restore health. Under the guidance of “physical-psychological-social-moral” concept, TCM rehabilitation targets at the overall recovery in these four aspects and emphasizes the harmonious relations of body and mind based on the thought that all disorders are the results of disharmony between body and mind. Apart from rehabilitation exercises, traditional sports, acupuncture and moxibustion, tuina, diet and medication, rehabilitation approaches with focus on emotions, psychology, entertainment and music are emphasized to improve or restore the functions in physical, psychological and social levels. TCM focuses more on the qi transformation rather than physical structure. Therefore, as a branch of TCM, the science of TCM rehabilitation has its own features and advantages on function recovery. Through supporting vital qi, promoting the circulation of qi and blood and restoring balance of qi transformation, the smooth

其二，是强调整体康复，长于功能康复的特点。康复的目的是最大限度地恢复健康，在中医超前的“生理-心理-社会适应性-道德”四位一体的健康观的根本指导下，中医康复学同样强调四位一体的整体康复，强调“形与神俱”的辩证和谐关系，认为任何疾患导致机体不得康复都是形神失调的结果。康复手段不离形神，除运用康复训练、传统体育、针灸、按摩、食疗、药疗等治形的康复方法外，更突出情志、心理娱乐、音乐等康复疗法的作用，力求使受损机体在生理机能、心理道德、社会适应诸方面得以改善或恢复正常。在对人体生理、病理的认识上，中

qi-blood circulation, construction-defence hormony and unity of form and spirit are achieved, and in turn, the purpose of rehabilitation is achieved.

医学本身具有详于气化功能而略于形质结构的特点。因此作为中医学分支的中医康复学,在功能康复方面,其思想和方法具有特色和优势。在康复治疗上强调功能的恢复,其作用的发挥均在于扶持正气、疏通气血、恢复气化平衡,以使气血通畅、营卫通达、形与神俱,达到康复目的。

Thirdly, worship nature and focus on self-recovery. TCM rehabilitation insists that the source of recovery lies in the nature, society and human body. Therefore, instead of passive rehabilitation, the rehabilitation approaches should conform to the nature, stem from society and rely on the capability of self-recovery. These approaches often take advantages of the necessities of life (such as air, sunshine, temperature and food) and daily activities (work, exercise, rest, sleep, clothing and entertainment), make full use of the exchange of "material-energy-information" between human and environment. Mind regulation and breathing exercises are emphasized so as to recover positively with pleasure.

其三,是崇尚取法自然,强调自我修复的特点。中医康复学自来坚持:康复之源存于自然之中,存于社会之中,存于人体自身。其康复方法崇尚取法于自然、取材于社会,强调依靠人体自身主动修复能力,而不只是被动的机械康复。常常利用人体生命活动中原本所需,如空气、阳光、温度、饮食等不可或缺的因素,劳作、运动、休息、睡眠、服饰、文娱等日常生活内容,充分利用人体与环境在进行"物质-能量-信息"交换过程中一切积极因素进行康复。强调认知心态调整、不良心理纠正,以及以意领气、以气导形的功法修炼等,使身心合一、主观能动、心情愉快地康复。

Fourthly, both the internal and external factors and comprehensive treatment are emphasized. Due

其四,是强调内外并重、综合调治的特点。中医康复

to the complexity of life, TCM rehabilitation should combine the external environment and individual conditions. Based on syndrome identification, approaches for both internal and external conditions are applied with acupuncture, tuina, exercises, daoyin, medication, diet and natural factors. Practicality is of top priority.

学充分认识到生命活动的复杂性，强调康复应从多维度进行，综合天时、地宜和个体具体情况，以辨证为依据，内外并进，杂合针灸按摩、功法导引、药治食疗、自然因子等多种方法，以实用为要，以实效为目的，综合应用，灵活施治。

2 Basic Theory and Methods

2 基本理论和方法

2.1 Theoretical Basis of TCM Rehabilitation

2.1 中医康复学的理论基础

As a branch of TCM, TCM rehabilitation inherits its theories from TCM theoretical system and deepens them. Therefore, the concepts, theories and methods of TCM are also reflected in TCM rehabilitation. For example, the holism, the concept of life, disease, identification, health preservation and prevention; the theories of yin and yang, five element, zang-fu organs, meridians and collaterals, qi and blood, essence, qi and spirit; the therapeutic methods like medicines, acupuncture and moxibustion, tuina, daoyin and herbal diet. Therefore, based on the subjects and targets of this discipline, the core theoretical bases are yin and yang, five elements, visceral manifestation, meridians and collaterals, qi, blood, essence and mind, and as well as emotions.

作为中医学分支学科的中医康复学，其学术理论秉承自中医学理论体系，将中医学相关理论学说汲取并加以深化，因此，中医康复学中随处可见中医学整体观、生命观、疾病观、辨证观、养生预防观等观点原则，阴阳、五行、脏腑、经络、气血、精气神等学说理论，以及药物、针灸、推拿、导引、食疗的方法。其中，以学科研究对象和目标为内在依据，主要以阴阳五行论、藏象经络论、气血精神论、情志论等，作为本学科认识和解决命题的核心理论基础。

The mutual restriction, dependency, promotion and transformation are the basis of TCM rehabilitation. In *Yellow Emperor's Inner Cannon* (Huang Di Nei Jing), the theory of yin and yang is clarified to interpret the principles regarding physiology, pa-

阴阳学说的权衡制约、互根互用、消长转化，是中医康复学的立论基础。早在《黄帝内经》中就运用阴阳学说的理论阐明人体的生理、

thology, diagnosis and treatment, thereby establish many important theoretical principles and concepts of rehabilitation. In conclusion, the theory of yin and yang is deeply reflected in the following aspects. First, balance yin and yang, which is the primary approach and the core for rehabilitation. Second, taking yang qi as the leading factor, functions need to be recovered first so as to impair the physical disorders. This is the rudimentary principle. Third, rehabilitation approaches are applied on the basis of syndrome identification and analysis so as to promote the balance of yin and yang. This is the fundamental way of rehabilitation.

病理、诊断和治疗的规律，创立了许多重要的康复理论原则和观点。概括起来，阴阳学说在中医康复学中的深化体现在以下几方面。其一，将调和阴阳，以平为期，恢复阴阳平衡作为康复的根本途径。这是中医康复认识论和方法论的核心。其二，以阳气为主导，首重功能康复，以功能康复带动（促进）形质修复。这是中医康复根本法则。其三，强调通过辨证分析，创造康复条件，使用康复手段，促进阴阳的互根、制约、消长、转化，从而促使病损向恢复方向转化，达到权衡以平的康复目的。这是中医康复根本路径。

Governed by the theory of yin and yang, five elements and visceral manifestations are also applied in TCM rehabilitation as the core basis. Other theories on meridians and collaterals, qi, blood, fluid and liquid, essence and spirit as well as emotions are the theoretical basis for specific approaches. As a matter of fact, many essential concepts, principles and methods of TCM rehabilitation are derived from these TCM theories. For example, preventive concept based on the generation, restriction, over-restriction and counter-restriction, the method of supporting earth to restrict wood, the approach of benefiting fire to supplement earth, emotion-restricting method and so on, rehabilitation approaches based on the five sounds, five directions and

阴阳学说统摄下的阴阳五行藏象学说，应用于中医康复学，是其具体认识问题和解决命题的核心基础。经络、气、血、津液、精神、情志等学说，应用于中医康复学，则是中医康复具体落实途径、着力点和方法的理论基础。许多重要的中医康复观念、原则、治法皆由此发展而来。例如：根据五行生克乘侮的预防康复观、扶土抑木法、益火补土法、以情制情法……根据藏象相应的五音、五方、五色等康复疗法，

five colors corresponding to visceral manifestations, meridians and collaterals, qi and blood circulation are dredged through exercises, acupuncture and tuina. In addition, exercises and daoyin focusing on coordination of body and mind, and occupational exercises are emphasized.

着力于流通经络血气运动锻炼、针刺推拿，着力于形神协调的功法导引、作业训练等。

2.2 Basic Concept of TCM Rehabilitation

2.2 中医康复学的基本观念

Inherited from the theoretical system of TCM, TCM rehabilitation shares the basic concepts and theories with TCM. But as an independent branch, it has special contents and tasks. Therefore, some basic concepts are preferred. In conclusion, there are five concepts, namely holism, pattern identification, function restoration, comprehensive rehabilitation and preventive rehabilitation.

秉承自中医学理论体系的中医康复学，其基本观点和基本理论与中医学一脉相承。但因其作为独立分支学科的特殊内容和任务需要，其学科基本观点有所侧重，概括起来主要有五，即整体康复观、辨证康复观、功能康复观、综合康复观和康复预防观。

According to the holism, there is a close relation between body and mind, human and nature, human and society. Rehabilitation approaches need to take advantage of these relations. Through conforming to nature, adapting to society and overall regulating, body and mind are integrated so as to satisfy the need of holism. It involves the integration among body parts, between body and spirit, human and nature, human and society.

整体康复观认为，人的形体与精神、人与自然、人与社会之间都是密切联系、相互影响的，康复医疗中必须利用形体与精神以及人与自然、人与社会之间的这种相互联系。通过顺应自然、适应社会、整体调治等手段，来达到人体的形神统一、整体康复的目的。其内容包括人体各部分相统一、形体与精神康复相统一、人体康复与自然环境相统一、人体康复与社会环境相统一。

Pattern identification is closely related to rehabilitation, for the former is the premise and

辨证康复观是建立在中医学辨证论治观念基础之上

evidence for the latter and the principles and approaches are identified based on the results of pattern identification. The rehabilitation approaches are identified based on the results of pattern differentiation. Rehabilitation treatment guided by the combination of pattern identification and disease differentiation is the main content.

的，它认为辨证与康复之间有着密切的关系，辨证分析是康复的前提和依据，康复则是根据辨证的结果确定相应的康复法则和方法。病同证异则康复亦异，病异证同则康复亦同，辨证与辨病相结合指导康复医疗，是辨证康复观的主要内容。

Established based on the concept of perpetual motion, function restoration focus on the general resumption of daily life and work. It contains the recovery of physiological functions of zang-fu organs and tissues, and the resumption of daily life and work.

功能康复观是建立在中医学恒动观基础之上的，它要求中医康复不单着眼于脏腑组织具体生理功能的恢复，更重要的是通过功能训练，从总体上促使患者日常生活和职业工作能力的恢复。其内容包括恢复脏腑组织生理功能及恢复生活和职业工作能力。

Based on pattern identification, comprehensive rehabilitation targets at different constitutions and disease conditions. Various rehabilitation approaches can be applied comprehensively to make the patients fully recovered. This important concept is unique and proved by practice.

综合康复观是以辨证论治为基础的，针对不同的体质和病情。综合运用多种康复方法，使患者全面康复，回归社会，是中医康复学独具特色而历经实践检验的重要康复观点之一，亦是“杂合以治”的具体体现。

Preventive rehabilitation is one of the important features of TCM rehabilitation. It involves three parts: prevention before the onset, prevention before transmission, rehabilitation after recovery. Different from the general disease prevention, preventive rehabilitation focuses more on the occurrence of diseases that might cause disabilities and

预防康复观是以中医“治未病”思想为基础的，是中医康复重要的特点之一，其基本观点主要包括“未病先防”“既病防变”和“瘥后防复”3 个方面的内容。康复预防不同于一般意义上的疾病

how to minimum these disabilities.

预防，其着眼点在于预防可导致残疾病变的发生以及将残疾降低到最低限度。

As the theoretical core of TCM rehabilitation, these five basic concepts guide clinical rehabilitation a lot.

以上 5 个基本观点是中医康复学的理论核心，对临床康复具有重要的指导作用。

2.3 Therapeutic Methods of TCM Rehabilitation

2.3 中医康复疗法

Guided by TCM theory, rehabilitation approaches refer to various methods and techniques adopted for recovery. They are unique, simple, effective, convenient and cheap. Through thousands of years' development, these approaches are enriched and proved effectively. With the improvement of techniques and changes of diseases, some traditional methods are seldom applied in modern times, such as Zhu You (witched-doctors treating diseases by prayer).

中医康复疗法是在中医理论指导下以疾病康复为目的而采取的各种措施和手段。中医康复疗法各具特色而疗效肯定，具有简便效廉的特点。通过几千年的不断积累发展，中医康复方法内容相当丰富，在实践中证明在其适用范围内行之有效；同时随着人文的变迁、疾病谱的改变、技术条件的改善，一些传统方法在现代运用较少，例如祝由康复法。

In summary, the current basic approaches that are used commonly are: psychological methods (emotion restriction, emotion guidance, behavior therapy, color therapy), herbs (for internal and external use), acupuncture and moxibustion (needling, moxibustion, skin scrapping, cupping therapy), tuina, exercise and daoyin, diet, nature therapy (spring, sunshine, air, sand, mud, forest, cave, mountains, direction), artificial physical therapy (cryotherapy, thermotherapy, wax therapy, magnetotherapy, aromatherapy), entertainment (music, songs, dances, painting and calligraphy, games) and nursing.

归纳起来，目前常用中医康复基本方法主要有：中医心理康复法（情志相胜法、情志导引法、行为疗法、色彩疗法）、中药康复法（中药内治法、中药外治法）、针灸康复法（针刺疗法、艾灸疗法、刮痧疗法、拔罐疗法）、推拿康复法、功法导引康复法、饮食康复法、自然康复法（矿泉疗法、日光疗法、空气疗法、砂疗、泥疗、森林疗法、洞穴疗法、高山疗法）、人工物理康复法(冷疗法、热疗法、蜡疗法、磁疗法、芳香疗法)、娱乐康复法(音乐疗法、歌咏疗法、舞蹈疗法、书画疗法、游戏疗法),以及护理康复等。

2.4 Assessment of TCM Rehabilitation

To make sure the rehabilitation approaches are correctly performed with good results, the conditions of patients and the aims of rehabilitation need to be identified before. Therefore, the assessment and treatment are of equal importance. Guided with TCM theory, the disabilities and impairments of patients are systematically and comprehensively assessed with four diagnostic methods. With pattern identification, the symptoms, signs, disease nature, disease location and prognosis are evaluated.

The assessment is an important basis for identifying the severity of functional disorders, making targeted measures, evaluating rehabilitation results and function recovery. It evaluates two parts: function and therapeutic effects.

Function assessment is to evaluate the nature and severity of impairment, the influence that have induced or might cause through a series of clinical examinations and tests, and to pave the foundation for periodic rehabilitation programs. Different

2.4 中医康复评定

康复疗法是康复目标得以实现的途径措施,而其方法得以正确实施并达成目的,须以对患者心身各方面的具体情况和可能达到的康复目标的正确拟定为前提。因此康复评定与康复治疗的意义同等重要。中医康复评定,是在中医理论指导下,以四诊为纲,突出病机辨证,根据康复对象的形体和精神损伤残障的特点,进行系统综合的评定。通过辨证掌握患者当时的诸如症状、体征、病性、病位、病势等,评估其病损程度与预后,评价康复后的效果。

中医康复评定是明确功能障碍程度、采用针对性康复措施、评估康复效果及功能恢复水平的重要依据。其评定内容相应地包括功能评定和疗效评定两方面。

中医康复学的功能评定,主要是通过对康复患者的临床检查和检测,了解其形神功能损伤的性质、程度,以及其已经造成的和可能造

hemiplesia are often presented with symptoms like the loss of voluntary movements of one side of the body, flaccid paralysis, even sensory loss, or hypertonicity and spasms of the limbs, dark purple tongue with or without stasis macules, greasy coating, string-like and rough pulse or slow and weak pulse.

为一侧肢体不能自主活动，肢体软瘫，甚至感觉丧失，或者肢体拘急痉挛，舌质正常或紫暗，或有瘀斑瘀点，苔腻，脉多弦涩或缓而无力。

1.2 Rehabilitation Evaluation

Evaluation will be made based on the improvements of systemic symptoms before and after the rehabilitation, muscular force, muscular tension, mobility and daily activities. The common evaluations include manual muscle test, muscular electrophysiology assessment, motor pattern quality test and functional independence measure. Motor recovery can be assessed according to the Brunnstrom Rating Scale. The rehabilitation assessment can be made every two or three weeks.

1.2 康复评定

主要根据康复治疗前后全身症状改善情况，以及患侧肢体肌力、肌张力、运动功能和日常生活能力的情况进行评估。常用评定方法有六级肌力评定、肌电生理学评定、运动模式质量测试评定，以及日常生活活动能力评定。运动功能恢复情况还可参照偏瘫功能六级评价表进行。康复评定一般2～3周1次。

2 Rehabilitation Treatments

Rehabilitation treatments should be given as early as possible, right after patients' regaining of consciousness. Generally speaking, the prompt treatments begin 3 days after the onset of ischemic stroke and 14 days after hemorrhagic stroke. The rehabilitation aims at restoring muscle forces, controlling spasms, maintaining the normal ROM, preventing contracture or spasticity and restoring mobility.

2 康复措施

偏瘫患者应当早期接受康复治疗。一般在中风后意识恢复即可开始进行，缺血性中风可在发病后3日开始，出血性中风则可以在14日后开始。康复目标是旨在恢复肌力、控制肌痉挛，保持正常范围的关节活动度，预防挛缩或强直，恢复肢体随意、协调运动功能。

2.1 Functional Training

Functional training includes passive exercise, active exercise and resistance exercise. In the early

2.1 功能训练

包括肢体的被动运动、主动运动和抗阻运动。早期

stage of rehabilitation, the passive exercise of the affected body plays an important role in preventing secondary impairment, bedsore and body contracture.

进行患侧肢体的被动运动对预防继发进行损害,如褥疮、肢体挛缩等有重要的意义。

Early passive exercise begins with the position in the bed. Four limbs should be in functional positions. The shoulder joints are at 50° abduction, 40° flexion and 15° intorsion. The elbows should be up to the level of chest and at 90° flexion. Forearms are at neutral position and wrists are at 30-45° dorsal extension with fingers slightly flexed and thumbs pointing to nose. Hip joints are straightened and sand packets or cushions can be placed laterally to legs to avoid abduction and extorsion of lower extremities. Knee joints are straightened or at 30° flexion and ankles are at 90° neutral position. Food board or "T"-shoes can be used for food drop prevention.

早期的被动运动始于患者床上体位的放置。使四肢摆放置于功能位。肩关节置于外展 50°,屈曲 40°,内旋 15°的体位;使肘与胸平,肘关节置于屈曲 90°的体位;前臂中立位,腕背伸 30～45°,各手指微屈曲,拇指指向鼻;髋关节伸直,腿外侧置放砂袋或枕,以防下肢外展、外旋;膝关节伸直或微屈 30°左右,踝关节呈 90°中立位,防足下垂,可用挡足板或"丁"字鞋。

After conditions are stabilized, gentle and small-range passive exercises can be acceptable. For example, abduct or flex shoulder joints within the range between 0-90°, and keep it within 120°. To prevent shoulder subluxation, do not pull shoulders with sudden force. Flex and extend the hip and knee at the same time and keep the ROM within 120° and the ankle at 90° neutral position during passive exercises. At first every session of exercises for each joint involve 5 to 6 times of movements and daily exercises involve 3 to 4 sessions. ROM and times of exercises can be gradually increased.

病情稳定后,对患侧上下肢可以进行动作轻柔、小范围的被动运动。如肩关节外展或屈曲运动,控制在 0～90°,不超过 120°,并且要避免猛力的拔拉,以防肩关节半脱位;髋膝关节可同时进行屈伸运动,运动范围在 0～120°之间,在被动运动中注意保持踝关节于 90°中立位。每次每个关节作 5～6 遍,每日 3～4 次,以后逐步增加活动幅度和重复次数。

In the early stage of motor recovery, associated reactions can contribute to the realization of voluntary movements of affected body. When a patient is

在肢体运动功能的恢复早期,患肢的随意动作可由健侧肢体的联合反应引出。

moving a certain joint, the muscles will contract voluntarily as synergists and form a fixed motion pattern. For instance, synergic movements of upper limb flexion include scapular adduction or elevation, shoulder abduction and external rotation, elbow flexion, forearm supination, and flexion of wrist and fingers. Among them, elbow flexion is the most notable motion and appears firstly, while shoulder abduction and external rotation are the weakest.

当病人活动某一关节时，整个肢体肌肉均按协同肌的形式出现自主性的收缩并形成一固定的动作模式。例如，上肢屈曲协同动作是肩胛骨内收或抬高、肩外展、外旋、肘屈曲、前臂旋后、腕和手指屈曲。在所有屈曲联合动作中，肘屈曲最为显著且常最早出现，肩的外展和外旋是最弱部分。

Synergic movements can also be induced by associated reactions of the opposite side of the body. For example, resistance flexion of the healthy upper limb can lead to flexion of hemiplegic upper limb.

肢体协同动作也可以作为对侧的联合反应而引出。例如，对健侧上肢的抗阻屈曲可引起患侧上肢的屈曲协同动作。

With decreased muscle tension, the affected body is flaccid in the early stage of hemiplesia. Therefore, the hemiplegic body can be triggered to move with synergic movements. However, once muscle tension is increased, precautions should be taken against spasms.

偏瘫早期，患肢肌张力低，呈软瘫状态，可以利用协同动作的特点诱发患肢运动，但一旦患肢肌张力增高，应预防痉挛。

For hemiplegic patients, upper limb often flexes as associated motions and lower limb often extends. Therefore, extension is encouraged for upper limb and flexion is for lower limb.

偏瘫患者的上肢动作常出现屈曲型联合动作，因此应鼓励多作伸展动作；下肢多出现伸展性联合动作，应鼓励多作屈曲活动。

Motor recovery should conform to the motor development of human beings, beginning with simple actions and then gradually advanced and complex movements. Training for joints should start from small joints to large joints, from the proximal to the distal, from single joint to associated joints. Exercises for muscle force should begin with passive

肢体运动机能的恢复，应遵循人类运动发育的规律，从下级简单动作开始，逐渐进入高级复杂的运功动作训练。关节活动度训练，早期也应从小关节开始，逐渐到大关节；由近端至远端，由

movements, assisted movements, and then active movements and resistance movements. Each stage of exercises should be taken for a period before progressing into the next one. Generally speaking, passive or assisted exercises are more favorable when muscle force is below level III, while active or resistance exercises are preferable when muscle force is above level III. Maximum resistance exercises are only for a short time and do not take endurance exercises. When spasms and stiffness occurs in joints, restore or increase training for joint ROM.

单一关节至联合多关节。肌力的训练,应从被动运动到助力运动,再到主动运动和抗阻运动。每个运动训练阶段应持续一定时期,然后进入下一个阶段。通常情况,肌力在 3 级以下者,以被动或助力运动为宜;肌力在 3 级以上者,可进行整肌群的主动或抗阻运动练习,但多采用短暂最大阻力法,不宜作耐力练习;当出现关节痉挛僵硬时,须作恢复和增进关节活动度练习。

Early functional training is mainly taken on the bed. At first repeatedly strengthen the muscles of trunk, head and neck while keeping the trunk straight by simple movements like turning over, sitting balance and alternation from sitting to lying. Then in order to keep joints stable and in balance when standing, gluteus and trunk muscles should be strengthened by exercises in kneeling position. Finally, to walk, the ability to carry weight and stand in balance should be acquired through exercises altering from sitting to standing.

早期功能训练,以床上运动为主,从最简单的床上翻身、坐位平衡、坐卧转换开始,反复加强躯干肌与头颈肌力量,保持躯干直立态。继而进行跪位训练,在增进躯干肌力量同时,增加臀肌力量,以保证患者后续站立时关节稳定平衡。最后进行由坐位到站位的转换联系,使其获得负重与站立平衡的能力后能顺利进入步行训练。

In the early stage of hemiplesia (2-3 weeks on average since the onset), muscle force and muscle tension of the affected limb is disappeared or decreased to a low level. Therefore, rehabilitation in this stage aims at increasing muscle force and muscle tension. 3 weeks after onset, most patients have spasticity with abnormally increased muscle tensions

偏瘫早期(平均 2～3 周),患侧肢体肌力和肌张力消失或很低,此期以提高肌力和增加肌张力为主。发病约 3 周后,多数患者进入痉挛期,患侧肌张力异常增高,被动运动阻力增加,常见上

and resistance against passive movements. The flexor of upper limbs and the extensor of lower limbs are often tensed into spasticity. When spasm occurs, the rehabilitation should aim at breaking this abnormal model and building a normal one with voluntary and coordinated movements. Blindly doing exercises to increase muscle force and joint ROM, like pull-down works of flexors of upper limbs and straight leg raising test, will lead to misuse syndrome.

肢屈肌与下肢伸肌紧张的痉挛模式，当肌体运动时出现以此为基础的异常运动模式，因此该阶段的康复训练原则则是要打破这种异常模式，建立具有各个关节自主和协调运动特征的正常运动模式。如果只是盲目进行增加肌力和增加关节活动度的训练，例如上肢屈曲运动的拉力训练和下肢直腿抬高训练等，容易错误地导致肢体出现“误用综合征”。

The functional training of upper limb mainly focuses on the recovery of shoulder girdle. For example, patients may be instructed to lift the arms straight up reaching toward the ceiling with thumbs crossed, elbow extended and forearm externally rotated. This exercise can be implemented in supine, sitting and standing position. When in supine position, to improve the strength of shoulder, shoulder girdle and trunk, patents may roll towards the laterals while lifting the arms. Functional training for lower extremities mainly involves alternating hip extension, knee flexion, ankle flexion and external rotation. Adduction and internal rotation of lower extremities can be combined with the trainings mentioned above.

上肢的功能训练，着重于肩胛带的功能恢复。例如，令患者练习两手拇指交叉，两肘关节伸展、前臂外旋上抬上举过头。仰卧、坐位、站立均可练习。以仰卧位练习时，可在保持两臂上举位同时，躯体向两侧翻滚，以加强肩部、肩胛带及躯干肌力量。下肢功能训练，以在床上进行伸髋、屈膝、踝背屈和外翻的交替运动训练为主。可配合下肢内收内旋的运动。

At the same time, sit-and-stand exercise and balance exercise while sitting and standing may be implemented. When the conditions are improved, sit-and-stand exercise can be performed. If patients can stand for 10 to 20 minutes, balance exercise can be initiated from dependence to independence,

上下肢功能训练的同时，当进行坐、站训练，以及坐位和立位的平衡训练。坐站练习时在患者一般情况好转时进行。当每次站立时间达到 10～20 分钟，即可开始

stand straddle position to standing position with feet together, double-feet standing to single foot standing. At first, patients should stand on flat and hard surface, and then on uneven and soft surface. Finally, various gestures of head, extremities and trunk can be added.

进行站立平衡训练。站立平衡训练应从有依靠到无依靠,由分腿站立到并脚站立,由双足站立到单足站立,站立地面由平到不平、由硬到软,最后进展到站立位作头、上肢、躯干以至下肢的各种动作。

Walking can be introduced when the standing balance is higher than level 3, the affected leg can bear 1/3 of weight, and hip, knee, ankle joints are able to flex and extend voluntarily. Patients should walk firstly with the aid of parallel bar, toddler car, walker or crutch and then independently. These exercises should focus on coordinating the flexion and extension of hip, knee and ankle, decreasing the tension of abductor muscle and remedying pathologic gait. In order to improve the ability of walking balance, individuals should start from walking on a wide surface, then a narrow surface, and finally along a line. To improve the balance, patients may walk at different speed and in various gaits, such as walking forward, backward, and transversely.

当站立位平衡达到 3 级以上,患腿负重达到体重 2/3 以上,髋、膝、踝关节具备自主协调的屈伸运动能力时,可进入步行训练。步行练习可在平行杆或学步车中进行,继而拄拐步行,逐步到弃拐扶行,最后单独步行。步行练习中须注意协调髋膝踝的屈伸,降低外展肌张力,尽可能纠正病理步态。步行的平衡训练,可规定步行路面宽度,逐渐变窄到沿直线行走;再用不同速度和步态行走,如前、后、侧向交替行走,以提高平衡能力。

Functional training aims at maximizing the remaining function and tapping potential capability. Therefore, training should be repeated to increase the input of normal sensory stimuli and build up the normal movement pattern. Patients may take those exercises step by step and choose the appropriate training program and frequency. Occupational therapy is also essential to improving the regaining of motor coordination and endurance.

功能训练的目的在于发挥患者残存功能和潜在能力,应强调反复学习、反复训练的原则,不断增加患者对正确运动感觉,强化正常运动模式。要把握循序渐进的原则,选择合适的运动量、活动项目、训练频度。应配合适当的作业治疗,促进患者运动协调能力和耐力的全面恢复。

2.2 Occupational Management

Mobility skills practice is conducive to restoring clients' coordination ability. For example, finger-to-nose and finger-to-finger practice, clapping, playing marbles, game bars, domino, stacking blocks, bunching beads, writing, painting, etc.

Activities of daily life (ADLs) training should also be included, such as bed transfer (supine to sit, bed to chair/wheelchair and back, sit to stand), dressing (upper body dressing, lower body dressing), eating (holding bowl and cup, using utensils, cutting food), steps, grooming (oral care, hair care, shave), toileting, etc.

To enrich spirit life and eliminate negative emotion, patients may be encouraged to take part in leisure activities, such as listening to music, singing songs, playing chess and cards.

2.3 Acupuncture

In stage of paralysis: The therapeutic principle is to free channels and network vessels and to harmonize and regulate blood and qi. Acupoints along Foot-Yangming meridian, Taiyang meridians and Shaoyang meridians can be selected. For example: Bai Hui (GV 20), Feng Chi (GB 20), puncturing Jian Yu (LI 15) towards Ji Quan (HT 1), Qu Chi (LI 11), He Gu (LI 4), Wai Guan (TE 5), Huan Tiao (GB 30), Yang Lingquan (GB 34), Zu Sanli (ST 36), Jie Xi (ST 41), Xuan Zhong (GB 39). If it is in the early stage, puncture the acupoints on the affected limb with drainage. If it is a long-time con-

2.2 作业康复

运动技能性动作练习用于促进患者协调能力的恢复。例如：睁眼（闭眼）状态下行手指指鼻练习；双手手指对指练习；鼓掌练习；摆弄玻璃球、游戏棒、积木、骨牌、插板、穿绳、套圈、写字、作图等。

进行日常生活动作练习。包括：床上翻身、起坐、移位、上下床；穿脱内外衣裤鞋袜；端碗、执杯、用筷、抓拿切割食物；跨门槛、上下楼梯；洗漱、梳头、剃须、如厕等。

宜用消遣性文娱活动丰富患者精神生活、消除不良情绪。如：听曲、歌咏、游戏、下棋、打牌等。

2.3 针灸康复

软瘫期：以疏通经络、和调血气为则。取穴可以足阳明经穴辅以太阳、少阳经穴。如：百会、风池、肩髃透极泉、曲池、合谷、外关、环跳、阳陵泉、足三里、解溪、悬钟等。初病取患侧，久病取两侧；初病以泄为主，久病以补为重。喑哑窍闭则兼以启闭开窍，可取任督辅以少阴经穴，如廉泉、风府、哑门、天突、灵道、复溜、然谷等。头针可取

dition, needle the acupoints of both limbs with supplementation. If voice is lost and orifices are blocked, acupoints in conception vessel, governor vessel and Shaoyin meridians can be selected to open orifices. For example: Lian Quan (CV 23), Feng Fu (CV 16), Ya Men (GV 15), Tian Tu (CV 22), Ling Dao (HT 4), Fu Liu (KI 7), Ran Gu (KI 2). For scalp acupuncture, motor area along Anterior Oblique line of Vertex-temporal, sensory area along Posterior Oblique line of Vertex-temporal, foot motor sensory area along Line 1 Lateral to Vertex may be selected. Tian Chuang (SI 16) and Bai Hui (GV 20) are necessary in moxibustion. To trigger the muscle tension, acupoints on the affected limb can be stimulated by low-frequency electroacupuncture.

顶颞前斜线的运动刺激区、顶颞后斜线的感觉刺激区、顶旁一线的足运动感觉区。艾灸可取天窗、百会。低频电针治疗可取患侧肌肉上 2 个相应穴位进行刺激，以诱发肌张力。

In the stage of spasm: Selected acupoints are the same as those chosen in the stage of paralysis, but the therapeutic principle is to diffuse and discharge. Pricking Wei Zhong (BL 40) and Qu Ze (PC 3) may also be available. Two acupoints adjacent to antagonistic spasmodic muscles can be stimulated by electroacupuncture. Through the strong contraction of antagonistic muscles, reciprocal inhibition of prime mover can be triggered to inhibit spasms.

痉挛期: 取穴参考软瘫期而治宜宣泄。还可在委中、曲泽处放血治疗。痉挛期电针，可在痉挛肌肉拮抗肌上局部取 2 穴进行刺激，通过拮抗肌的强烈收缩而引起原动肌的交互抑制，从而抑制痉挛。

2.4 Tuina

In the early stage of hemiplegia, tuina the affected limb to improve the circulation of qi and blood, prevent phlebitis, bedsore and muscle atrophy and to promote the restoration of functions. At this stage, it is better to tuina from the distal to the proximal. For delayed hemiplesia, deep and strong manipulations are necessary, such as short-term digital acupoint pressure. Spasmodic hemiplesia is of-

2.4 推拿康复

偏瘫早期，对患肢进行按摩可改善气血运行、预防静脉炎和褥疮、防止肌肉萎缩，促进功能的恢复。此期按摩宜从远端向近端推进。迟缓性偏瘫的按摩，应采用较深而有力的手法，可运用点穴法，时间宜短。痉挛性

ten treated with gentle and slow manipulations, such as kneading and rubbing. The manipulations should be administrated for a long time to relax the spasmodic muscle group.

偏瘫则多采用较轻缓的手法，如揉、摩、擦手法，治疗时间宜长，以使痉挛肌群松弛。

2.5 Medication

The treating principle is to boost qi and quicken the blood. Bu Yang Huan Wu Tang (*Supplementing-yang Restoring-five Decoction*) is the basic formula. For severe blood stasis, add Shui Zhi (*Hirudo*), Sang Zhi (*Ramulus Mori*), Wu Gong (*Scolopendra*) to strengthen the blood quickening and stasis transforming. For severe phlegm-turbidity, add Chang Pu (*Rhizoma Acori Tatarinowii*), Yu Jin (*Radix Curcumae*), Yuan Zhi (*Radix Polygalae*) and Tian Nan Xing (*Rhizoma Arisaematis*) to flush phlegm and orifices. If dizziness is accompanied, add Gou Teng (*Ramulus Uncariae cum Uncis*) and Tian Ma (*Rhizoma Gastrodiae*). If palpitation is accompanied, add Gui Zhi (*Ramulus Cinnamomi*) and Zhi Gan Cao (prepared *Rudix Glycyrrhizae*). With rigidity and spasm, use large dose of Di Long (*Pheretima*) and Gou Teng. With flaccidity, add Sang Ji Sheng (*Herba Taxilli*), Xu Duan (*Radix Dipsaci*), Niu Xi (*Radix Achyranthis Bidentatae*), Rou Cong Rong (*Herba Cistanches*) to supplement and boost liver and kidney.

2.5 药物康复

治以益气活血为主要原则。可以补阳还五汤为基础方辨证加减。瘀血重者，加水蛭、桑枝、蜈蚣等以加强活血化瘀之力；痰浊重者，加菖蒲、郁金、远志、天南星等以涤痰利窍；兼眩晕者，加钩藤、天麻；兼心悸，加桂枝、炙甘草；肢体强直痉挛者，重用地龙、钩藤；肢体瘫软无力者，加桑寄生、续断、牛膝、肉苁蓉等补益肝肾。

2.6 Mental Rehabilitation

Function regaining for hemiplesia takes time and severe condition can easily leads to lifetime disability. Therefore, patients are easily to be negative. In addition, patients with stroke often develop cognitive dysfunction and react abnormally to the environment around them. They are usually pessimistic, desperate, anxious, nervous or worried.

2.6 精神康复

偏瘫功能恢复时间长，病变严重则易致终身残疾。因此，患者容易出现不良情绪反应。且中风易造成患者感知功能障碍，也容易导致患者对周围人事、家庭、社会环境产生异常心理反应，常

Therefore, physicians should take effective measures to eliminate patients' mental disorders, such as explanation and empathy. Patients should be actively involved in the rehabilitation exercises. To build confidence, physicians should frequently encourage patients and let them feel the happiness of improvement.

有悲观、绝望、焦虑、紧张、忧愁等情绪。因此医护人员在采取有效治疗措施同时，应注意说理开导、谈心释疑、移情等方法的运用，消除患者心理障碍。在进行肢体运动康复训练同时，注意调动其积极性和主动参与度；多用鼓励，让患者体验到康复治疗后的功能恢复进展，以增强其信心。

2.7 Diet and Daily Life

Patients with hemiplesia should be more careful in temperature changes, in order to prevent re-attack of external pathogenic factors and aggravation. In the early stage, patients in bed should frequently be turned over to prevent bedsore. In remission, patients should have adequate rest and lead a leisure life to prevent recurrence. Light but nutritious diet should be maintained. Eat more laxative vegetables and fruits and keep away from cigarette and liquor. Herbal diet should be given based on pattern identification. For example, those with qi deficiency and blood stasis may have porridge made of 30 g of Huang Qi (*Radix Astragali seu Hedysari*), 30 g of Shan Zha (*Fructus Crataegi*) and 200 g of Jing Mi (*Seme Oryzae*) every morning and night. Patients with insufficiency of liver and kidney can have porridge made of 30 g of Shan Yao (*Rhizoma Dioscoreae*), 30 g of Gui Jia (*Carapax et plastram Testudinis*) and 200 g of Jing Mi every morning and night. Individuals with spleen deficiency and severe dampness-turbidity may have porridge that consists of 60 g of Yi Yi Ren (*Semen Coicis*), 30 g of Bai

2.7 膳食起居

偏瘫患者应特别注意适寒温，严防外邪再袭而加重病情。早期卧床患者，为防止褥疮，应注意经常翻身。恢复期患者要注意节劳逸、闲情志，以防复发。饮食以清淡为主，但要保证充足的营养。适当多进食可润肠通便的蔬菜水果，禁烟忌酒。可根据不同证候，辨证处以药膳食疗。如：气虚血瘀者，可用黄芪 30 克，山楂 30 克，粳米 200 克，煮粥服食，早晚服用；肝肾不足者，可用山药 30 克，龟板 30 克，粳米 200 克，煮粥服食，早晚服用；脾虚而湿浊重者，可用薏苡仁 60 克，白扁豆 30 克，粳米 200 克，煮粥服食，早晚服用。

Bian Dou (*Semen Lablab Album*) and 200 g of Jing Mi.

2.8 Exercises

Relaxation Exercise can lower the tension of spasmodic muscles, while Strengthening Exercise can induce internal qi to circulate through the four limbs and promote recovery. Breathing exercises (Nei Yang Gong) and Six-word qigong (Liu Zi Jue) have the function of securing root and cultivating the source, strengthening the coordinating role of five viscera in qi transformation. Once patients are able to walk, Taiji Quan and Eight-brocade Exercise (Ba Duan Jin) may be necessary in promoting the full recovery.

2.8 功法锻炼

可练习放松功以降低痉挛肌的肌张力;练习强壮功诱导内气流行四肢,以促进恢复;练习内养功、六字诀,可固本培元,增强五脏气化协调功能;能行走后,坚持练习太极拳、八段锦等,可促进其全面康复。

Section 2 Arthralgia Syndrome

第2节 痹证

Arthralgia syndrome is a condition characterized by soreness, pain, numbness, heaviness in the muscles and joints, impairment of flexion and extension with stiffness as well as swelling and burning sensation of joints. It results from pathogenic wind, cold, dampness, heat obstructing the exterior and the meridians. The main pathogenesis is the obstructed flow of qi and blood causing sinews and joints deprived of nourishment.

痹证是指人体机表、经络因感受风、寒、湿、热等引起的以肢体关节及肌肉酸痛、麻木、重着、屈伸不利,甚或关节肿大灼热等为主症的一类病证。其主要病机是气血痹阻不通,筋脉关节失于濡养。

1 Rehabilitation Diagnosis and Evaluation

1.1 Rehabilitation Diagnosis

Diagnosed with arthralgia syndrome, patients with one of the following symptoms can be treated: ① joint pain aggravated with cold, soreness and heaviness, swelling and numbness of joints; ② diffi-

1 康复诊断与评定

1.1 康复诊断

临床确诊痹证,日久出现下列情况之一,即宜进行康复治疗。①关节疼痛,遇寒加重。或酸痛重着,关节

culty in flexion and extension as well as functional disturbances; ③ joint deformation and stiffness, bone enlargement

1.2 Rehabilitation Evaluation

Evaluation should be made once a month according to the joint function, redness, swelling and pain of the joint and the systemic condition.

2 Rehabilitation Treatments

2.1 Medication

Oral medication is mainly for those with lingering pathogenic wind, cold and dampness. Moving impediment can be treated by dispelling wind and freeing the network vessels, dispersing cold and eliminating dampness. Modified Fang Feng Tang (*Saposhnikovia Decoction*) is the major formula. For depressed heat with joint swelling, modified Gui Zhi Shao Yao Zhi Mu Tang (*Cinnamon Twig, Peony, and Anemarrhena Decoction*) is available. Pain impediment can be treated by dispersing cold and relieving pain, dispersing wind and eliminating dampness. Wu Tou Tang (*Aconite Main Tuber Decoction*) is the major formula. For pains mainly in joints of upper limbs, add Qiang Huo (*Rhizoma et Radix Notopterygii*), Gui Zhi (*Ramulus Cinnamomi*), Bo He (*Herba Menthae Heplocalycis*) and Jiang Huang (*Rhizoma Curcumae Longae*). For pains mainly in joints of lower limbs, add Du Huo (*Radix Angelicae Pubescentis*), Niu Xi (*Radix Achyranthis Bidentatae*) and Mu Gua (*Fructus Chaenomelis*). For severe lower back pain, add Du Zhong (*Cortex Eucommiae*) and Sang Ji Sheng (*Herba Taxilli*). Fixed impediment can be treated by eliminating dampness and freeing the network

肿大、麻木。②关节屈伸不利、功能障碍。③关节变形、骨节增大、关节强直畸形。

1.2 康复评定

根据关节功能、红肿、疼痛及全身情况辨证评估，一般每月1次。

2 康复措施

2.1 药物康复

内服药物康复主要用于风寒湿邪未尽者。行痹宜祛风通络、散寒除湿，可用防风汤为基础方加味；关节肿大、邪郁化热者，可用桂枝芍药知母汤加减。痛痹宜散寒止痛、祛风除湿，可用乌头汤为主加味；疼痛以上身关节为主者，加羌活、桂枝、薄荷、姜黄等；以下身关节为主者，加独活、牛膝、木瓜等；腰脊疼痛明显，加杜仲、桑寄生。着痹宜除湿通络、祛风散寒，可用薏苡仁汤加味；若肌肤麻木不仁，加用海桐皮、豨莶草、威灵仙、蜈蚣等。若邪从热化而成热痹者，宜散热通络、疏风胜湿，可用蠲痹汤为基础加减。

vessels, dispelling wind and dispersing cold. Yi Yi Ren Tang (*Coicis Semen Decoction*) is the major formula. For numbness, add Hai Tong Pi (*Cortex Erythrinae*), Xi Xian Cao (*Herba Siegesbeckiae*), Wei Ling Xian (*Radix Clematidis*) and Wu Gong (*Scolopendra*). If evils are transformed into heat and lead to heat impediment, Juan Bi Tang (*Impediment-Alleviating Decoction*) can be used as the major formula to disperse heat and free network of vessels, course wind and overcome dampness.

External treatment can be applied with oral medication. For example, bathe with mugwort leaf decoction; fumigating and washing joints with decoction of Hai Tong Pi, Gui Zhi, Hai Feng Teng (*Caulis Piperis Kadsurae*), Lu Lu Tong (*Fructus Liquidambaris*), Wu Tou (*Aconiti Radix*) and so on. Apply hot compress with cloth pocket filled with wine-fried cotton seed and silkworm droppings or directly compress fried Hui Xiang (*Fructus Foeniculi*), Shu Jiao (*Zanthoxyli Pericarpium*) and salt. Embrocate medicinal liquor prepared with Wu Tou, Fu Zi (*Radix Aconiti Lateralis Preparata*), Nan Xing (*Rhizoma Arisaematis*) and, Ban Xia (*Rhizoma Pinelliae*) Qing Feng Teng (*Sinomenii Caulis*) on affected joints.

内治的同时可以配合外治。可用艾叶煎汤热浴；海桐皮、桂枝、海风藤、路路通、乌头等，煎水趁热熏洗关节。可用棉花籽、蚕沙以酒炒热，装入布袋热敷患处；茴香、蜀椒、大盐炒热外敷亦可。可用乌头、附子、南星、半夏、青风藤等药为主配制药酒外用涂擦患处。

2.2 Acupuncture

Acupoints can be selected based on systemic pattern identification. For wind-cold-dampness impediment, Da Zhui (GV 14), Qi Hai (CV 6), Guan Yuan (CV 4) and Shen Que (CV 8) are main acupoints. For heat impediment, Da Zhui (GV 14), Shen Zhu (GV 12) and Qu Chi (LI 11) are main acupoints. Other acupoints around the treated joints can also be selected. Jian Yu (LI 15), Jian Liao (TE

2.2 针灸康复

全身辨证取穴，风寒湿痹者可选大椎、气海、关元、神阙为主；热痹者可取大椎、身柱、曲池。配合根据关节表现局部取穴：肩关节可取肩髃、肩髎、巨骨、曲池；肘关节可取曲池、尺泽、曲泽、少海、手三里；腕关节可取阳

14), Ju Gu (LI 16) and Qu Chi (LI 11) are to treat shoulder joint. Qu Chi (LI 11), Chi Ze (LU 5), Qu Ze (PC 3), Shao Hai (HT 3) and Shou Sanli (LI 10) are for elbow joint. For wrist, Yang Chi (TE 4), Yang Xi (LI 5), Da Ling (PC 7), He Gu (LI 4) and Wai Guan (TE 5) are available. For metacarpophalangeal joints, Ba Xie (EX-UE 9), He Gu (LI 4), San Jian (LI 3) and Hou Xi (SI 3) are useful. Si Feng (EX-UE 10) can be chosen to treat interphalangeal joints. For hip joint, Huan Tiao (GB 30), Ju Liao (GB 29) and Yang Lingquan (GB 34) are selected. Xi Yan (EX-LE 4), Liang Qiu (ST 34), Wei Zhong (BL 40), Xi Yang Guan (GB 33), Qu Quan (LR 8) and Yang Lingquan (GB 34) can be chosen to treat knees. Kun Lun (BL 60), Tai Xi (KI 3), Jie Xi (ST 41), Qiu Xu (GB 40) and Ran Gu (KI 2) are for ankle. For metatarsophalangeal joints, Ba Feng (EX-LE 10), Nei Ting (ST 44) and Tai Chong (LR 3) are useful. For spine, Da Zhui (GV 14), Shen Zhu (GV 12), Yao Yang Guan (GV 3) and the corresponding Hua Tuo's paravertebral acupoints can be selected. According to the number of the affected joints and patient's tolerance, choose 6 to 10 acupoints for each time and then alter to other acupoints for the next time. Balanced supplementation and drainage combined with moxibustion are for wind-cold-damp impediment. Combined with three-edged needle pricking to bleed, moderate and strong drainage is mainly for heat impediment.

池、阳溪、大陵、合谷、外关；掌指关节可取八邪、合谷、三间、后溪；指间关节取四缝；髋关节可取环跳、居髎、阳陵泉；膝关节可取膝眼、梁丘、委中、膝阳关、曲泉、阳陵泉；踝关节可取昆仑、太溪、解溪、丘墟、然谷；跖趾关节可取八风、内庭、太冲；脊柱关节可取大椎、身柱、腰阳关和相应节段的华佗夹脊穴。根据受累关节多少和患者耐受力，每次选用6～10穴为宜，交替使用。风寒湿痹用平补平泻，可配合灸法；热痹宜用中强度泻法为主，可配合病变局部三棱针点刺出血。

Before cupping, cutaneous needle is used to tap the acupoints near the affected joints or the place with severe swelling. If many joints are swelled, pricking and cupping therapy can be done in batches and each joint will be treated at the interval of 2 to

刺络拔罐，可在病变关节取穴或在肿胀明显处为穴，以皮肤针重叩出血，然后加拔火罐使少量出血；如全身多关节肿胀，可分批次交

4 days.

替刺络拔罐，一般间隔 2～4 日可在原位上重复。

Hydro-acupuncture with injection is also helpful for local lesions. Shen Men, Sympathetic Nerve and other corresponding tenderness points can be selected for ear-acupuncture. 3 to 6 acupoints should be chosen every time for strong manipulation and 15 to 20 minutes' needle retention or needle embedding.

在病变局部，亦可选用穴位进行穴位注射的水针法。耳针可取神门、交感，以及相应肢体反应区压痛点。每次取 3～6 穴，强刺激留针 15～20 分钟，或用埋针法。

2.3 Tuina

2.3 推拿康复

Guided by the principle of soothing the sinews and freeing the network vessels as well as quickening the blood and relieve pain, the main therapies are spine pushing, acupoint tuina as well as joint exercises. Spine pushing mainly involves horizontal pushing with thumbs or finger kneading from cervical to lumbar for several times. It should be modest so that patients can feel soreness and swelling. Selected acupoints can refer to those treated with acupuncture. Manipulation therapies like pushing and kneading with the tip of thumb, pressing with middle finger nail, rubbing and kneading with palms are selected on the basis of the anatomical structures and the specific symptoms of swelling and pain. Choose proper tuina therapies according to the degrees of joint dysfunctions. Generally speaking, relax the local muscles by kneading, rolling and pushing and then apply passive exercises. For example, bounching pressure is for lower back; distraction is for dysfunctional joints and pulling is for deformed joints in upper limbs; rocking the extending is for dysfunctional joints in lower limbs. For passive exercises, manipulation therapies should be gentle, quick and flexible. Don't be violent or in haste.

以舒筋通络、活血止痛为原则，施术的大法常以推脊、穴位按摩为主，加以活动关节。推脊以拇指平推或指揉法，常由上往下反复数遍，力道宜稳重，使患者感觉酸胀为好。穴位选取可参考针刺，视局部解剖结构和肿痛症状，灵活选用拇指尖推揉、中指掐按、掌指搓揉按摩等手法。根据关节功能障碍程度不同，选取适当强度的被动按摩活动手法。一般先用揉、㨰、推等手法放松局部肌群，然后施以被动活动。如：腰部可用弹动性按压法；上肢可牵伸障碍关节，扳拔畸形关节；下肢可摇动引伸障碍关节。作被动手法，应把握手法的轻巧、快速而带弹性，切不可暴力，亦不能急于求成。

After joint activities are recovered, patients

在初取成效，患者关节

can do some tuina for functional exercises rehabilitation by themselves. For example, press, knead, rub the local joints and acupoints around them, pinch ten fingers, press Feng Chi (GB 20), rub Yao Yan (EX-B 7) and so on.

活动有所好转的基础上，患者可进行日常自我推拿配合功能锻炼康复。如：病变局部关节及周围穴位的按揉搓摩、捻十指、按风池、擦腰眼等。

2.4 Diet and Daily Life

Live in a warm place with ample light. Stay away from damp places to avoid wind-cold-damp attack. For prolonged impediment pattern with essential qi deficiency, avoid long-time seeing, walking, sitting, standing and lying for they will damage essence. Eat more vegetables and lean meat. Hot meals are more proper. Sheng Jiang (*Rhizoma Zingiberis Recens*), Ba Jiao Hui Xiang (*Fructus Anisi Stellati*), La Jiao (*Fructus Capsici*) and Rou Gui (*Cortex Cinnamomi*) can be added to dispel cold and damp. Avoid cold, greasy food for they will induce phlegm and cause damp. However, acrid food wears qi and damages liquid. Therefore, take a small amount of acrid food, especially for patients with heat arthralgia, acrid food should be completely avoided.

Patients should frequently have food like eels, Yi Yi Ren (*Seed Coix*), cherry and water chestnut, for they can dispel wind-damp and alleviate arthralgia. Elderly patients with yang deficiency should have mutton and dog meat, for they can warm yang, disperse cold and strengthen sinews and bones. It has been proved that traditional herbal diets have therapeutic effects on rehabilitation of impediment pattern. For example, Yi Yi Ren Porridge in *Emergency Prescriptions to keep up one's sleeve* (Zhou Hou Bei Ji Fang), Su Zi Porridge and

2.4 膳食起居

居住环境应保持温暖、光线充足，注意防潮避湿，慎防风寒湿外邪侵袭；痹证日久脏腑精气亏虚，应注意避五劳伤精。饮食宜多食菜蔬瘦肉；以热食为宜，副食中可适量添加姜、茴香、椒、桂皮等帮助驱散沉寒湿邪；禁生冷、肥厚油腻等生痰碍湿之品。但同时应注意，辛燥食物有耗气伤津之弊，不宜过量，特别是于热痹患者当禁忌。

鳗鱼、鳝鱼、薏苡仁、樱桃、菱角等食材本身有祛风湿、蠲痹痛之功，常食之宜；老年阳气匮乏者，羊肉、狗肉可温阳散寒强筋骨，宜食之。传统药膳食疗方于痹证康复确有良效，例如：《肘后备急方》的薏仁粥，《太平圣惠方》的苏子粥、牛膝叶粥，《食医心鉴》的乌鸡汤等，可辨证施膳。

Niu Xi (*Achyranthis Bidentatae Radix*) Leave Porridge in Sagelike prescriptions from the *Taiping Era* (Tai Ping Sheng Hui Fang) and Silkie Soup in *Experiences on Herbal Diet* (Shi Yi Xin Jian). Take the diet on the basis of pattern identification.

2.5 Exercises

Choose proper exercises according to the specific condition of dysfunctions. For systemic exercises, Tai Ji, Eight Trigram Boxing (Ba Duan Jin), Five-animal Boxing (Wu Qin Xi) are available. For local joints function recovery, some movements in exercises mentioned above can be strengthened by combing active and passive exercise. For example, tiger imitating and deer imitating exercises are to promote joint ROM; ape imitating exercise is for agility. Based on patients' interests, choose handcraft, writing and painting or abacus to develop the agility and coordination of small joints.

2.5 功法锻炼

针对功能障碍的具体情况，选用适当的体育功法锻炼。全身性运动功法可选用太极拳、八段锦、五禽戏等。局部关节功能锻炼，根据其受累情况选择主动和被动运动相结合的方式，强化选练上述功法中的某些动作。如为发展关节活动度为主可强化练虎戏和鹿戏，为发展肢体灵活度可强化练习猿戏。可视患者自己的兴趣，酌情选择工艺、书画、珠算等作业练习，以强化小关节灵活协调能力。

2.6 Natural Factors

For patients in inactive stage and with self-care ability, they can live in rehabilitation resort with mild climate, mineral spa or desert instead of humid coastal areas. Guided with the principle of warming and freeing, spa, sunbath, hot mud therapy and sand therapy are helpful. Sulfur spa, hydrogen sulphide spa and radon spa with temperature between 38 and 40 degrees centigrade are helpful. Take the spa twice a day and each time is for 30 minutes. A course involves 12 to 16 times of treatments. Keep the room ventilated when taking hydrogen sulphide spa to prevent poisoning. The temperature of the

2.6 自然因子

生活能自理的非活动期患者，可选择气候温和，有矿泉、沙漠的地方作为康复疗养地，不宜去湿度较大的海滨或湖滨地域。以温通为原则，可选用温泉浴、日光浴、热泥疗、砂疗等方法。矿泉温泉浴，可选择硫磺泉、硫化氢泉、氡泉，水温 38～40 ℃，每日 2 次，每次 30 分钟，12～16 次为 1 个疗程。硫化氢温泉浴时要特别注意通风，防

mud should be controlled at 37 to 43 degrees centigrade. The mud therapy should be taken every day or every two days. A course is about 10 to 15 times. Systemic or local sunbath is acceptable. It should be taken about half an hour every time for 10 to 15 days as a course.

止硫化氢中毒。泥疗泥温控制在37～43 ℃为宜，每日或间日一次，10～15日为1个程。日光浴可全身或局部照射，每次约半小时，15～20日1个疗程。

2.7 Mental Rehabilitation

2.7 精神康复

Patients often feel depressed, despair, pessimistic, irritated and anxious due to the lingering pain that is difficult to relieve and progressing activity limitation. Mutual restraining of emotions, enlightening, color therapy and aromatherapy can promote rehabilitation by comforting patients and making them feel happy.

本病因疼痛久治不效，活动日益受限而容易出现精神忧郁、悲观失望、郁怒烦躁等不良情绪。可以采用情志相胜法以平之，开导转移之。可采用色彩疗法、芳香疗法等舒畅情志，以促进病情康复。

Section 3 Flaccidity Syndrome

第3节 痿证

Flaccidity syndrome is a condition characterized with flaccid sinews and bones, thin muscles, numb skin and weakness in hands and feet. It is often caused by sinews and vessels deprived of nourishment due to lung heat damaging fluids, damp-heat infiltration, deficiency of spleen and stomach and deficiency of liver and kidney. The condition may affect lung, spleen, liver and kidney.

痿证是指筋骨痿软，肌肉瘦削，皮肤麻木，手足不用的一类疾患。中医学认为，痿证主要由肺热津伤、湿热浸淫、脾胃虚弱、肝肾亏虚等，导致肢体筋脉失养而引起。病位与肺、脾、肝、肾四脏关系较为密切。

1 Rehabilitation Diagnosis and Evaluation

1 康复诊断与评定

1.1 Rehabilitation Diagnosis

1.1 康复诊断

The condition is mainly featured by flaccid sinews and vessels and weakness. Besides, it is also characterized by inability to hold, to stand independently, to walk steadily and even to move. Sometimes toes are the only parts in the body that

肢体筋脉弛缓、软弱无力为主要特征。上肢不能持物、握力下降；下肢不能独立稳站行走，甚至不能活动，或仅有足趾轻微活动；重者关

can move. Stiff and deformed joints, inability to stand and walk and atrophied muscles can be seen in severe conditions. Patients with stroke history and impediment symptoms should be excluded. In western medicine, the condition is also diagnosed as polyneuritis, acute myelitis, progressive muscular atrophy, myasthenia gravis, periodic paralysis, muscular dystrophy and flaccidity after central nervous system infection.

节僵硬畸形，步履全废，大肉尽脱等。且排除中风病史，无痹证关节表现。现代医学常诊断为：多发性神经炎、急性脊髓炎、进行性肌萎缩、重症肌无力、周期性麻痹、肌营养不良、中枢神经系统感染后软瘫等。

1.2 Rehabilitation Evaluation

The once-a-month evaluation should be made mainly based on the degree of flaccidity, especially the flaccidity of lower limbs, sensation of four limbs and the systemic symptoms. Patients with flaccid and weak lower limbs, atrophied muscles, decreased muscle force, declined cutaneous sensation, and systemic symptoms like fever, vexation and thirst, anorexia and epigastric stuffiness are in the stage of treatment. Those with improved flaccidity of four limbs with muscle force above level IV, ability to stand and walk with occasional and mild flaccidity and normal cutaneous sensation are in the stage of rehabilitation.

1.2 康复评定

主要从四肢痿软程度，尤其是下肢痿疲程度，四肢感觉情况，以及全身症状，进行综合辨证评估，每月评定 1 次。患者四肢尤其下肢痿疲无力，不能任地或见大肉进行萎缩、肌力进减、皮感减低，伴见发热、烦渴、纳呆脘痞等全身症状等，归属治疗康复期；四肢痿疲改善稳定，肌力四级以上，可行走站立或偶发轻微软瘫，皮知觉基本常者，归属疗养康复期。

2 Rehabilitation Treatments

2 康复措施

2.1 Medication

Oral medication differs according to the pattern identification of external contraction and internal damage. For lung heat, modified Qing Zao Jiu Fei Tang (*Dryness-Clearing Lung-Rescuing Decoction*) is helpful by clearing heat and nourishing lung, engendering liquid and moistening sinews. For damp-heat infiltration, modified Jia Wei Er Miao San (*Supplemented Mysterious Two Powder*) can be used to clear

2.1 药物康复

药物内治康复应分辨外感或内伤，辨证区别处置。肺热叶焦者，治以清热养肺、生津润筋，可以清燥救肺汤为主加减。湿热浸淫者，治以清利湿热、攘利筋脉，可以加味二妙散为主加减。脾胃虚弱者，治以健脾益气、通经

heat, remove damp and clear sinews and vessels. For deficiency of spleen and stomach, modified Center-Supplementing Bu Zhong Yi Qi Tang (*Qi-Boosting Decoction*) can be taken to fortify spleen and boost qi, free the channels and quicken the network vessels. For deficiency of liver and kidney, Jian Bu Hu Qian Wan (*Steady Gait Hidden Tiger Pill*) can be used to supplement kidney and nourish liver, foster yin and clear heat. For deficiency of qi and blood and deprivation of nourishment in sinews and vessels, Dang Gui Bu Xue Tang (*Chinese Angelica Blood-Supplementing Decoction*) combined with Tao Hong Si Wu Tang (*Peach Kernel and Carthamus Four Agents Decoction*) or modified Bu Yang Huan Wu Tang (*Supplementing-yang Restoring-five Decoction*) can be taken to supplement qi and blood, free vessels and nourish sinews.

活络,可以补中益汤为主加减。肝肾亏虚者,治以补肾养肝、育阴清热,可以健步虎潜丸为主加减。气血亏弱、筋脉不和者,治以补益气血、通脉养筋,可以当归补血汤合桃红四物汤加减,或以补阳还五汤为主加减。

External treatment is guided by the principle of warming and freeing. Steamed Cang Zhu (*Rhizoma Atractylodis*), Huang Bai (*Cortex Phellodendri*), Niu Xi (*Radix Achyranthis Bidentatae*), Shou Wu (*Radix Polygoni Multiflori*) and Hei Xiao Dou (Bean Black) are used for hot compress. Boil the herbs that can quicken blood and free vessels for washing or bathing twice a day. Each time is for 15 to 20 minutes. The decoction dregs can be steamed for hot compress.

药物外治康复以温通为要。可用苍术、黄柏、牛膝、首乌、黑小豆等蒸热热敷。可选用活血通脉药物,煎水外洗或热浴,每日 2 次,每次 15～20 分钟;药渣可分包交替蒸热热敷。

2.2 Acupuncture

Acupoints in Yangming meridian, governing vessel and Hua Tuo's paravertebral acupoints are mainly selected for acupuncture. Da Zhui (GV 14) and Zu Sanli (ST 36) are major acupoints. To treat upper limbs, Jian Yu (LI 15), Qu Chi (LI 11), He Gu (LI 4) and Yang Xi (LI 5) are helpful. Bi Guan

2.2 针灸康复

体针取阳明经、督脉经穴和华佗夹脊穴为主。大椎、足三里常为基础穴;上肢可取肩髃、曲池、合谷、阳溪等;下肢可取髀关、梁丘、解溪等;督脉可取身柱、命门、

(ST 31), Liang Qiu (ST 34) and Jie Xi (ST 41) can be added to treat lower limbs. Shen Zhu (GV 12), Ming Men (GV 4) and Yao Yang Guan (GV 3) in governing vessel can be chosen. For lung heat, Chi Ze (LU 5), Qu Chi (LI 11), Wei Zhong (BL 40), Ba Feng and Ba Xie are helpful. For prolapsed hands and feet, add Yang Lao, Wai Guan (TE 5), Xuan Zhong (GB 39) and Qiu Xu. Qiu Xu can treat strephenopodia and Zhong Feng and Shang Qiu can treat strephexopodia. For lower limbs that can flex instead of extending, Yao Yang Guan (GV 3) can be added, while for lower limbs that can extend instead of flexing, Qu Quan (LR 8) is helpful. To treat toes which can't lift, add Xing Jian (LR 2). With low-grade fever and night sweating, Fu Liu (KI 7) and Yin Xi (HT 6) can be added. With anorexia and abdominal distension, add Zhong Wan (CV 12) and Tian Shu (ST 25). Manipulate moderately with balanced supplementation and drainage. When manipulating the needles at acupoints in governing vessel and Hua Tuo's paravertebral acupoints, make sure the needle sensation directs at sacrococcygeal joints and hypochondrium. If the condition progresses slowly, administer acupuncture once a day; if quickly, twice or three times a day. If muscle is atrophied without excessive heat, acupuncture combined with moxibustion or warm needling moxibustion is helpful.

腰阳关。肺热叶焦者,可加尺泽、曲池、委中、八风、八邪等;手足下垂,可加养老、外关、悬钟、丘墟等;足内翻可加丘墟,足外翻可加中封、商丘;下肢能屈不能伸可加膝阳关,能伸不能屈可加曲泉;足趾不翘加行间;伴低热盗汗,可加复溜、阴郄;纳呆腹胀,可加中脘、天枢。常用中等刺激,平补平泻;督脉经腧和华佗夹脊穴,应使针感向尾骶、胸胁放射;病情进展缓慢时,可每日一次,进展迅速可每日 2～3 次。肌肉萎缩而无实热者,可针灸并用,或用温针灸法。

Cutaneous acupuncture mainly focuses on tapping and pricking the Hand-Yangming meridian combined with acupoints in affected areas. Manipulate the needle moderately and tap the skin until hyperemia or even slight bleeding. Cutaneous acupuncture therapy should be given once a day or ev-

皮肤针可以手阳明经为叩刺重点,并结合患部腧穴叩刺;中等强度,叩至皮肤明显充血或略有出血,可每日或隔日 1 次。耳针可取神门、交感,以及相应反射区耳

ery two days. With ear acupuncture, Shen Men, Sympathetic Nerve and other auricular acupoints in corresponding reflex zones can be selected. Manipulate them strongly with 15 to 20 minutes' retention. It should be given once a day. Motor area, sensory area and corresponding reflex zones can be treated with scalp acupuncture through twirling. Manipulate the needles for 0.5 to 1 minute every 5 to 10 minutes. The total retention time is about 30 to 60 minutes. Qu Chi (LI 11), Wai Guan (TE 5) and He Gu (LI 4) in upper limbs and Zu Sanli (ST 36), Yang Lingquan (GB 34) and Jie Xi (ST 41) in lower limbs can be selected for electric acupuncture. Each time choose 2 to 4 acupoints and apply dilatational wave or discontinuity wave for 15 to 20 minutes. It should be given every two days. For hydro-acupuncture, Qu Chi (LI 11), Wai Guan (TE 5), He Gu (LI 4), Zu Sanli (ST 36), Xuan Zhong (GB 39) and Tai Chong (LR 3) are helpful.

穴;以强刺激,留针 15～20 分钟,可每日 1 次。头针可取运动区、感觉区和患部相应反射区穴位,捻转刺激,间歇运针,每隔 5～10 分钟加强捻转 0.5～1 分钟,总留针时间可 30～60 分钟。电针,上肢可取曲池、外关、合谷,下肢可取足三里、阳陵泉、解溪;穴位交替使用,每次 2～4 穴,用疏密波或间断波,15～20 分钟,隔日 1 次。也可选用曲池、外关、合谷、足三里、悬钟、太冲等穴位,作水针穴位注射。

2.3 Tuina

Tuina mainly applies to acupoints in governing vessel, back transport acupoint and acupoints in Yangming meridians. Acupoints near the affected areas can be selected and passive exercise of joints can be combined. The manipulation should be gentle and slow. The treatment should be given once a day for 15 days as a course.

For upper limbs, grasp Jian Jing (GB 21), knead and pinch Bi Nao, Shou Sanli and muscles and sinews near He Gu (LI 4), and rub muscles of arms. For lower limbs, grasp Yin Lian (LR 11), Cheng Shan (BL 57) and Kun Lun (BL 60), knead and pinch Fu Tu (ST 32), Cheng Fu (BL 36) and muscles and sinews around Yin Men (BL 37), press

2.3 推拿康复

以穴位推拿为主,可取督脉、背俞、阳明经穴为主,结合局部取穴和关节被动运动,手法宜轻柔和缓,可每日 1 次,15 次为 1 个疗程。

上肢可拿肩井,揉捏臂臑、手三里、合谷部肌筋,点肩髃、曲池等穴,搓揉臂肌肉。下肢可拿阴廉、承山、昆仑,捏揉伏兔、承扶、殷门部肌筋,点腰阳关、环跳、足三里、委中、犊鼻、解溪、内庭,

Yao Yang Guan (GV 3), Huan Tiao (GB 30), Zu Sanli (ST 36), Wei Zhong (BL 40), Du Bi (ST 35), Jie Xi (ST 41) and Nei Ting (ST 44), rub muscles of thighs and knees. Besides, knead auricle, press reflex zones of Shen Men, Jiaogan, subcortex, spleen, spine, stem, liver and kidney in ears.

搓揉股膝肌肉。此外可按揉耳廓，点按神门、交感、皮质下、脾、脊髓、脑干、肝、肾等耳部反应部位。

2.4 Diet and Daily Life

Live in a quiet and clean place with fresh air and ample light. Keep warm and avoid wind and cold. Be careful during daily activities and exercises.

Have something light, healthy, rich in nutrition and easy to digest. For example, vegetables like bean sprouts, spinach, Chinese cabbage, radish and tomato, fruits Shan Zha (*Fructus Crataegi*), Da Zao(*Fructus Jujubae*) and tangor. People with habit of drinking can have a small amount of fruit wine. Avoid food damaging liquid and impairs stomach and spleen. Herbal diet like Ren Shen(*Radix Ginseng*) porridge, Shan Yao (*Rhizoma Dioscoreae*) Porridge, Porridge with *Magnetitum* (Ci Shi) and pig kidney, Pig Kidney Porridge, Huang Qi(*Radix Astragali seu Hedysari*) and Da Zao(*Fructus Jujubae*) Porridge, Tao Ren(*Semen Persicae*) Porridge, Shan Zha Porridge, wonton wrapped with chicken, Dang Gui (*Radix Angelicae Sinensis*) with chicken soup, Lu Jiao(*Cornu Cervi*) wine is also available based on pattern identification.

2.4 膳食起居

起居环境应安静清洁、空气清新、光线充足。注意保暖，避免外邪风冷侵袭。日常活动和锻炼时，应加以监护、注意安全，防止跌倒意外。

饮食宜清淡，富营养而易于消化。宜多食豆芽、菠菜、白菜、萝卜、西红柿等蔬菜；水果宜多食山楂、枣子、广柑等；有饮酒习惯者宜少量饮用果酒为佳；忌服伤津耗液及伤胃损脾之品。可辨证选用相关药膳。如人参粥、山药粥、磁石猪腰粥、猪腰子粥、黄芪大枣粥、桃仁粥、山楂粥、鸡肉馄饨、当归母鸡汤、鹿角酒等。

2.5 Exercises

Operational and functional exercises are chosen based on the condition. If the condition is severe, take a seat or lie on the back, play Five-animal Boxing (Wu Qin Xi) or Eight-vessel Running Boxing

2.5 功法锻炼

视病患肢体功能状况选择相应的功法作业及功能锻炼。肢体痿疲较重时，可平坐或仰卧位，选练五禽戏动

(Ba Mai Yun Xing Fa). Patients without hypertension can play will-control qigong. If the condition is improved, play Relaxing and Calming Exercises (Song Jing Gong) and Breathing Exercises (Nei Yang Gong).

功或八脉运行法;如无高血压,可选练意气功;肢体功能情况好转后,逐渐以练习松静功、内养功为主。

To recover joint function, improve muscle force and prevent malformation, functional exercises should be taken as soon as possible. It should be played step by step, beginning from passive and assisted exercises to active and resistance ones. Keep the movements slow and joint ROM as large as possible. Patting is proper for patients with flaccidity. Pat the left limbs with right palm or fist and right ones with left palm or fist, from the upper to the lower in every aspect.

功能锻炼宜尽早实行,以恢复肢体关节功能、锻炼肌力、防止畸形。运动量由被动运动→助力运动→主动运动→抗阻力运动,循序渐进,动作宜缓慢、关节活动范围宜尽量大。拍打健身功法对痿证患者康复比较适宜。可由患者自己或医疗工作者施术,先用右掌或拳拍打左上肢体的四面,从上而下、前后左右,每面拍打;然后用左手掌或握拳拍打右上肢,方法同前;再用左手掌或握拳拍打左侧大腿和小腿,从上往下拍打上、下、内、外四面,以右手拍打右侧大腿小腿,方法与拍左腿相同。

Besides, on the basis of disease condition combined with personal interests, living conditions and occupations, operational exercises like knitting, typing, carpentering, carving, sewing, embroidering and repairing can be selected to improve muscular agility and tolerance. Increase the level of challenges gradually to prevent mechanical injury caused by sensory disturbance.

此外,后期可根据患者病情,结合其个人兴趣、生活条件、职业特性等,选择相关的作业训练。如进行编织、打字、木工、雕刻、缝纫、刺绣、修理器械等。从而增加肌群协调灵活度和肌肉耐受力。作业练习应注意逐渐增加难度和实践,防止由于感觉障碍引发机械性损伤。

2.6 Mental Rehabilitation

Patients often feel depressed, pessimistic, and anxious due to the inability to move. Some patients lose their confidence in life and strong will to combat disease. Choose proper mood regulating therapies to eliminate pessimistic moods and stay optimistic. For example, method of mutual restraining of emotions is for pessimistic and anxious patients. Enlighten and encourage those without confidence. Aromatherapy like will-stabilizing Formula is for those without determination. Color therapy like Happy Color Formula is helpful too. Proper entertaining activities also help.

2.6 精神康复

由于肢体痿弱失用，患者容易产生悲观、忧郁、急躁等不良情绪。有的患者对生活与战胜疾病缺乏信心和坚强意志。可根据其精神特点，选择适当的调摄情志康复方法，以排除消极情绪，保持乐观，增强抗病心理。例如：以说理开导的同时，对悲观急躁者运用情志相胜法；对缺乏信心者说理鼓励；意志不定者配合运用芳香疗法的定志方，色彩疗法的喜色方；选择适当的娱乐等怡情逸性等。

Section 4 Fracture

第 4 节 骨折

Fracture refers to complete or partial break of bone structures. It can affect one bone or several bones simultaneously. Most patients may regain the functions after proper treatment. For those who may not, or with degrees of sequel, rehabilitation is encouraged.

骨折是指骨结构的连续性完全或部分断裂，常见于一个部位，少数为多发性。骨折经及时恰当治疗，多数病人能恢复原来的功能。对于少数不能正常愈合者，或遗留有不同程度的后遗症者，须配合康复治疗。

1 Rehabilitation Diagnosis and Evaluation

1.1 Rehabilitation Diagnosis

Rehabilitation for fracture only applies to those who don't recover beyond the average healing dura-

1 康复诊断与评定

1.1 康复诊断

骨折康复是针对外伤骨折后已超过平均愈合时间仍

tion. It can be divided into three conditions according to the modern diagnostic methods.

One is prolonged recovery. The fracture doesn't recover after conventional treatment and the impaired limbs can't sustain loads. Examination shows the skin temperature of injured limbs is higher than the healthy ones, and mobility and tenderness still occurs in broken ends. Callus is shown in the imaging checkup, but it is not enough for recovery.

The second is disconnection. The broken ends still can't connect after conventional treatment. Physical checkup indicates flaccid and weak limbs, round broken ends that don't induce pain while moving and are presented as pseudarthrosis. The imaging checkup shows atrophied and rounded broken ends, scare callus, enlarged spatium, osteosclerosis and closed medullary cavity.

The third is malfunction after healing. The fracture heals after conventional treatment, but joints are still stiff and can't function properly or sustain a heavy load.

未正常愈合者。结合现代诊断手段,包括以下三种情况:

其一是骨折延迟愈合:经过常规治疗后,超过平均愈合时间,伤肢仍不能正常负重;检查伤肢皮温较健侧稍高,骨折断端仍可查及轻微活动和压痛;影像学检查骨折虽有骨痂生长,但未达到愈合标准。

其二是不连接症:经过常规治疗后,已超过平均愈合时间,但骨折处仍无连接,检查伤肢软弱无力,骨折处圆滑活动无疼痛,呈假关节状;影像学检查提示骨折断端萎缩尖圆,骨痂稀少,间隙增大,骨质硬化,髓腔封闭等。

其三是愈合后功能失常者:经过常规治疗,虽然骨折对位愈合良好,但患处附近关节僵直,失去正常活动功能;或功能恢复不完全,存在功能障碍;或关节活动尚可但不能完全任重者。

1.2 Rehabilitation Evaluation

Comprehensive evaluation should be made every month or every one and a half month, based upon the symptoms of poorly-recovered fracture, malfunction and systemic symptoms. The local indications of the fracture in limbs are pain, percussion pain, abnormal motions, joint ROM, images and time of fracture.

1.2 康复评定

主要根据患者骨折愈不良的诊断表现、功能障碍情况和全身伴随表现进行综合辨证评定,通常1个月到1个半月评定一次。骨折患肢局部评定指针主要有:疼痛、叩击痛、异常活动、关节活动程度、影像学表现、折伤时间等。

2 Rehabilitation Treatments

2.1 Osteopathy

Manipulation or operation should be re-performed aiming at causes of poor recovery. For those with malunion fracture, break the bone with manipulation or through operation and then relocate and fix it. If the recovery is prolonged due to improper fixing, re-fix it; if it is caused by over-pulling, lighten the load. For fractures without union, bone grafting helps.

2.2 Medication

Oral medication differs according to the pattern identification. For deficiency of liver and kidney, supplement with modified Jin Gui Shen Qi Wan (*Golden Coffer Kidney Qi Pill*) and modified Jian Bu Hu Qian Wan (*Steady Gait Hidden Tiger Pill*). If yin is severely deficient with poor formation of callus, add Du Zhong (*Cortex Eucommiae*), Chuan Duan (*Radix Dipsaci*), Gu Sui Bu (*Rhizoma Drynariae*), Duan Long Gu (*Processed Os Draconis*) and Duan Mu Li (*Processed Oyster Shell*). For insufficiency of qi and blood, supplement qi and blood with Ba Zhen Tang (*Eight-Gem Decoction*). With slow recovery, add large dose Huang Qi (*Radix Astragali seu Hedysari*), Huai Niu Xi (*Radix Achyranthis Bidentatae*) and Gu Sui Bu; with qi deficiency of spleen and stomach and symptoms like anorexia and epigastric stuffiness, lassitude of limbs and fatigue, add Mu Xiang (*Radix Aucklandiae*), Sha Ren (*Fructus Amomi*), Ban Xia (*Rhizoma Pinelliae*), Chen Pi (*Pericarpium Citri Reticulatae*) and Huai Shan Yao (*Rhizoma Dioscoreae*). For phelgm-stasis obstructing network vessels, transform stasis,

2 康复措施

2.1 整骨康复

针对产生不良愈合的局部原因，重新施以手法或手术。畸形愈合者，可手法折骨或手术凿断，重新整复固定；延迟愈合因为固定不当者，重新手打后行固定；过度牵引所致者，立即减轻重量；不愈合者，可行植骨术。

2.2 药物康复

药物内治，对于肝肾虚弱者，宜补益肝肾，可用金匮肾气丸、健步虎潜丸加减；如真阴亏损较甚，骨痂形成不良者，可加杜仲、川断、骨碎补、煅龙骨、煅牡蛎等。对于气血不足者，宜补益气血，可以八珍汤加减；如骨折愈合缓慢，加重黄芪、怀牛膝、骨碎补等；如脾胃气虚较甚，伴见脘痞纳呆、肢倦乏力者，可加木香、砂仁、半夏、陈皮、怀山药等。痰瘀阻络者，宜化瘀祛痰透络，可以跌打丸加减，成药可用接骨丹。

expel phlegm and free network vessels with Die Da Wan (*modified Knocks and Falls Pill*) or patent drugs like Jie Gu Dan (*Bone-Joining Elixir*).

External treatment mainly focuses on soothing sinews and quickening blood, using Jie Gu Xu Jing Gao (*Bone and Sinew Joining Plaster*) or fumigating and washing with decoctions of Hai Tong Pi (*Cortex Erythrinae*), Shen Jing Cao (*Herba Lycopodii*), Tou Gu Cao (*Herba Speranskiae seu Impatientis*), Sang Zhi (*Ramulus Mori*), Cang Zhu (*Rhizoma Atractylodis*) and Hong Hua (*Flos Carthami*).

外用中药以舒筋活血，如外贴接骨续筋膏药，可用海桐皮、伸筋草、透骨草、桑枝、苍术、红花等，煎水每日熏洗。

2.3 Acupuncture

In the early stage of fracture, acupuncture only aims at relieving pain and dispersing swelling and it should be seldom used. In the later stage and period of sequela healing, acupoints around broken ends and those of the affected meridians, mainly at the four extremities, may be selected for acupuncture. For example, He Gu (LI 4), Yu Ji (LU 10), Nei Guan (PC 6) and Wai Guan (TE 5) are for upper limb fracture, and Nei Ting (ST 44), Tai Chong (LR 3), Sanyin Jiao (SP 6), Tai Xi (KI 3), Zu Sanli (ST 36), Yang Lingquan (GB 34) and Cheng Shan (BL 57) are for lower limb fracture. Yin Men (BL 37), Cheng Shan (BL 57) and Wei Zhong (BL 40) are for thoracolumbar fracture. If atrophied muscles or stiff joints are seen near the fracture, local acupoints should be selected for acupuncture with drainage. Moxibustion may be used for warming and freeing. For deficiency of liver and kidney, add Shen Shu (BL 23), Ming Men (GV 4), Guan Yuan (CV 4), Sanyin Jiao (SP 6), Tai Xi (KI 3) and Tai Chong (LR 3). For insufficiency of qi and blood, add Pi Shu (BL 20), Xin Shu (BL 15),

2.3 针灸康复

早期骨折，少用灸，只针对疼痛肿胀以止痛消肿；后期及愈合后遗症，针灸可取穴于骨折附近结合循经取穴。循经取穴以四梢远端为主，如上肢骨折可取合谷、鱼际、内关、外关；下肢骨折可取内庭、太冲、三阴交、太溪、足三里、阳陵泉、承山；胸腰椎骨折可选殷门、承山、委中等。患处附近肌肉萎缩或关节僵直者，可以局部取穴为主，多以泄法，可配合灸法以温通。辨证肝肾虚弱者，可加肾俞、命门、关元、三阴交、太溪、太冲等；气血不足者，可加脾俞、心俞、足三里、气海、神门等，针用补法。

Zu Sanli (ST 36), Qi Hai (CV 6) and Shen Men (HT 7) for acupuncture with supplement.

2.4 Tuina

In the early and middle stage of fracture, tuina is forbidden because it will cause further displacement. It is only acceptable when swelling and pain occurs in distal end and during the rehabilitation of atrophied muscles and malfunctioned joints in the later stage. Tuina at the distal end of fracture aims at dispersing swelling, quickening blood, transforming stasis and relieving adhesions. The manipulations should be gentle and focus on pressing and kneading to avoid displacement and local impairment due to the pulling of the muscles. If the swelling is severe, manipulate along the circulation of qi and blood. For atrophied muscles and malfunctioned joints, to avoid aggravating local injury and pain, tuina manipulations, mainly focusing on kneading, pressing, pushing and sinew-separating, should be slow at first and then gradually increase the range of passive exercises. For those with long-time bed rest, perform systemic tuina to accelerate fracture healing by promoting qi and blood circulation and safeguarding healthy qi.

2.5 Exercises

Proper exercises not only accelerate function recovery of affected limbs, but also strengthen fixation of fracture and promote connection of broken ends. Small splint fixation, designed for limbs fracture under the guidance of TCM theory on combination of motion and tranquility, is conducive to functional activities at early stage.

2.4 推拿康复

推拿禁用于骨折早期和中期，以防骨折再移位，仅适用于远端有肿胀疼痛部位，以及对后期患处肌肉萎缩和关节功能障碍的康复。骨折远端推拿以消除肿胀、活血化瘀、解触粘连为目的，注意手法轻柔、柔中寓刚，以按揉为主，避免因肌群牵引联合反射造成骨折移位和局部损伤；肿胀较甚者，推拿应注意沿气血正常流行方向进行。对损伤附近肌肉萎缩及关节功能障碍的推拿，初始手法宜慢，被动活动范围逐步增大，避免加重局部损伤和患者痛苦，手法宜揉、按、推为主，结合分筋。长久卧床者，也可进行全身按摩，以促使气血运行，护养正气，加快骨折愈合。

2.5 功法作业

正确地运用功法功能锻炼，既可以促进患肢的功能恢复，也可增强骨折处的固定，促进骨折断端良好对位和愈合。特别是中医“动静相合”治疗思想指导下的针对四肢骨折的小夹板固定法，为早期的功法功能锻炼提供了方便。

Rehabilitation exercises for patients whose four limbs are fixed with small splint emphasize on restoring physiological functions, such as the ability to grip and to walk with load. Depending on the stability of the fracture, range of motion exercises may be started 1 to 2 weeks after treatment and progressed to strengthening exercises. Exercises that are unfavorable for healing should be avoided. Activities should be suitable for the recovery. To make the movements smooth and balanced, the healthy limb may be started first to initiate the affected one.

四肢骨折小夹板固定患者的康复练功，以恢复生理功能为主，上肢以增强握力为主，下肢以增强负重步行能力为主；练功时要注意循序渐进；一般在骨折处理后1～2周即可开始，根据骨折部位的稳定程度，逐步增加活动量和范围，并避免进行对骨折愈合不利的活动方式；具体练功方法应切合不同的愈合阶段，注意以健肢带动患肢，使动作协调，相称自如。

Hematoma organization begins 1 to 2 weeks after fracture. At this stage, pain and swelling still lingers. Exercises aims at promoting blood circulation, eliminating swelling, prevent muscle atrophy and joints adhesion and stiffness. Upper limbs activities focus on clenching a fist, suspending arms, lifting shoulders and joints extension and flexion like cloud hands and bend arms backwards is for radius and ulna fracture. Lower limbs activities emphasize on dorsally extending ankles, contracting quadriceps femoris to drive the lower limb muscles into motion and then relaxing. Exercises for tibia and fibula fracture should focus on lifting legs and flexing knees.

在骨折后1～2周的血肿机化期，骨折处疼痛肿胀仍较明显，练功以促进血脉流通、消除肿胀，防止肌肉萎缩和关节粘连僵硬为目的。上肢以练习握拳、吊臂、提肩和一定范围的关节伸展活动为主，如桡、尺骨骨折可练习云手、反转手。下肢可作踝关节的背展，股四头肌的收缩运动，带动整个下肢的机头活动，然后再放松；胫、腓骨骨折后的练功以抬腿、屈膝为主。

3 weeks after fracture, primary callus forms, and pain and swelling disappears with slight tenderness and dysfunction. At this stage, patient may clench with strength, fix and extend joints, walk slowly with the aid of walking stick.

骨折后3周左右，原始骨痂形成，骨折处肿胀疼痛基本消失，或仅有轻微压痛和障碍，上肢可用力握拳，进行关节伸展活动；下肢可下床练习扶拐杖缓慢步行。

Fracture gradually heals at 5 to 10 weeks after break. Large joints can move gradually and 7 weeks after fracture the patient can do gymnastics exercises. Patient with upper limb fracture can play simplified Tai Ji boxing and repeat upper limbs movements like cloud hands and forearm rollings on both sides 5 weeks after fracture. For patient with lower limb fracture, exercises may start when patient is able to walk without help 7 weeks after fracture and then progress to strengthening exercises. After healing, patient can resume activities like climbing.

骨折后5～10周，骨折逐渐愈合，可逐步进行大关节活动，到7周后可进行形体体操功法活动。上肢伤者，在骨折5周后可选练简化太极拳，反复练习上肢招式，如云手、倒卷肱等；下肢伤者，一般需要7周脱拐行走后开始练习，运动量和运动范围由小到大；下肢功能基本恢复后可行攀登等动作训练。

After fixation for fracture reduction and during bed rest, the patient may play static exercises or relaxation exercises and concentrate minds on the affected limb, which can alleviate pain, supplement healthy qi and promote blood circulation.

另外，骨折复位固定后，早期卧床阶段，可练习气功导引法，采用静功或放松功，意念集中患部，有助于减轻骨折疼痛、培补正气、流通血脉。

2.6 Diet and Daily Life

For elderly and weak patients who need bed rest, complications like bedsore, hypostatic pneumonia and urinary system infection should be prevented and make sure the urination and bowel movement are normal. Have something rich in nutrition and easy to digest. At the early stage of fracture, have something that can quicken blood and transform stasis, disperse swelling and relieve pain, such as ginger, green onion, shepherd's purse and Xie Bai (*Allium macrostemon*). At the middle and later stage, have something that can supplement blood and qi and enrich and supplement kidney and liver, such as Gou Qi Zi (*fructus Lycii*), Long Yan Rou (*Arillus Longan*), Chinese chestnut, black soy bean, mutton and beef, quail and pigeon. Diet

2.6 膳食起居

对于年老体弱卧床患者，要注意防范褥疮、坠积性肺炎、泌尿系感染等并发症，应注意保持二便通畅。饮食上应尽可能营养丰富而易于消化；骨折初期可选择具有活血化瘀、消肿止痛功效的食物，如姜、葱、荠菜、薤白等；中后期可选择具有补益血气、滋补肝肾功效的食物，如枸杞子、龙眼肉、板栗、黑豆、牛羊肉、鹌鹑、鸽子等。食疗方可选用骨头汤、脊髓粥等以促进骨修复。

therapies, like bone soup and spinal cord porridge, are to promote bone healing.

2.7 Mental Rehabilitation

Patients with fracture, especially with severe fracture, always worry about their future work and daily life. They are irritable due to the pain and dysfunction after fracture. To promote early recovery, it is important for treating physicians to regulate patients' emotions and stimulate their initiatives. Through enlightening, patients can be informed of their condition and be positive about the rehabilitation. For those over restless, it is imperative to guide patients to regulate and relax on their own.

2.7 精神康复

骨折患者,特别是伤势较重者,常有一定思想负担,担心以后的生活工作能力,随着骨折后疼痛和功能障碍,情绪容易烦躁不安。应注意调治患者精神情志,激发患者最大的主观能动性,以促进早日康复。通过解释开导的方法,使患者能正确清醒地认知病情,从而乐观对待、积极配合康复治疗;对于情绪过于烦躁者,应引导其自我调节放松。

Section 5 Sinew Damage

第5节 伤筋

Sinew damage refers to the injury due to violence or chronic strain. It corresponds to soft tissue injury in western medicine. Sinew damage can be divided into sprain and bruise according to forms, and into acute and chronic sinew damage according to the disease course.

凡因各种暴力或慢性劳损等原因造成筋的损伤,称为伤筋或筋伤,相当于现代医学的软组织损伤。按不同形式,伤筋可分为扭伤、挫伤两类;按不同病程,伤筋可分为急性伤筋及慢性伤筋。

1 Rehabilitation Diagnosis and Evaluation

1.1 Rehabilitation Diagnosis

With a definite history of sinew damage, the individual has lingering pain and swelling, and a certain degree of dysfunction after symptoms like swelling and bruise fade away. Sinew damages occur

1 康复诊断与评定

1.1 康复诊断

有明确的伤筋史,但肿胀和皮肤青紫等症状在伤筋消退后,仍留有局部疼痛肿胀,伴有一定的功能障碍者。

in one place repeatedly and are hardly cured for a long time.

在同一部位多次反复出现伤筋，日久不愈者。

1.2 Rehabilitation Evaluation

1.2 康复评定

Comprehensive evaluation should be evaluated every 15 days on pain, tenderness, swelling, dysfunction and systemic conditions. It mainly focuses on the improvement of dysfunction.

常根据疼痛程度、压痛情况、肿胀情况、功能障碍程度，以及全身状况进行综合辨证评估；其中以功能障碍改善情况为核心，一般每 15 日评估一次。

Patients with soreness or dull pain, mild swelling, severe tenderness in the joint and unable to make daily activities are in stage Ⅰ; those with mild dull pain, swelling and tenderness, or feeling pain only in motion and whose daily activities are affected are in stage Ⅱ; in the stage of rehabilitation, patients have slight pain, no swelling and tenderness and are able to do daily work in the inactive time, but due to change of weather or overwork, pain or dull pain occurs and joint functions are slightly affected.

如关节损伤部位疼痛酸楚或隐痛，轻度肿胀，压痛明显，局部功能受限，难以胜任日常工作者，属于康复治疗Ⅰ期；损伤部位稍有隐痛，或仅于活动时疼痛，肿胀压痛不明显，功能轻度受限，难以完全胜任日常工作者，属康复治疗Ⅱ期；患者损伤部位疼痛不明显，无肿胀压痛，功能基本正常，能胜任日常工作，但于天气巨变及劳累，损伤部位仍出现疼痛或隐痛，伴轻度功能受限者，属疗养康复期。

2 Rehabilitation Treatments

2 康复措施

2.1 Acupuncture

2.1 针灸康复

Nearby Ashi acupoints and remote acupoints along the meridians are often selected together. The selection of acupoints differs according to the sinew damage. Qu Chi (LI 11), Da Zhui (GV 14), Tian Zhu (BL 10), Jian Waishu (SI 14), Jue Gu (GB 39) and Hou Xi (SI 3) are selected if sinew of neck is damaged. Jian Yu (LI 15), Jian Liao (TE 14), Jian

取穴以局部和远端相结合，局部多取阿是穴，远端多循经取穴，不同伤筋部位取穴不同。颈项处伤筋，可取曲池、大椎、天柱、肩外俞、绝谷、后溪等；肩部可取肩髃、肩髎、肩贞、臑俞、外关等；肘

Zhen (SI 9), Nao Shu (SI 10) and Wai Guan (TE 5) are chosen for shoulder sinew damage. Qu Chi (LI 11), Xiao Hai (SI 8), Tian Jin (TE 10) and He Gu (LI 4) are for elbow sinew damage. Yang Chi (SJ 4), He Gu (LI 4), Yang Gu (SI 5) and Wai Guan (TE 5) are for wrist damage. For lumbar damage, Shen Shu (BL 23), Dachang Shu (BL 25), Yao Yangguan (GV 3), Yin Men (BL 37), Wei Zhong (BL 40) and Tai Xi (KI 3) are selected. For thigh damage, Huan Tiao (GB 30), Zhi Bian (BL 54) and Cheng Fu (BL 36) are chosen. Liang Qiu (ST 34), Xi Yan (EX-LE 5), Xi Yangguan (GB 33), Kun Lun (BL 60), Tai Xi (KI 3), Qiu Xu (GB 40) and Jie Xi (ST 41) are for knee damage. With ankle damage, Jie Xi (ST 41), Kun Lun (BL 60) and Qiu Xu (GB 40) are selected. The manipulation should be under the guidance of balanced supplement and drainage, but with severe pain, manipulate the needle with drainage. With local pain, soreness and aversion to cold, gentle moxibustion, warm needling moxibustion or cupping helps. Twice-a-week cutaneous needle tapping till slight bleeding, combined with pricking and cupping, is also helpful.

部可取曲池、小海、天井、合谷等;腕部可取阳池、合谷、阳池、阳谷、外关等;腰部可取肾俞、大肠俞、腰阳关、殷门、委中、太溪等;髀部可取环跳、秩边、扶承等;膝部可取梁丘、膝眼、阳关、昆仑、太溪、丘墟、解溪等;踝部可取解溪、昆仑、丘墟等。针刺以平补平泻为主,剧烈疼痛者可用泻法;如局部疼痛酸楚畏寒明显者,可配合温和灸,温针灸,或者拔火罐。刺络拔罐可以皮肤针重叩至局部微出血,加以火罐,每周 2 次。

2.2 Tuina

Tuina mainly focuses on the acupoints nearby or along the meridians. For old injury, manipulations like pushing, grasping, kneading and pinching are strengthened. For mild injury, manipulations should be gentle. For damaged sinews which aren't broken, plucking damaged sinews, tendons and vessels are emphasized. If sinews of joints in four limbs are damaged, flexion, extension and rotation are combined to promote the healing. The manipula-

2.2 推拿康复

推拿以受损局部为主,可采用循经或局部穴位点按。宿伤者的手法宜重,伤筋部位可加强推、拿、揉、捏等;轻症者,则宜采用轻柔手法;只伤筋无断裂者,着重拨正受损筋络、经筋、筋腱。四肢关节伤筋者,可配合屈伸旋转手法以协助恢复其功

tions should be slow and be progressed step by step to avoid causing new injury. Tuina therapy may be given every day or every two days. A course involves 10 times of treatment.

Patients in rehabilitation stage can perform tuina on their own to supplement kidney and liver, strengthen sinews and bones and harmonize qi and blood. Manipulations like pressing, kneading and rubbing are for local joints. Rotating, flexing and extending, shaking joints, rubbing lumbar, pushing downward three yangs, pushing upward three yins and grasping shoulder and neck are also helpful.

能，注意手法缓慢、活动范围逐渐增大，避免形成局部新损。推拿可每日或间日一次，每10次为1个疗程。

疗养康复期患者，可进行自我推拿以补肝肾、强筋骨、和气血。如对局部关节运用按、揉、摩等手法；旋转、屈伸、抖动关节，擦腰，推下三阳，推上三阴，拿肩颈等。

2.3 Exercises

With the function of extending and soothing sinews, plucking bones and quickenging network, traditional exercises is significant to restoring and strengthening local functions of damaged sinews. Apart from Taiji Quan, Eight-brocade Exercise (Ba Duan Jin), Sinew-transformation Exercise (Yi Jin Jing), other exercises targeted at different locations are also conducive to restoring sinew functions and preventing local adhesions and cramps. For example, for patients with sinew damage in neck, movements like looking around, crane dapping on water, pulling neck forward are advised; with sinew damage in shoulder, patients can play movements like drawing the bow on both sides, lifting sky with hands, circling the arms, pulling the sword from the back, parting the wild horse's mane on both sides, red phoenix spreading the wings and cloud hands; in elbow, movements like carrying baskets with elbow spread, rotating elbow and bending wrist, pulling, blocking and pounding are necessary; with sinew damage in wrist, patients can play movements like

2.3 功法锻炼

传统功法有很好的伸筋拔骨、舒筋活络作用，对恢复伤筋局部功能和巩固意义重大。除选练太极拳、八段锦、易筋经等一般性功法外，可根据不同部位选用不同的有针对性的小功法以强化伤筋局部的功能锻炼恢复、防治局部粘连痉挛。例如，颈项部伤筋，可选练左顾右盼、仙鹤点水、与项争力等；肩部伤筋可选练左右开弓、双手托天、轮转辘轳、九鬼拔马刀、野马分鬃、丹凤展翅、云手等；肘部伤筋者可选练展肘挎篮、旋肘拗腕、搬拦捶等；腕部伤筋可选练怒目攥拳、拧拳反掌、上翘下钩、单鞭式、单鞭下势等；腰髀伤筋可选练摩肾腰、攥腰推碑、掌插华山、双手攀足、翻身披身捶

clenching fists with staring eyes, clenching fists and turning hands, dorsal extension and ventral flexion, single whip, single whip with squatting; in lumbar and thigh, movements like rubbing lumbar region, pushing through the lateral side of waist, palms thrusting into the Mount Hua, hands climbing the legs and turning to pound are necessary; with sinew damage in knees, patients can play movements like arhat arresting tiger, squatting with straight back and bending and kicking towards four directions. Each movement can be repeated for 20-25 times for a session, and it can be taken for 2-3 times a day.

等;膝部伤筋可选练罗汉伏虎、行者下坐、四面摆莲等。单一动作功法练习可每20～25次为一组,每日可练2～3次。

2.4 Medication

Oral medication differs according to the pattern identification. For wind-cold-damp obstructing meridians and network vessels, modified Da Huo Luo Dan (*Major Network-Quickening Pill*) can be used to dispel wind, disperse cold and eliminate damp. Modified Du Huo Ji Sheng Tang (*Pubescent Angelica and Mistletoe Decoction*) is for lumbar sinew damage with cold and damp attack. For insufficiency of kidney and liver combined with phlegm and stasis obstruction, modified Bu Shen Huo Xue Tang (*Kidney-Supplementing Blood-Quickening Decoction*) is used for supplementing liver and kidney, transforming phlegm and expelling stasis. For kidney yang insufficiency presented with sore lumbar and knees as well as cold and weak limbs, Jia Wei Shen Qi Wan (*Supplemented Kidney Qi Pill*) is helpful. With torn fascia, modified Zhuang Jin Xu Gu Dan (*Sinew-strengthening and Bone-joining Elixir*) can be used to supplement liver and kidney, strengthen sinews and bones and nourish qi and blood. Jian Bu Hu Qian Wan (*Steady Gait Hidden*

2.4 药物康复

药物内治,风寒湿邪痹阻经络者,宜祛风散寒除湿,可以大活络丸加减;腰部伤筋兼寒湿外侵者,可用独活寄生汤加减;肝肾不足、痰瘀阻结者,宜补益肝肾、化痰逐瘀,可以补肾活血汤加减;肾阳不足、腰膝酸软、肢冷无力者,可以加味肾气丸;筋膜撕裂者,宜补肝肾、强筋骨、养血气,可以壮筋续骨丹加减;肢体痿软无力者,可以健步虎潜丸。

Tiger Pill) is for patient with flaccidity and weakness.

External treatments like fumigation and washing, medicine external application are also helpful in recovery. The formulae should be guided by the principle of quickening blood and transforming stasis, eliminating swelling and relieving pain, warming meridians and freeing network vessels, such as Eight Immortals Free Wandering Decoction (Ba Xian Xiao Yao Tang), liquid medicine for sinew damage, bone-setting liquid, Dampness Damage Pain-Relieving Plaster and other plasters.

熏洗、熨帖、外敷等外治法均可运用于本病的康复，组方以活血化瘀、消肿止痛、温经通络为原则。如八仙逍遥汤、伤筋药水、正骨水、伤湿止痛膏、狗皮膏、万应膏等。

2.5 Diet and Daily Life

Patients with sinew damage should protect its local damage and also avoid new damage caused by cold and damp attack. According to the condition, avoid being in a posture for a long time while sitting, lying, standing, walking and working. For example, with neck damage, do not bend over desks working or look up for a long time. Pillows should be flexible, warm-keeping, and of medium height and hardness. With lumbar damage, keep the right posture and avoid long-time standing and sitting. If necessary, squat more and stoop less while working.

2.5 膳食起居

筋伤患者，在起居作息时应注意对创伤局部的保护，避免寒湿邪气侵袭和形成新创伤。根据病变部位，其坐、卧、立、行、劳作时，均应注意体态姿势、且避免长时间保持一种姿势。例如：颈项部损伤者，不宜长时间伏案或仰头，枕头不宜过高，枕头软硬要适中且有一定弹性和保暖性。腰部筋伤者，则要注意保持正确的腰部用力姿势和力平衡，避免长时间站、坐，避免过久弯腰或剧烈弯腰用劲，劳作时应尽量屈膝下蹲用力而减少弯腰。

Patients with sinew damage should avoid acrid drinks that consume qi, such as cigarette, liquor, coffee and strong tea, for they can aggravate qi and blood obstruction. Eat less greasy and sweet food, for they can produce phlegm and obstruct qi and

伤筋者，不宜烟、酒、咖啡、浓茶等味辛气烈耗气之品，以免加重气血郁阻；肥甘厚味易生痰浊而阻碍气血运行，也不宜多食；宜多食蔬

blood circulation. Eat more vegetables and fruits that can regulate qi, such as celery, eggplant, tomato, and radish.

菜、水果，如芹菜、茄子、番茄、萝卜等理气之品。

Chapter 2 Rehabilitation for Diseases of Internal Medicine of Traditional Chinese Medicine

第2章 中医内科诸症康复

This chapter only lists internal diseases that closely related with rehabilitation, such as vertigo, chest impediment and heart pain, asthma and lung-distension, dissipation-thirst. TCM Rehabilitation only applies to the remission stage of these diseases or daily prevention and self-care if coordinated with TCM health preservation.

中医内科病种较多，本章仅列举与康复关系密切者，如眩晕、胸痹心痛、哮喘肺胀、消渴等。中医康复多用于这些病的缓解期，或配合中医养生，用于日常预防及自我保健。

Section 1 Vertigo

第1节 眩晕

Vertigo is a condition characterized by dizziness and blurred vision. Those with mild vertigo may stop spontaneously by closing their eyes for a while. Those with severe vertigo may feel like sitting in a boat or car, spinning, inability to stand over a long time or with symptoms such as nausea, vomiting, or even sudden collapse. In TCM, vertigo is often induced by ascendant hyperactivity of liver yang, deficiency of qi and blood, insufficiency of kidney essence, phlegm obstruction.

眩晕即指头晕眼花，轻者闭目即止，重者如坐车船，不能站立，伴恶心、呕吐，甚则昏倒等症状。中医认为，眩晕多由肝阳上亢、气血亏虚、肾精不足、痰浊中阻所致。

1 Rehabilitation Diagnosis and Evaluation

1 康复诊断与评定

1.1 Rehabilitation Diagnosis

1.1 康复诊断

Diagnosis is made based on main symptoms like

主要依据反复发作的目

recurrent dizziness and blurred vision. To be specific, symptoms are recurrent dizziness and blurred vision, spinning objects, feeling like sitting in a boat or car, possibly complicated with tinnitus, nausea, vomit, sweating and flaccid limbs.

眩和头晕为主症确立诊断。即反复发作头旋眼花、眼前昏黑、天旋地转感、如坐舟车感，或兼见耳鸣、恶心、呕吐、汗出、肢软等症。

1.2 Rehabilitation Evaluation

Evaluate the patient with scale or counting method according to the frequency and the degree of the main symptoms. If it is severe and affects daily life, Activity of Daily Living Scale (ADL) may be applied.

1.2 康复评定

根据临床主要症状的发作频率和程度，采用数法或量表法作辨证评估；病情严重，影响日常生活者，应进行日常生活活动能力评估。

2 Rehabilitation Treatments

2 康复措施

2.1 Medication

Patients with ascendant hyperactivity of liver yang may take modified Tian Ma Gou Teng Yin (*Gastrodia and Uncaria Beverage*) and Shi Jue Ming Mu Li Tang (*Haliotidis Concha and Oyster Shell Decoction*) to calm the liver and subdue yang. With yin deficiency of liver and kidney, modified Qi Ju Di Huang Wan (*LyciumBerry, Chrysanthemum, and Rehmannia Pill*) and modified Lian Shen Tang (*Nelumbinis Stamen and Mori Fructus Decoction*) are useful in nourishing kidney and moistening liver. To treat qi deficiency and phlegm turbidity, modified Xiang Sha Liu Jun Tang (*Costusroot and Amomum Six Gentlemen Decoction*), Ban Xia Bai Zhu Tian Ma Tang (*Rhizoma Pinelliae, Atractylodes and Rhizoma Gastrodiae Decoction*) and Zhe Jue Qi Wei Yin (*Haematitum and Cassiae Semen Seven Ingredients Beverage*) can be used to boost qi and flush phlegm. With stasis obstructed internally, Xue Fu Zhu Yu Tang (*House of Blood Stasis-Expelling Decoction*) can be used to quicken blood and dispel

2.1 药物康复

肝阳上亢者，治宜平肝潜阳，可以天麻钩藤饮、石决明牡蛎汤加减；肝肾阴虚者，治宜养肾滋肝，可以杞菊地黄丸、莲椹汤加减；气虚痰浊者，治宜益气涤痰，可以香砂六君汤、半夏白术天麻汤、赭决七味饮等加减；瘀血内阻者，治宜活血祛瘀，可用血府逐瘀汤加减。

stasis.

Traditional formulae with single ingredient are effective in treating dizziness. For example, decoction with 10 g of Sang Zhi (*Ramulus Mori*) and 10 g of Ai Ye (*Folium Artemisiae Argyi*) is helpful in treating ascendant hyperactivity of liver yang. Herbal tea with 15 g of Xi Gua Cui Yi (*Exocarpium Citrulli*) and 15 g of Cao Jue Ming (*Semen Fetid Cassia*) may treat all kinds of dizziness. Niu Bang Gen (*Root Arctii*) can prevent dizziness with internally stirring liver wind. Decoction with banana's flower may treat dizziness complicated with numb fingers.

传统单验方对眩晕亦有较好效果。例如：桑枝 10 克，艾叶 10 克，水煎服，用于肝阳上亢者；西瓜翠衣 15 克，草决明 15 克，煎汤代茶饮，可用于各种眩晕；牛蒡根适量煎汤服，可防治肝风内动型眩晕；香蕉花煎水服，可治疗眩晕伴手指麻木者。

2.2 Acupuncture

Feng Chi (GB 20), Tai Yang (EX-HN 5), Tou Wei (ST 8), Yin Tang (GV 29) and He Gu (LI 4) are major acupoints. Other acupoints may be added according to the pattern identification. For example, Tai Chong (LR 3) may be selected to treat ascendant hyperactivity of liver yang; Shen Shu (BL 23), Gan Shu (BL 18) and Tai Xi (KI 3) are to treat yin deficiency of liver and kidney. Zu Sanli (ST 36) and Feng Long (ST 40) are for qi deficiency and phlegm obstruction. Ge Shu (BL 17) and Sanyin Jiao (SP 6) are for blood stasis. In general, needles are retained for 20 to 30 minutes and treatment is given every day or every two days. A course involves 7 times of treatments.

Bai Hui (GV 20), Feng Long (ST 40), Pi Shu (BL 20) and Zu Sanli (ST 36) may be selected for moxibutstion. It may be given until the skin of acupoints turn red and warm without burning. In general, each acupoint is moxibusted every two days and each time is for 5 to 7 minutes. A course in-

2.2 针灸康复

体针可选风池、太阳、头维、印堂、合谷等为主穴，根据辨证配穴：肝阳上亢者，可加太冲；肝肾阴虚者，可加肾俞、肝俞、太溪；气虚痰阻者，可加足三里、丰隆；瘀血阻滞者，可加膈俞、三阴交。一般留针 20～30 分钟，每日或间日 1 次，每 7 次为 1 个疗程。

可取百会、丰隆、脾俞、足三里等行艾条灸，灸至局部红晕、温热、无灼伤为度。通常每穴灸 5～7 分钟，间日 1 次，10 次为 1 个疗程。

volves 10 times of treatments.

If patients are presented with severe dizziness, spinning objects, nausea and vomiting, Feng Chi (GB 20), Tai Yang (EX-HN 5), He Gu (LI 4), Nei Guan (PC 6), Zu Sanli (ST 36) may be chosen for electronic acupuncture with dilatational wave impulses at the frequency of 1 to 2 hertz. It is proper to perform medium-tolerance needle manipulation for 20 to 30 minutes. It may be given every day until symptoms disappear.

如眩晕剧烈、天旋地转、恶心呕吐发作者,可以电针风池、太阳、合谷、内关、足三里等穴,选用频率 1～2 赫兹的脉冲疏密波,针感以中等耐受量为度,时间 20～30 分钟,每日 1 次,症状消失后停止。

2.3 Tuina

Press Bai Hui (GV 20) at the onset of dizziness. Push with thumb from Yin Tang (GV 29) straight towards hair line for 4 to 5 times, and then from Yin Tang (GV 29) to Si Zhu Kong (TE 23) along eyebrows for 4 to 5 times, and finally push from Yin Tang (GV 29) to Jing Ming (BL 1) and then circle eye socket for 3 to 4 times for both sides respectively. Push or knead from one Tai Yang (EX-HN 5) to the other Tai Yang (EX-HN 5) along the forehead for 3 to 4 times. At last, quickly rub the head along the gallbladder meridian from the anterosuperior to posteroinferior for 20 to 30 times.

Patients can also do tuina on their own with manipulations like kneading Cuan Zhu (BL 2), rubbing nose, covering ears with palms and tapping occipital bone with fingers, combing hair with fingers, kneading Tai Yang (EX-HN 5), rubbing forehead, pressing and kneading the back of the head, covering face with hands after rubbing, kneading Yao Yan (EX-B 7), rubbing Yong Quan (KI 1) and so on.

2.3 推拿康复

眩晕发作时,可点按百会穴;用一指禅推法从印堂直线上推至发际,往返四五次,再从印堂沿眉弓推至丝竹空,往返四五次,然后从印堂至睛明、绕眼眶,双侧交替进行各三四次;亦可用揉法,在额部从一侧太阳穴至另一侧太阳穴,往返三四次,然后用扫散法在头侧沿胆经循行部位,自前上向后下 20～30 次。

患者可行自我康复推拿,如揉攒竹、擦鼻、鸣天鼓、手梳头、揉太阳、抹额、按揉脑后、搓手浴面、揉腰眼、擦涌泉等。

2.4 Exercises

Patients with dizziness may heal by itself

2.4 功法锻炼

眩晕患者可选择太极

through exercises like Taiji Quan and Eight-brocade Exercise (Ba Duan Jin) as they can strengthen body and harmonize qi and blood, or breathing exercises (Nei Yang Gong) and Six-character Chant (Liu Zi Jue) Exercise as they can free meridian qi by regulating body and spirit. The onset of dizziness is often closely associated with qi and blood of liver, so patients can play conduction exercise targeted for liver to regulate qi circulation.

拳、八段锦等功法锻炼,使体质增强、气血调和,则眩晕自愈;亦可选用内养功、六字诀等气功功法,以调和形神、流畅经气;眩晕的发作往往与肝脏气血关系密切,患者可有针对性练习肝脏导引法以舒调其气机。

Long-term and recurrent dizziness can affect daily life, so proper operation may be performed for rehabilitation. For example, rotating balls with fingers is to free meridians and network vessels, regulate blood and qi and relieve dizziness by finger movements; with wood comb massaging the head, combing hair therapy is to improve dizziness by regulating meridians, relaxing nerves and promoting local blood and qi circulation.

病程长,反复发作,影响正常工作学习者,可选择适当的作业进行康复治疗。例如:弄球疗法,通过手部细小关节的活动,达到疏通经络、调和血气、减缓眩晕的作用;梳头疗法,通过木梳的梳理按摩作用,调节经络功能、松弛神经、促进局部血气流通,从而改善眩晕状况。

2.5 Diet and Daily Life

During the active stage of vertigo, patient should stay in bed with head in prostration and avoid turning head. Keep the room from noise and strong light. Develop a balanced routine life. Avoid staying up late, late rising, long-time traveling and working. Take more outdoor exercises.

2.5 膳食起居

眩晕发作期,应卧床休息,选择头颈平卧位,尽量避免头颈左右前后的转动;应保持卧室安静,避噪声干扰和强光刺激。平时应注意保持良好的作息规律,避免熬夜、懒床、长途舟车、长时闭户伏案等,应多参与户外活动。

Patients with vertigo may eat more eggs, lean meat, fresh vegetables and fruits instead of greasy, sweet, pungent and spicy food. Herbal diets like bamboo shoots fried with Gou Qi (*Fructus Lycii*), fish head stewed with Tian Ma (*Rhizoma Gastrodiae*), chicken

眩晕患者,忌食肥甘辛辣之品;宜进食蛋类、瘦肉等,多食新鲜蔬菜水果。可选择竹笋枸杞头、天麻鱼头、首乌煨鸡等药膳调养。

stewed with Shou Wu (*Radix Polygoni Multiflori*) are also helpful.

2.6 Mental Rehabilitation

Dizziness is closely related with liver, for liver governs anger and easily gets stagnated. Thus, patients should stay optimistic, strong and open-minded. Pleasure and stable emotion are significant to its rehabilitation. Therefore, patients may participate in some activities to improve their mental state and avoid negative emotions like anger and depression.

2.6 精神康复

眩晕与肝脏关系密切，肝主怒而又容易气郁，因此，注意培养患者乐观、坚强的性格，保持心胸宽广、心情舒畅、情绪稳定，对该病的康复意义重大。可通过参加一些雅趣活动陶冶情操、改善精神状态，避免忧郁恼怒等不良情绪刺激。

Section 2 Chest Impediment and Heart Pain

第2节 胸痹心痛

Chest impediment and heart pain is a condition characterized with paroxysmal feeling of oppression and pain in Dan Zhong (CV 17) or left chest. It is mainly induced by phlegm, stasis, qi stagnation, heart vessels obstructed with cold due to deficiency of healthy qi, improper diet, emotional disorders, and attack of cold.

胸痹心痛是以膻中或左胸部发作性憋闷、疼痛为主要临表现的一种病证，多由于正气亏虚，触冒饮食、情志、寒邪等因素，引起痰浊、瘀血、气滞、寒凝痹阻心脉而致。

1 Rehabilitation Diagnosis and Evaluation

1.1 Rehabilitation Diagnosis

Diagnosis can be made based on typical symptoms of chest impediment and heart pain and modern tests. The typical symptom is paroxysmal pain at Dan Zhong (CV17) or left chest. Those with mild condition may present with suffocated chest stiffness and difficulty in breathing, and those with severe conditions may present with pain radiating to

1 康复诊断与评定

1.1 康复诊断

依据胸痹心痛的典型症状，并借助现代检查手段确立诊断。其典型症状为：突发性膻中或左胸膺部位疼痛，轻则胸痛如窒、呼吸不畅，重者胸痛彻背、背痛彻心；疼痛可向咽部、左侧肩

the back and the back pain radiating to the chest. In some cases, pain may also radiate to pharynx, left shoulder, back, sternum, and hypochondrium. Other symptoms include palpitation, shortness of breath with inability to lie flat, and a pale complexion. Pain may persist for 2 to 3 minutes or several hours. During inactive stage, ECG results are normal or indicate previous myocardial infarction. The changes of nonspecific ST segment and T waves may also be revealed. With onset of heart pain, pathological Q waves, down-sloping ST depression (>1 mm), T inversion or pseudo-normal T waves develop on the ECG. Rehabilitation only applies to conditions except heart failure, persistent hypertension and shock.

臂、背部、剑突下、胁下放射；常伴见心悸、气短，甚则喘息不得平卧、面色苍白等症；疼痛时间可持续 2～3 分钟或数小时不等。心电图检查：平时可呈正常心电，或为陈旧性心肌梗死表现，或见非特异性 ST 段和 T 波改变，或见有房早、室早；心痛发作时，可见异常 Q 波、ST 段下移 1 毫米以上，或 T 波倒置，或 T 波假性正常化。排除诊断心衰、持续性高血压、休克等情况，归康复治疗范畴。

1.2 Rehabilitation Evaluation

Evaluation can be made on the basis of incidence rate, pain, abnormal results of tests, and systemic condition. The condition can affect daily life, therefore, Activity of Daily Living Scale and Occupational Activity Scale may be necessary to assess improvements.

1.2 康复评定

根据患者心痛发作频率、疼痛程度以及相关检查指标异常度，结合全身情况进行综合辨证评估。由于患者发病后，其生活职业能力常有受损。应同时评估其日常生活能力、职业活动能力，其改善状况也应作为康复疗效的评价指标。

2 Rehabilitation Treatments

2.1 Medication

Oral medication differs according to the pattern identification. With blood stasis obstructing heart, modified Xue Fu Zu Yu Tang (*House of Blood Stasis-Expelling Decoction*) and Dan Shen Yin (*Salvia Beverage*) are necessary to quicken blood and transform stasis, free the vessels and relieve pain. With

2 康复措施

2.1 药物康复

药物内治，心血瘀阻者，治宜活血化瘀、通脉止痛，可用血府逐瘀汤、丹参饮加减。痰浊痹阻者，治宜通阳泄浊、豁痰开痹，可以瓜蒌薤白半夏汤加减；寒痰痹阻气机甚

phlegm obstruction, modified Gua Lou Xie Bai Ban Xia Tang (*Trichosanthes, Chinese Chive, and Pinella Decoction*) may be taken to free yang and remove turbidity. If with cold phlegm, Gan Jiang (*Rhizoma Zingiberis*), Gui Zhi (*Ramulus Cinnamomi*), Chen Pi (*Pericarpium Citri Reticulatae*), Kou Ren (*Semen Myristicae*) and Tan Xiang (*Lignum Santali Albi*) can be added to regulate qi and sweep phlegm, warm heart and free yang. With phlegm and stasis binding together, add Dan Shen (*Radix Salviae Miltiorrhizae*), Chuan Xiong (*Rhizoma Chuanxiong*) and Hong Hua (*Flos Carthami*). With heat caused by depressed phlegm, Huang Lian Wen Dan Tang (*Coptis Gallbladder-Warming Decoction*) with Yu Jin (*Radix Curcumae*), Gua Lou (*Fructus Trichosanthis*), Chang Pu (*Rhizoma Acori Tatarinowii*) and Dan Shen is helpful. With cold obstruction chest-yang, formulas like Gua Lou Xie Bai Bai Jiu Tang (*Trichosanthes, Chinese Chive, and White Liquor Decoction*), Gua Lou Xie Bai Zhi Shi Tang (*Tichosanthes, Chinese Chive, and Unripe Bitter Orange Decoction*) and Gua Lou Xie Bai Gui Zhi Tang (*Trichosanthes, Unripe Bitter Orange, and Cinnamon Twig Decoction*) and herbs like Dan Shen, Tan Xiang and Sha Ren (*Fructus Amomi*) will help in warming yang and dispersing cold, freeing impediment and relieve pain. If phlegm invades the lung due to yang deficiency, add Sheng Jiang (*Rhizoma Zingiberis Recens*), Fu Ling (*Poria*), Xin Ren (*Semen Armeniacae Amarum*) and Chen Pi to move qi and transform phlegm. For severe yin-cold retention, Su He Xiang Wan (*Storax Pill*), Xin Tong Wan (*Heart Pain Pill*) and Kuan Xiong Wan (*Chest-soothing Pill*) are necessary to open with

者,可加干姜、桂枝、陈皮、蔻仁、檀香等理气豁痰、温心通阳;如痰瘀互结者,加入丹参、川芎、红花等;痰浊郁结化热者,可与黄连温胆汤加郁金、瓜蒌、菖蒲、丹参等味。寒凝心脉、胸阳痹阻者,治宜温阳散寒、通痹止痛,可以瓜蒌薤白白酒汤、瓜蒌薤白枳实汤、瓜蒌薤白桂枝汤等,酌加丹参、檀香、砂仁等理气通脉止痛之品;若阳虚痰饮上犯者,可加生姜、茯苓、杏仁、陈皮等行气化痰;如阴寒凝滞甚者,可用苏合香丸、心痛丸、宽胸丸等以温开。心肾阴虚者,治宜滋阴补肾、养心安神,可以左归饮加减。气阴两虚者,治宜益气养阴、活血通络,可以炙甘草汤、生脉饮加减。阳气虚衰者,治宜温阳益气、活血通络,可以参附汤加味;如心阳欲脱者,可重用红参、制附片、龙骨、牡蛎以回阳救逆。

warmth. For deficiency of heart-yin and kidney-yin, modified Zuo Gui Yin (*Left-Restoring Beverage*) will aid in enriching yin and supplementing kidney, nourishing heart and quieting spirit. For deficiency of qi and yin, modified Zhi Gan Cao Tang (*Honey-Fried Licorice Decoction*) and Sheng Mai Yin (*Pulse-Engendering Beverage*) are necessary to boost qi and nourish yin, quicken blood and free network vessels. For debilitation of yang-qi, modified Shen Fu Tang (*Ginseng and Aconite Decoction*) will aid in warming yang and boost qi, quicken blood and free network vessels. For yang qi on the verge of desertion, Hong Shen (*Radix Ginseng Rubra*), sliced processed Fu Zi (*Radix Aconiti Lateralis Preparata*), Long Gu (*Os dracoris*), Mu Li (*Oyster shell*) can restore yang from collapse.

Some medications can also be applied externally. For example: Heart-freeing Plaster can be applied to Xin Shu (BL 15), Jueyin Shu (BL 14) and Dan Zhong (CV 17). Coronary Pain-relieving Plaster can be applied to Dan Zhong (CV 17), Xin Shu (BL 15) and Xu Li.

可选用药物外治康复。例如:以通心膏贴敷心俞、厥阴俞、膻中;冠心止痛膏贴敷膻中、心俞、虚里。

2.2 Functional Training

With medication, appropriate functional training can improve the cardiac function and promote early resumption of daily activity and work.

2.2 功能训练

在接受药物康复的同时进行适当的功能训练,可明显改善心脏的功能,使患者日常生活能力和职业能力得以早日康复。

Within a week after onset, if conditions are well-controlled and no complications occur, activities with 1-2 METs are necessary, such as dining on bed, washing face, drinking, passive movements of limbs, using chamber pot or moving from bedside to chairs. During the activities, physicians should ob-

在发病1周内,患者临床病情控制后且无并发症,可进行1～2 METs(代谢用量)的活动。如床上进餐、洗漱、饮水、肢体被动活动、床上使用便器、床旁坐椅子等。

serve the patients carefully. If abnormal cardiac functions are triggered, patients should stop the training immediately for a rest. 2 to 3 weeks after onset, if conditions are stable, exercises can be strengthened under the surveillance. Functional training with 2 to 3 METs are acceptable, such as dressing, washing face while standing, dining on its own, indoor activities, and sweeping. 4 weeks after onset, if conditions are significantly improved, training at the METs of 3 to 5 are available, such as walking 4 kilometers every hour, showering, going upstairs and downstairs and gardening. Through training, the patients may resume daily living activities and be capable of working.

训练时应注意观察患者状况,如诱发心功能明显异常,应暂停活动,保持静息。在发病第 2～3 周,患者病情平稳后,可在监护下稍增大活动量,进行 2～3 METs 的功能训练。如穿衣、站立洗漱、自行进食、室内或廊道活动、小范围扫地等。注意活动前后要充分休息,禁止进行负重练习,活动前后应作心脏指标检测,如出现不良反应,应减少甚至暂停训练。发病第 4 周以后,患者状况明显改善,可进行 3～5 METs 的功能训练,如:每小时 4 公里左右的散步、淋浴、上下楼梯、园艺活动等。力求经过训练,能毫无困难地生活自理,并胜任适当的职业活动。

2.3 Acupuncture

Xin Shu (BL 15), Jueyin Shu (BL 14), Dan Zhong (CV 17), Nei Guan (PC 6), Xi Men (PC 4) and Zu Sanli (ST 36) are main acupoints. With heart yin deficiency, add Sanyin Jiao (SP 6), Tai Chong (LR 3) and Tai Xi (KI 3). For heart yang deficiency, add Su Liao (GV 25), Da Zhui (GV 14) and Guan Yuan (CV 4). For heart qi deficiency, add Su Liao (GV 25) and Lie Que (LU 7). For internal congestion of phlegm, add Feng Long (ST 40), Chi Ze (LU 5) and Pi Shu (BL 20). For heart vessel obstruction, add Sanyin Jiao (SP 6), Lie Que (LU 7) and Ge Shu (BL 17). Rotation may be combined with lifting and thrusting under the guidance

2.3 针灸康复

可取心俞、厥阴俞、膻中、内关、郄门、足三里为主穴;心阴虚则可配三阴交、太冲、太溪;心阳虚则可配素髎、大椎、关元;心气虚则可配素髎、列缺;痰浊内壅可配丰隆、尺泽、脾俞;心脉痹阻可配三阴交、列缺、膈俞。捻转结合提插,平补平泻,视情况留针 5～20 分钟,注意行针引气。阳虚、气虚者,可配合温和灸、温针灸法。通常每日或间日针灸 1 次,10 次

of balanced supplementation and drainage. Needles may be retained for 5 to 20 minutes and physicians should be careful in manipulating needles and guiding qi. With yang deficiency and qi deficiency, gentle moxibustion and warm needling moxibustion are necessary. In general, acupuncture should be given every day or every two days. A course involves 10 times of treatment. The following course is given after an interval of 5 days.

为1个疗程，间隔5日后可进入下1个疗程。

With ear acupuncture, auricular acupoints like Heart, Shen Men, Sub-cortex, Kidney, Sympathetic Nerve, Endocrine and Zhen are necessary. 3 to 4 acupoints may be selected every time. Needle-embedding or auricular plaster with Wang Bu Liu Xing (Vaccariae Semen) may be applied for every 5 days.

耳针可选心、神门、皮质下、肾、交感、内分泌、枕等穴位，每次取3～4穴，双侧同时取穴，可埋针，也可用王不留行籽贴压，5日左右更换1次。

2.4 Tuina

2.4 推拿康复

For yin deficiency and stasis, push, knead and press the acupoints like Shen Shu (BL 23), Gan Shu (BL 18), Xin Shu (BL 15), Xinbao Shu (BL 14), Sanyin Jiao (SP 6) and Tai Xi (KI 3). If with deficiency of both qi and yin, add Zu Sanli (ST 36) and Qi Hai (CV 6). For yang deficiency and stasis, press and knead Ming Men (GV 4), Pi Shu (BL 20), Xin Shu (BL 15), Xinbao Shu (BL 14) and Nei Guan (PC 6) and rub Shen Shu (BL 23), Dachang Shu (BL 25) and Ming Men (GV 4). In addition, rub auricle and press auricular acupoints of Heart, Chest and Shen Men. For patients with long-time bed rest, systemic tuina may be performed to free blood vessels to prevent venous thrombosis and bedsore.

阴虚瘀阻者，可选肾俞、肝俞、心俞、心包俞、三阴交、太溪等穴位，行推、揉、按手法；气阴不足者，在此基础上，加足三里、气海等穴。阳虚瘀阻者，可取命门、脾俞、心俞、心包俞、内关等穴，行按揉手法，并在肾俞、大肠俞、命门加用擦法。另可按摩耳廓，注意点按心、胸、神门等部位。对于较长时间卧床者，可行适当全身按摩，以疏通周身血脉，预防静脉血栓和褥疮等。

If possible, patients can do tuina on their own twice or three times a day. ① Pressing chest: Press the hypochondrium and then rub it from the superi-

有条件行自我按摩者，可每日自我按摩2～3次：①按胸肋。右手贴于左胸

or to the inferior with left hand with the right hand placed on left chest. Then press the other side. Each side is for 9 times; ② Pressing Ming Men (GV 4): two thumbs are placed on the chest with other fingers rested on the back and then press and knead Ming Men (GV 4) for 18 to 36 times; ③ Tapping Nei Guan (PC 6): Pull Nei Guan (PC 6) for 100 times with index finger, middle finger and ring finger rested on Nei Guan (PC 6), Shen Men (HT 7) and Lie Que (LU 7) respectively; ④ Rubbing Yong Quan (KI 1): rub left Yong Quan (KI 1) with the right hand for 18 to 36 times and vice versa.

前，左手按于相应后胁腋部位，自上而下反复按摩，然后换至对侧，左右各9次；②按命门。双手大拇指置于胸前，四指指尖贴于后背，呈反手叉腰姿势，然后用四指微用力按揉18～36次；③叩内关。两手相对，食指、中指、无名指指尖扣在对侧腕部内关、神门、列缺穴上，叩动内关100次左右；④擦涌泉。先用左手擦右侧涌泉，再用右手擦左侧涌泉，各18～36次。

2.5 Mental Rehabilitation

Emotion disorder, like anxiety, thought and anger, is one of the factors that lead to heart pain. Patients always have mental disorders of varying degrees, for example, anxiety and depression due to the fear of losing living ability and work. Severe conditions will affect the rehabilitation. Therefore, it is important to regulate moods, for it can sooth qi circulation and harmonize qi and blood, free meridians and network vessels. To make sure active cooperation in rehabilitation treatment, physician should inform patients and their families of the condition and healing process, the aim and function of treatment. For patients with depression, therapy of happiness is necessary to regulate emotion; for anxious and nervous patients, doubt-explaining and empathy are useful. Patients may be guided to relax and avoid heart pain caused by negative emotions; for patients without confidence, group lectures may be held to share experiences and give encouragement among them.

2.5 精神康复

忧思恼怒是心痛的致病因素之一，且心痛患者常伴有不同程度的心理障碍，如害怕丧失生活工作能力、害怕突然死亡，因而焦虑、忧郁等。情志异常严重影响患者的康复，因此，调畅情志以疏导气机，使血气和调、经络通利是康复的重要方面。应针对患者具体情况，作好解释工作，使患者及其家属正确认知病情和病愈过程、康复治疗的目的和作用，使其积极配合康复。对抑郁者，宜采用喜疗法以调畅情志；对易于焦虑、紧张者，多用释疑法、移情法调治，并指导患者学会自我放松，避免不良情绪诱发心痛；对于信心不足者，可采用集体座谈方式，通过患友经验交流,生动有力地给予鼓励。

2.6 Exercises

Traditional exercises will aid in supporting healthy qi, regulating blood vessels and quieting emotions. Simple rest in bed or functional exercises may be more helpful. Static exercises like Relaxing and Calming Exercises (Song Jing Gong) should be started and played once or twice a day and each time for 15 to 20 minutes. Later, exercises combining motion with stillness is acceptable, such as Heart-soothing and Blood-calming Exercise, one of conduction and health-keeping exercises. At last, exercises like Tai Ji Quan, Eight Trigram Boxing (Ba Duan Jin), Five-animal Boxing (Wu Qin Xi) are available. Start with single movement, and then progress into half set or the whole set according to the condition.

Exercises should be chosen by patients according to their own personal interests and conditions. Seek the combination of body with spirit and progress step by step during playing. If patients feel tired or have the sign of heart pain, reduce the duration of exercises or stop it.

2.6 功法锻炼

传统功法练习,有助于扶助正气、调畅血脉、安定情志。较单纯的静卧休息或功能运动锻炼更有益。开始可以静功为主,如选练松静功,每日1～2次,每次15～20分钟,逐渐增加练功时间。之后可选择动静结合功法,如选择导引养生功的舒心平血功。之后可选择动中有静的功法,如选练太极拳、八段锦、五禽戏之类;可从单式开始练习,随后根据康复情况练习半套或全套路,再根据情况增加练习遍数。

功法修炼要注意根据患者病情结合个人兴趣和条件选择安排,力求心身合一,不可勉强;应注意循序渐进,量力而行;总以自觉练功后舒适为佳,如行功后出现疲劳过度或心痛征兆,则应减量或暂停练习。

2.7 Diet and Daily Life

Patient should stay in quiet places and have adequate sleep with noon break. Temperature changes can affect the condition, so patients should be careful and avoid external pathogenic factors, especially in winter when getting up in the morning or going to bathroom at night. Overwork also easily triggers heart pain, so patients should alternate work with

2.7 膳食起居

应注意保持环境安静,睡眠充分,午间适当休息。寒温变化对本病影响较大,衣着、被盖、动静之类,皆应注意适寒温、防外邪。特别是在寒冬季节,清晨起床或夜间如厕时更要加以留意。

rest and avoid five exertion. During bowel movements, do not force too much. Patients with constipation should regulate with diet or medicine.

过劳容易诱发心痛，应注意劳逸结合，慎防五劳。排便时不可屏气或过分用力，如有便秘者应通过食药调理以保持大便通畅。

To guarantee nutrition without increasing burden to heart, patients with heart pain should have more meals a day but less food at each, have a rest after meal for 0.5 to 1 hour. Overweight patients should eat less, especially for supper, and don't eat before sleeping. Greasy and sweet food easily produces phlegm and turbidity, obstructing network vessels. Therefore, eat more fruits and vegetables. Strong tea, coffee, liquor and cigarette should be forbidden. Herbal meals based on pattern identification may be necessary for rehabilitation. For example, for patients with qi stagnation, porridge with Jing Mi (*Oryzae Seme*) is necessary to move qi and soothe chest, free yang and disperse binds. For patients with phlegm impediment, Shan Zha (*Fructus Crataegi*) porridge will help in soothing chest, transforming phlegm and precipitating qi. Yu Zhu (*Rhizoma Polygonati Odorati*) and Shan Zha Porridge is for patients with yin deficiency. Xie Bai (*Bulbus Allii Macrostemonis*) and Tao Ren (*Semen Persicae*) porridge is for yang deficiency. Ren Shen (*Radix Ginseng*) and Bai He (*Bulbus lily*) porridge is for deficiency of both qi and yin.

心痛患者，切忌暴饮暴食，应少食多餐，既保证营养又不增加心脏负担。餐后宜静息半小时到 1 小时，然后再活动；形体肥胖者更应控制食量，尤其晚餐应注意节制，临睡前不能进食。膏粱厚味易生痰浊而阻滞脉络，故宜多食瓜果蔬菜，少食肥甘。忌饮浓茶、咖啡、烈酒，吸烟对本病危害较大，应主动戒烟。可辨证选用合适药膳配合康复治疗。如：气滞者可给予能行气宽中、通阳散结的粳米粥；痰痹者可与宽胸化痰下气的山楂粥；阴虚者可用玉竹山楂粥；阳虚者可与薤白桃仁粥、气阴两虚者可与人参百合粥等。

Section 3 Asthma and Lung-distention

第 3 节 哮喘肺胀

Asthma is a paroxysmal condition characterized

"哮"指哮病，是由于宿

by rapid and difficult breathing, wheezing sound in the throat, or inability to lie flat. The pathogenesis is as follows: stimulants or external pathogenic factors trigger hidden phlegm and obstruct airway, causing impaired depurative downbearing of the lung and phlegm-qi mixture. Wheezing (Chuan) is a condition featured by difficulty in breathing, or even breathing with raised shoulders and open mouth, flaring nostrils and inability to lie flat. Lung-distension is condition presenting with dyspnea, cough with phlegm, chest stuffness and fullness. Patients with long-time condition may have cyanosis in nails and lip, palpitation and edema. With contraction of external pathogenic factors or inappropriate treatment, coma, convulsion and collapse may occur. It is often caused by many advanced chronic lung diseases. As these three conditions are lung diseases with similar pathology, etiology and pathogenesis, they are introduced together.

痰伏肺,遇诱因或感邪引触,以致痰阻气道,肺失肃降,痰气搏击所引起的发作性痰鸣气喘疾患,发作时喉中哮鸣有声,呼吸气促困难,甚至喘息不能平卧为主要表现;“喘”指喘证,是以呼吸困难,甚至张口抬肩,鼻翼煽动,不能平卧为特征的一种肺系疾病;“肺胀”,是以“喘、咳、痰、胀”,即喘息气促,咳嗽,咳痰,胸部膨满,胀闷如塞等为主要临床特征的病证,病久可见唇甲发绀、心悸、浮肿等症。兼外邪或调治不当,其变证坏病可见昏迷、抽搐以至喘脱等,为多种慢性肺系疾病后期转归而成。哮、喘、肺胀,三者的病理表现、病因病机有相似之处,且均为肺系疾病,因此合于一节讨论。

1 Rehabilitation Diagnosis and Evaluation

1.1 Rehabilitation Diagnosis

The rehabilitation also applies to some diseases in Western medicine such as chronic obstructive pulmonary diseases and pulmonary heart disease in remission, such as chronic bronchitis, bronchial asthma, emphysema. Related clinical diagnosis criteria may be referred.

1.2 Rehabilitation Evaluation

Evaluation can be made based on the course of disease, the degree of dyspnea and systemic condition. In addition, it is advisable to assess high risk

1 康复诊断与评定

1.1 康复诊断

凡现代医学诊断为慢性支气管炎、支气管哮喘、肺气肿等慢性阻塞性肺病的缓解期及肺心病缓解期,均归属本病康复范畴。具体可参见临床医学相关诊断标准。

1.2 康复评定

主要根据患者病程,呼吸困难程度,结合全身体质状况进行辨证评估。同时应

factors, patients' to lerance, the organs involved and their functions, activity of daily living and capability of working.

评定其诱发加重高危因素，及患者耐受能力；累及的脏腑及其功能状况；以及日常生活自理能力和职业承担能力。

2 Rehabilitation Treatments

2 康复措施

2.1 Medication

2.1 药物康复

Based on the condition, constitution and the course of disease, medication focusing on treating lung should be given. For lung deficiency with insecurity of defense qi, modified Gui Zhi Huang Qi Tang (*Cinnamomi Ramulus and Astraglalus Decoction*) and Yu Ping Feng San (*Jade Wind-Barrier Powder*) are necessary to supplement lung and secure the exterior. Medication should be moderate. For spleen deficiency with hidden phlegm, modified Yi Gong San (*Special Achievement Powder*) and Liu Jun Zi Tang (*Six Gentlemen Decoction*) are necessary to supplement spleen and boost lung, transform phlegm and guiding qi downward. For kidney failing to receive qi, modified Mai Wei Di Huang Wan (*Ophiopogon and Rehmannia Pill*) and Jin Gui Shen Qi Wan (*Golden Coffer Kidney Qi Pill*) are necessary to supplement kidney and receive qi. For qi and yin deficiency of heart and lung, modified Sheng Mai San (*Pulse-Engendering Powder*) combined with Yu Ping Feng San (*Jade Wind-Barrier Powder*) is available to nourish heart and supplement lung, boost qi and free vessels.

应根据病情轻重、体质强弱及病程长短，以肺为核心辨证调理康复。肺虚卫气不固者，治宜补肺固表，可以桂枝黄芪汤、玉屏风散加减；调理上宜守不宜攻，宜缓不宜峻。脾虚痰浊内伏者，治宜补脾益肺、化痰顺气，可用异功散、六君子汤加减；肾虚不能纳气者，治宜补肾纳气，根据肾虚阴阳偏颇情况选用麦味地黄丸、金匮肾气丸加减；心肺气阴两虚者，治宜养心补肺、益气通脉，可以生脉散合玉屏风加减。

Traditional formulae with single ingredient are available: ①Di Long (*Pheretima*) powder, 3 times a day and 3 g each time; ②20 g of Yan You (*Limacidae*) and 15 g of Zhe Bei Mu (*Bulbus Fritillariae Thunbergii*) are

传统单验方可选：①广地龙粉，每次 3 克，每日 3 次；②蜒蚰 20 克，浙贝母 15 克，捣烂晒干为末制丸，每次 3

mashed, dried and then made into pills. 3 g of pills are taken for 3 times a day; ③60 g of Zi He Che (*Placenta hominis*) powder, 45 g of Ge Jie (*Gecko*) powder and 24 g of Wu Wei Zi (*Fructus Schisandrae Chinensis*) are made into pills. 5 g of pills are taken for twice a day; ④10 He Tao Ren (*Semen Juglandis*) may be taken with salty water before sleep; ⑤ 12 to 15 g of Wan Nian Qing Gen (*Rhizoma et Radix Rohdeae*) and 5 Da Zao (*Fructus Jujubac*) are decocted and taken once a day.

克,每日3次;③紫河车粉60克,蛤蚧粉45克,五味子粉24克,制丸,每次5克,每日2次;④胡桃仁10个,每晚临睡前细嚼,淡盐水送服;⑤万年青根12～15克,红枣5枚,煎服,每日1次。

2.2 Acupuncture

Da Zhui (GV 14), Fei Shu (BL 31), Pi Shu (BL 20), Shen Shu (BL 23), Gao Huang (BL 43), Qi Hai (CV 6), Zu Sanli (ST 36), Lie Que (LU 7), Tai Yuan (LU 9), Yu Ji (LU 10), Tai Xi (KI 3), Sanyin Jiao (SP 6) and Ming Men (GV 4) are helpful. 3 to 5 acupoints may be selected every time for manipulation with supplementation. Needles can be retained for 15 to 20 minutes. Acupuncture may be given every day or every two days. A course involves 10 times of acupuncture treatments. Auricular acupoints like Lung, Spleen, Kidney, Heart, Windpipe, Throat, Shen Men, Triple Jiao and Endocrine can be selected for ear acupuncture. 3 to 5 acupuncture are chosen for needle embedding or 5-minute pressing. Needles should be replaced every week.

Da Zhui (GV 14), Feng Men (BL 12), Fei Shu (BL 31), Dan Zhong (CV 17), Shen Shu (BL 23) and Qi Hai (CV 6) may be selected for cone moxibustion with 3 to 5 cones for each acupoint each time. Moxibustion may be given every 10 days and a course involves 3 times of treatment. Moxibustion in three hot periods of summer are more effective.

2.2 针灸康复

可取大椎、肺俞、脾俞、肾俞、膏肓、气海、足三里、列缺、太渊、鱼际、太溪、三阴交、命门等穴。每次选取3～5穴,补法留针15～20分钟,每日或间日1次,10次为1个疗程。耳针可取肺、脾、肾、心、气管、咽喉、神门、三焦、内分泌等,每次埋针3～5穴,每日按压3～5次,每次5分钟,1周换针。

艾灸可取大椎、风门、肺俞、膻中、肾俞、气海等穴,用艾炷灸,每穴每次灸3～5壮,10日灸1次,3次为1个疗程。冬病夏治的三伏天灸法对本病康复效果明显。可于每年夏天三伏分三次,敷

Under the guidance of treating winter disease in summer, apply medicines to Fei Shu (BL 31), Gao Huang (BL 43) and Bai Lao (EX-HN 14) for 3 to 4 hours. The fundamental formula includes 3 g of Bai Jie Zi (*Semen Sinapis Albae*) powder, 2 g of Gan Sui (*Radix Kansui*) powder, 0.5 g of Xi Xin (*Asarum*) powder and 3 g of Gui Zhi (*Cinnamomi Ramulus*) powder. Add Sheng Jiang (*Rhizoma Zingiberis Recens*) juice with the powder. The formula can also be modified based on pattern identification. For example, for wind-phlegm, add Ku Fan (*Calcined Alum*); for kidney failing to receive qi, add Wu Bei Zi (*Sumac gallnut*) and Wu Wei Zi (*Fructus Schisandrae Chinensis*); for deficiency of kidney yang, add garlic, sulphur and Rou Gui (*Cortex Cinnamomi*).

贴肺俞、膏肓、百劳等穴位，3～4 小时取下。常用三伏贴基础方为白芥子 3 克，甘遂 2 克，细辛 0.5 克，桂枝 3 克，共研细末，调用姜汁。敷贴配方也可辨证加减，如：风痰甚者，可加枯矾；肾不纳气者，可加五倍子、五味子；肾阳虚惫者，可加大蒜、硫磺、肉桂。

2.3 Exercises

Traditional exercises can strengthen body, for they can significantly improve the coordination and integrity of body, qi and mental powers. Through the correct way of breathing, patients can save strength to achieve the correct postures and improve respiratory functions and tolerance. Exercises like Relaxing and Calming Exercises (Song Jing Gong), Strengthening Exercises (Qiang Zhuang Gong), Breathing Exercises (Na Qi Gong), Tai Ji, Eight Trigram Boxing (Ba Duan Jin), Five-animal Boxing (Wu Qin Xi) are available.

The focus of the rehabilitation is to restore breathing functions, so patients should be guided to master the correct breathing method. To start with, inhale with nose and exhale with mouth. Then gradually progress to deep and long breathing. To learn abdominal respiration and whistling respiration, pa-

2.3 功法锻炼

传统功法可以增强体质，特别是其强调形、气、意，通过锻炼可明显提高三者的协调统一，使患者能正确运用呼吸配合形体动作，学会节省力气以完成形体动作的正确姿势和方法，可改善患者呼吸功能和耐受能力。可根据身体情况选练松静功、强壮功、纳气功、太极拳、五禽戏、八段锦等功法。

以肺部呼吸功能康复为核心，患者应特别注意训练掌握正确的呼吸方法。首先应做到鼻吸口呼，其次是逐步锻炼使呼吸深长。应让患者掌握腹式呼吸和吹哨呼吸

tients should first experience the movements of abdominal muscle, thorax and diaphragm, then practice it in static exercises and then in moving exercises. Finally patients should get used to breathing in different positions and in stillness and movements.

法，令患者注意体会腹肌、胸廓、膈肌的运动，可先在静功中练习该呼吸，然后结合到动功训练中，进而逐渐习惯在不同体位、动静状态下均运用此呼吸方式。

Step-by-step walking and running are helpful in rehabilitation. Patients should start walking at 60 to 80 steps per minute and then progress to 80 to 100 steps per minute. At first, rest at the intervals of 15 to 16 minutes and then gradually lower the frequency of rests. After being used to fast walking, patients can initiate running from interval running, that is 30-second jogging and then 30-second walking. Gradually patients may progress to more jogging and less walking, and finally to jogging all the way.

步行和健身跑对本病患者也很有益，应掌握循序渐进的原则，最初用 60～80 步/分钟的慢速，以后逐渐增加大 80～100 步/分钟的中速甚至更快；每次步行 15～16 分钟，开始时可暂行暂息，以后逐渐减少休息次数和时间。快速行走耐受后，可进一步行健身跑，从间隙跑开始，即慢跑 30 秒步行 30 秒，逐步延长慢跑时间，缩短步行时间，然后过渡到全程慢跑。

2.4 Diet and Daily Life

Patients should lead a routine life, take more exercises to strengthen the body and live in a place with mild climate, ample sunlight and fresh air. Rooms should be clean and tidy. Patients should avoid exposure to polluted environment, for noxious gases do harms to airway. Patients with allergic constitution should live in a room with simple layout, no plants and pets. Avoid external pathogenic factors and sexual indulgence. Quit smoking.

2.4 膳食起居

保持规律的生活作息，鼓励积极锻炼身体以增强体质。居住环境以气候温和、阳光充足、空气清新、居室整洁清爽为宜。空气中有害气体对呼吸道损伤大，应尽量做好自我防护，避免暴露在污染环境之下；过敏特殊体质者，居室布置应简单以减少尘螨聚积，不宜放置花卉和饲养宠物。应注意适寒温，避免外邪侵袭。应节制房事并坚决戒烟。

Nutritional and light diet is appropriate. Eat more lean meat, vegetables, agaric, kelp and animal's lungs. Avoid strong tea, greasy and sweet food, for they will generate damp and increase phlegm. Avoid food that patients are allergic to. The following herbal diets are available: ① Huang Qi (*Radix Astragali seu Hedysari*) Porridge: 20 g of Huang Qi, 60 g of Jing Mi (*Oryzae Seme*). Small-dose sugar can be added; ②Egg Porridge with Four kernels: grind ginkgo and apricot kernel (one portion respectively) and walnut and peanut (two portions respectively) into powders and decoct 20 g of powder with an egg and 50 g of Jing Mi (*Oryzae Seme*); ③Ren Shen porridge: 6 g of Ren Shen powder, 5 slices of Sheng Jiang (*Rhizoma Zingiberis Recens*), 100 g of Jing Mi, twice or three times a day; ④Beverage with fresh Mao Gen (*Rhizoma Imperatae*) and fresh lotus root: 15 g of Mao Gen and 200 g of fresh Ou (*Nelumbinis Rhizomatis Nodus*).

饮食宜清淡而富营养的食物。忌油腻荤腥和怪味；宜多食瘦肉、蔬菜、木耳、海带、动物肺脏等；忌食肥甘、浓茶，以免生湿助痰；对明确过敏的食物应禁食。下列食疗方可根据情况选择运用：①黄芪粥。黄芪 20 克，粳米 60 克，煮粥加少量糖食用。②四仁鸡子粥。白果仁、甜杏仁各一份，胡桃仁、花生仁各两份，按比例打粉，每晨 20 克，鸡蛋 1 枚，粳米 50 克，煮粥服。③人参粥。人参粉 6 克，生姜 5 片，粳米 100 克，煮粥，每日 2～3 次。④二鲜饮。鲜茅根 15 克，鲜藕片 200 克，煎汁代茶水饮。

2.5 Tuina

Tuina is mainly for supporting right and securing root, soothing chest and regulating qi. Manipulations like grasping back, rubbing chest, pressing and rubbing hypochondrium, kneading Feng Chi (GB 20) and Ming Men (GV 4), grasping He Gu (LI 4) and kneading Xue Hai (SP 10) are available. Pressing acupoints in the chest is more effective. Acupoints below the margins of sternal rib 1 to 5 are main acupoints. Other sensitive acupoints at chest are also available. Press 7 to 15 minutes every time and three times a day. A course involves 10 times of treatment.

2.5 推拿康复

以扶正固本、宽胸理气为主。可提拿背脊、擦胸、按摩胁下、揉风池、揉命门、捏合谷、揉血海等。胸部穴位按压效果明显，常以 1～5 胸肋下缘对称穴位为主穴，配以其他胸部敏感按点，每次按压 7～15 分钟，每日 3 次，10 日为 1 个疗程。

Patients can perform tuina manipulations as followed on their own once or twice a day. ①rub-

可以按下法每日自我按摩 1～2 次：①抹胸。两手交

bing chest: rub obliquely from shoulder to subcostal angle for 10 times at each side; ②patting lungs: pat along the thorax from supraclavicular fossa for 10 times with each hand; ③beating back with a fist for 10 times: while inhaling, bend the back and beat it from the medial to the inferior; while exhaling, stretch the back and beat it from the lateral to the medial; ④rubbing Dan Zhong (CV 17): press Dan Zhong (CV 17) with palms and rub it clockwise and anticlockwise for 36 circles at each direction.

替从一侧肩部由上向下呈斜线抹至肋下角，各重复 10 次。②拍肺。两手至上缺盆开始沿胸廓自上而下拍打各 10 次。③捶背。两手握空拳置于背部，呼气时背稍向前屈，同时由内向下捶打；吸气时挺胸，同时由外向内捶打，重复 10 次。④摩膻中。用手掌按于膻中穴，作顺逆时针按摩各 36 圈。

2.6 Mental Rehabilitation

Patients can easily be irritated, anxious and sad, because lung's function of governing qi and governing management and regulation is impaired and patients will focus more on the affected body and have strong dependency. Physician should communicate frequently with patients to satisfy their needs for dependency and care and to wipe away their depression and loneliness. Impaired breathing causes anxiety and in return anxiety will aggravate difficulty in breathing, so physicians should talk with patients and guide patients to change their negative attitude. Observe carefully and once potential body-spirit abnormal changes emerge, physicians can regulate through empathy, encouragement and explanation. Suicidal tendencies due to severe dyspnea should be avoided.

2.6 精神康复

患者由于肺主气和主治节的功能下降，容易情绪激惹、烦躁、悲伤、焦虑等，其活动能力下降容易对躯体过度关注并产生较强的依赖性。应多与患者交流，适度满足其依赖心理、对爱的需求，消除其抑郁、孤独心理；应注意对其进行语言疏导，改变其消极态度，协助其摆脱因呼吸功能下降导致焦虑和因焦虑加重呼吸困难的恶心循环；注意观察，及时发现其潜在的“身-心”关联异常变化倾向，及时运用制情、移情、鼓励、解释等方法以及早调整，应防范其因严重呼吸困难而绝望甚至于自杀倾向的行为。

Section 4 Consumptive Thirst

第 4 节 消渴

Consumptive thirst is a condition characterized

消渴，是以多饮、多尿、

by polyuria, polydipsia, polyphagia, debility, emaciation and sweet odor of the urine. Its treatment can also applies to diabetes in Western medicine. The condition mainly affects lung, stomach and kidney. The basic pathogenesis lies in insufficiency of yin-fluids and prevailing of dryness-heat. The common patterns are lung-dryness damaging fluids, exuberance of stomach-heat and deficiency of kidney-yin.

多食及消瘦、疲乏、尿甜为主要特征的综合病证，相当于现代医学之糖尿病。本病主要病变部位在肺、胃、肾，基本病机为阴津亏耗，燥热偏盛，常见证型有肺热津伤型、胃热炽盛型、肾阴亏虚型。

1 Rehabilitation Diagnosis and Evaluation

1 康复诊断与评定

1.1 Rehabilitation Diagnosis

Rehabilitation applies to patients diagnosed with diabetes by Western medicine but with mild condition (FBG < 10 mmol/L), with or without complications like cataract, night blindness, deafness and abscesses (Swelling or flat).

1.1 康复诊断

现代临床主要针对诊断为糖尿病的患者。其经过临床治疗，病情减轻，伴或不伴白内障、雀目、耳聋、痈疽等并发症，只要空腹血糖在10毫摩尔/升以内者，均可进行康复治疗。

1.2 Rehabilitation Evaluation

Evaluation can be made based on the course, blood glucose and systemic condition. In addition, patient's tolerance, the organs involved and their functions, daily living activities and capability of working should also be assessed.

1.2 康复评定

主要根据患者病程，血糖情况，结合全身体质状况进行辨证评估。同时应评定患者耐受能力，累及的脏腑及其功能状况，以及日常生活自理能力和职业承担能力。

2 Rehabilitation Treatments

2 康复措施

2.1 Diet and Daily Life

In general, this condition is lingering and closely associated with life style. Therefore, self-management is essential. Patients should lead a routine life, avoid anxiety, nervousness and sexual indulgence, and prevent external pathogenic factors. Pa-

2.1 膳食起居

消渴病程缠绵，其病情与生活习惯关系密切。因此，患者的自我管理非常重要。日常生活中，应避免焦虑紧张的情绪，应建立良好

tients with this condition always have yin deficiency of zang-fu organs. Due to disordered qi transformation, weak constitution and poor resistance, patients are vulnerable to pathogenic factors. Therefore, patients should be more careful in personal hygiene, frequently taking baths, changing clothes and brushing teeth. For women, keep the vulva clean. Due to poor circulation of qi and blood and stasis obstruction in vessels, feet will be insensitive to cold, heat and pain. Therefore, it is important to protect the feet. Check the shoes before putting them on and exam feet every day. Deal with blister, cutaneous fissure, gall, clavus, callus, paronychia and onychomycosis timely when they are presented. Do not use sharp nail scissors. Have a foot bath every day with moderate temperature. Shoes should be comfortable, soft and with fine air permeability. Nails shouldn't be cut too short.

的生活制度，慎起居、节房劳，适寒温以防外邪侵袭。消渴患者“脏腑阴虚”，内在气化紊乱，体质弱、抵抗力差，极易受秽浊之邪侵袭，应特别注意个人卫生，勤洗澡、勤换衣，注意口腔卫生，尤其是女性患者，要保持外阴清洁。足部保护十分重要，病程久者，由于气血不畅，络脉瘀阻，其对冷、热、疼、痛等感觉不灵敏，穿鞋前必须检查有无异物，每天检查足部情况，发现有水疱、皮裂、磨伤、鸡眼、胼胝、甲沟炎、甲癣等，应及时处理。不可用锐利刀剪自行修剪。每天用温水泡脚，水温不可过热，鞋要宽松舒适，袜子要松软，透气性好。指甲不要剪得太短。

Onset of Consumptive thirst is closely associated with improper diet. Therefore, diet is significant to the rehabilitation. Conditions of elderly patients with obese diabetes can be improved through regulating the diet. Cigarette, liquor, salty, greasy, sweat food and food with high calorie should be avoided. Eat less, especially staple food. It is traditionally believed that sweat food easily causes disease. Modern medicine also proves that sugar controlling is the core of rehabilitation. Reduce the amount of staple food sharply or gradually. At the beginning, patients will feel hungry. Eat more vegetables or have more meals but little food at each. When conditions are relieved and more exercises are taken, increase

消渴发病与食饮不节关系密切，因此，饮食康复是其他一切康复的基础，特别是老年肥胖型糖尿病患者，往往通过饮食调节即可缓解。应不吸烟、不饮酒、少吃食盐和富含糖类、油脂以及热量高的食物。食量特别是面食应注意节制，传统认为过食甘甜容易致病，现代医学证实其核心是控制糖的摄入。主食的限制可采取骤降法或递减法，在控制初期如饥饿感明显，可适当增加绿叶蔬

the amount of staple food with less than 50 grams each day. If simple diet controlling fails, other rehabilitation treatments should be added.

Eat more Yi Yi Ren (*Coix Seed*), bran, beans and pumpkins as staple food, and celery, cabbage, leek, Chinese cabbage, spinach, wax gourd, tomato and mushrooms as non-staple food. According to traditional experiences and modern research, turtle, eel, onion, bitter gourd and agaric can treat this condition. Herbal diet of TCM also helps, such as pork vertebrae porridge, steamed crucian carp. If dryness-heat is prevailing, Five-juice Beverage is helpful; for qi deficiency of spleen and stomach, pork pancreas soup is available; if abscess is complicated with severe heat-toxin, mung bean porridge will aid; if abscess is ulcerated and toxins are not eliminated, Yi Yi Ren porridge is necessary.

The following herbal diet can be selected based on pattern identification: ① fried onion: 250 g of onions for frying or 50 to 100 g of onions for poaching; ② lean meat stewed with corn silk: 30 g of cork silk, 100 g of lean meat. Boil them until they are cooked. Remove the corn silk. This diet can't apply to patients with kidney-yang deficiency; ③ clam and bitter gourd soup: 250 g of bitter gourd, 100 g of clam meat. Keep the living clam in clean water for 2 days and then obtain the meat. Boil them with bitter gourd, and finally add oil and salt.

菜，有时间者可采用少吃多餐的方法。当病情减轻，运动量较大时，则可适当增加主食，但一般一天增加量不超过 50 克。应注意，如单纯饮食控制不能抑制病情时，不能无限制过度节食，而应增加配合其他康复疗法。

主食中宜多食薏苡仁、麸子、豆类、南瓜等；副食宜多食芹菜、卷心菜、韭菜、小白菜、菠菜、冬瓜、西红柿、菌类等；传统经验和现代研究都认为甲鱼、鳝鱼、洋葱、苦瓜、木耳等对消渴有特殊效果，可常食之。中医药膳食疗在这方面积累了丰富经验，一般可食用猪脊羹、清蒸鲫鱼等；燥热明显，可用五汁饮；兼脾胃气虚者，可用猪胰汤；如并发痈疽，热毒甚者，可常食绿豆粥；痈疽已溃，毒邪未清者，可食薏苡仁粥。

平时，下列简单药膳食疗方剂均可辨证选用：①炒洋葱：取洋葱 250 克，用家常烹调法制成菜肴，随饭食用；或取洋葱 50～100 克，水煮 1～2分钟后服食。②玉米须煲瘦肉：取玉米须 30 克，瘦猪肉 100 克，加水共煮汤。待熟后去玉米须，饮汤食肉。偏于肾阳不足者则不宜本方。③蚌肉苦瓜汤：用苦瓜

This diet only applies to patients with stomach-heat and yin deficiency; ④rabbit meat stewed with Gou Qi Zi (*Lycium Fructus*): 15 g of Gou Qi Zi, 250 g of rabbit meat. Stew them with mild heat, and finally add flavors. It only applies to patients with yin deficiency of liver and kidney, intestinal dryness and stomach heat; ⑤herbal tea with Huang Qi (*Radix Astragali seu Hedysari*) and Shan Yao (*Dioscoreae Rhizoma*): 30 g of Huang Qi, 30 g of Shan Yao. It only applies to patients with deficiency of spleen and stomach, insufficiency of lung-qi. Those with lung and stomach dryness-heat or with external contraction shouldn't be treated with this tea; ⑥Shan Yao and Yi Yi Ren porridge: 60 g of Shan Yao, 30 g of Yi Yi Ren. After taking the porridge, patients should decrease staple food intake. The diet is more suitable for those with deficiency of spleen and stomach, and those who easily get thirsty and hungry.

2.2 Exercises

It has been found that stillness with less motions is a factor driving this condition. According to *Origins and Outcome of Diseases* which was written in Sui Dynasty, conduction, walking and exercises are recommended to promote recovery. Therefore, exercises based on proper diet is the fundamental way to achieve complete recovery.

Exercises, such as Breathing Exercise (Nei Yang Gong), Tai Ji Qi Gong, Relaxation Exercise (Fang Song Gong), Xu Ming Gong and Circulating Healthy Qi (Zhen Qi Yun Xing Fa), can be chosen according to the condition and taken once to three times a day and each time for 15 to 30 minutes. It is better to take exercises in the morning after getting

250克,蚌肉100克。将活蚌放清水中养2日,漂后取蚌肉,与苦瓜共煮汤,熟后酌加油盐调味,即可服食。适用于糖尿病之偏于胃热阴虚者。④枸杞子炖兔肉:取枸杞子15克,兔肉250克,加水适量,文火炖熟后加盐调味,饮汤食兔肉。该方适用于肝肾不足者,肠燥胃热者不宜。⑤黄芪山药煎:生黄芪30克,怀山药30克。煎水代茶饮。适用于脾胃虚弱及肺气不足者,对肺胃燥热或兼外感者不宜。⑥山药薏米粥:怀山药60克,薏苡仁30克,共熬粥食。本方食后有饱腹感,可减少饭量,尤以脾胃虚弱而口渴善饥者更佳。

2.2 功法锻炼

中医很早就认识到"静而少动"是本病的重要促发因素,早在隋代的《诸病源候论》中就主张以导引、行走练功等予以康复。节饮食的基础上配合功法锻炼是本症康复的根本途径。

可根据患者情况,选练内养功、太极气功,配合放松功、虚明功及真气运行法等。每日1～3次,每次15～30分钟,以晨起和近子午,体内阴阳气机交换时尤宜。姿势可取卧式或坐式均可,以腹式

up, at noon or at midnight when qi movements of yin and yang are exchanged. It can be taken while sitting or lying with abdominal breathing. If dry mouth is severe, conduction recorded in *Health-Keeping Secrets* (Bao Shen Mi Yao) is available. If cataract and night blindness are complicated, Five Wheels Rolling (Wu Lun Yun Zhuan Fa) is helpful.

呼吸为主。如口干明显者，可选作《保生秘要》口干导引法；如并发白内障、雀目等，可选作五轮转动法。

Exercises should focus on stillness. With spirits guiding internal qi, yin deficiency of five viscera and disordered qi transformation are rectified. Correspondingly, movements can generate yang and promote smooth circulation of blood and qi. Therefore, moving exercises can strengthen qi transformation of bowels and viscera, ascend the clear and descend the turbid, boost original qi and eliminate yin fire. Taiji quan, Eight Trigram Boxing (Ba Duan Jin) and Health-keeping Exercise are available. In addition, walking, jogging, swimming, canoeing, riding bikes and other exercises like table tennis, badminton are also helpful. Among them, walking is the easiest one. The speed of walking should be based on the condition. It is better to walk in a place with fresh air in the morning, at night, before or after meals or during breaks. Traditional breathing method can be applied during walking.

以静为主的功法修炼，核心在以人神导内气，修复纠正五脏阴虚、气化紊乱的病理。相对应地，动则生阳，动则血气流畅，以形体运动为主的动功，能强化脏腑气化功能，升清降浊，益元气而消阴火。可选练太极拳、八段锦、保健操等功法。也可坚持步行、慢跑、游泳、划船、骑自行车，以及一些非比赛性的乒乓球、羽毛球等运动锻炼。其中步行是非常生活化而易于坚持的常用方法，根据患者具体情况，可采用不同的步行速度，步行最好在空气新鲜的地方，于早晚进行，也可在饭前后或工间休息时进行，可配合以传统行走功呼吸法进行。

The following are the issues which patients should be aware during exercises: ①The amount of exercises should be increased gradually to avoid overexertion; ②It is traditionally held that exercises should be taken correspondingly to the transformation of exuberance and debilitation of qi and blood. According to the modern medicine, exercises may

在进行运动锻炼时，应注意以下几个问题：①运动量应适当，应因人而异，逐渐增加，避免过度疲劳。②练功应适时，传统认为应配合经脉气血盛衰转化而行，现代则认为根据自身胰岛分

be taken correspondingly to the rhythm of pancreas islet excretion and glucose metabolism; ③ Be safe and prevent hypoglycemia. It is necessary to regularly examine the blood glucose to regulate the exercises.

泌、糖代谢的节律而行。③运动中应注意安全，结合现代认识，应防备低血糖发生，定期检查血糖以调整运动负荷。

2.3 Medication

Oral medication: Patients with impaired liquid due to lung heat may be treated through clearing heat and moistening lung, engendering liquid and allaying thirst with modified Xiao Ke Fang (*Wasting-Thirst Formula*); those with impaired qi and yin of lung may be treated by boosting qi and engendering liquid, clearing heat and moistening dryness with modified Er Dong Tang (*Ophiopogon and Asparagus Decoction*); exuberant stomach heat may be managed by clearing stomach and discharging fire, nourishing yin and increase humor with modified Yu Nü Jian (*Jade Lady Brew*). Those with stomach heat with impaired liquid and bowel repletion can be treated by clearing heat and engendering liquid, moistening dryness and freeing bowels with modified Zeng Ye Cheng Qi Tang (*Humor-Increasing Qi-Coordinating Decoction*) and Ren Shen Bai Hu Tang (*Ginseng White Tiger Decoction*). Deficiency of middle jiao and spleen failing to disperse liquid can be managed by boosting qi and fortifying spleen, engendering liquid and relieving thirst with modified Qi Wei Bai Zhu San (*Atractylodes Powder with Seven Ingredients*). For yin deficiency and dryness-heat, modified Di Huang Yin Zi (*Rehmannia Drink*) may be helpful in enriching yin and supplementing blood, clearing deficiency-heat and moistening dryness. For deficiency of both yin and yang, modified Shen Qi Wan (*Kidney Qi Pill*) and Zuo

2.3 药物康复

药物内治：肺热津伤者，治宜清热润肺、生津止渴，可以消渴方加减；肺气阴两伤者，治宜益气生津、清热润燥，可以二冬汤加减；胃热炽盛，治宜清胃泻火、养阴增液，可以玉女煎加减；胃热津伤腑实者，宜清热生津、润燥通腑，可以增液承气汤合人参白虎汤加减；中焦虚弱、脾不散津者，治宜益气健脾、生津止渴，可以七味白术散加味；阴虚燥热者，治宜滋阴补血、清虚润燥，可以地黄饮子加减；阴阳两虚者，治宜温阳化气、补肾养阴，可以肾气丸合左归饮加减。

Gui Yin (*Left-Restoring (Kidney Yin) Beverage*) may be necessary in warming yang and transforming qi, supplementing kidney and nourishing yin.

The following single-ingredient formulae are available: ①Boil paste with 7 pieces of chopped and steamed pig pancreases and 50 g of honey. Take it twice to three times a day and each time for 15 g; ②30 g of pumpkin powder each day for 1 to 3 months; ③3 to 9 g of dried Ren Shen (*Radix Ginseng*) every day for decoction or herbal tea; ④Decoct 2 000 ml water with 30 g of Shan Zhu Yu (*Fructus Corni*), 20 g of Wu Wei Zi (*Fructus Schisandrae Chinensis*), 20 g of Wu Mei (*Fructus Mume*) and 20 g of Cang Zhu (*Rhizoma Atractylodis*) to 1 000 ml and take it once a day for three days.

下列传统单验方可选择使用：①猪胰7具，切碎煮熟，加蜂蜜500克熬膏，每次15克，每日2～3次。②南瓜粉，每天30克，坚持1～3个月。③生晒参3～9克每天，煎服或泡水代茶饮。④山茱萸肉30克，五味子20克，乌梅20克，苍术20克，加水2 000毫升，煮取至1 000毫升，分3次温服，每日1剂。

2.4 Acupuncture

Body acupuncture: To treat those with impaired fluid due to lung heat, needle Shao Fu (HT 8), Xin Shu (BL 15), Tai Yuan (LU 9), Fei Shu (BL 13), Pi Shu (BL 20), Chi Ze (LU 5), Qu Chi (LI 11), Lian Quan (CV 23), Cheng Jiang (CV 24), Zu Sanli (ST 36) and Sanyin Jiao (SP 6). For exuberant stomach heat, puncture Pi Shu (BL 20), Wei Shu (BL 21), Zu Sanli (ST 36), Sanyin Jiao (SP 6), Nei Ting (ST 44), Zhong Wan (CV 12), Yin Lingquan (SP 9), Qu Chi (LI 11) and He Gu (LI 4). For yin deficiency and dryness-heat, select Shui Gou (GV 26), Cheng Jiang (CV 24), Lian Quan (CV 23), Qu Chi (LI 11), Lao Gong (PC 8), Tai Chong (LR 3), Xing Jian (LR 2), Shang Qiu (SP 5), Ran Gu (KI 2), Yin Bai (SP 1), Sanyin Jiao (SP 6), Shen Shu (BL 23) and Sanjiao Shu (SP 6). For depletion of both yin and yang, needle Ming Men (GV 4), Guan Yuan (CV 4), Qi Hai

2.4 针灸康复

体针：肺热津伤者，可取少府、心俞、太渊、肺俞、脾俞、尺泽、曲池、廉泉、承浆、足三里、三阴交等穴；胃热炽盛者，可选脾俞、胃俞、足三里、三阴交、内庭、中脘、阴陵泉、曲池、合谷等穴；阴虚燥热者，可取水沟、承浆、廉泉、曲池、劳宫、太冲、行间、商丘、然谷、隐白、三阴交、肾俞、三焦俞等穴；若阴阳两亏，可取命门、关元、气海、肾俞、三阴交、太溪、复溜等。烦渴口干甚，常加金津、玉液；大便秘结，常加天枢、支沟；小便频数，常加中极；视物模糊，常加太冲、光明。

(CV 6), Shen Shu (BL 23), Sanyin Jiao (SP 6), Tai Xi (KI 3) and Fu Liu (KI 7). With severe vexation and dry mouth, add Jin Jin (EX-HN 12) and Yu Ye (EX-HN 13). With constipation, add Tian Shu (ST 25) and Zhi Gou (TE 6). With increased urination, add Zhong Ji (CV 3). With blurred vision, add Tai Chong (LR 3) and Guang Ming (GB 37).

With no skin infection or ulcer, moxibust Cheng Jiang (CV 24), Yi She (BL 49), Guan Chong (TE 1) and Ran Gu (KI 2) according to *Universal Salvation Formulary* (Pu Ji Fang), or moxibust Cheng Jiang (CV 24), Tai Xi (KI 3), Zhi Zheng (SI 7), Yang Chi (SJ 4), Zhao Hai (KI 6), Shen Shu (BL 23), Xiaochang Shu (BL 27) and tip of little finger and toe once a day and each acupoint for 5 to 10 cones according to *Classics on Effective Acupuncture* (Zhen Jiu Shen Ying Jing).

如无皮肤感染溃疡者，可取《普济方》载承浆、意舍、关冲、然谷，施以艾灸；或《针灸神应经》所载承浆、太溪、支正、阳池、照海、肾俞、小肠俞、手足小指尖，每穴每次灸5～10壮，每日1次。

Auricular acupuncture: 3 to 5 points among Pancreas, Endocrine, Kidney, Triple Jiao, Root of Ear Vagus, Shen Men, Heart and Liver can be selected for 20 minutes ear acupuncture. It could be given every two days and 10 times of auricular acupuncture treatments are regarded as a course. Alternatively, 5 to 6 points among those major ones like Pancreas, Gallbladder, Kidney, Liver, Central Rim, Inter-tragal Notch, Sympathetic Nerve and Inferior Tip of Tragal and accessory ones like Triple Jiao, Thirst Point and Hunger Point may be selected each time for ear acupuncture given every two days for both ears. A course involves ten times of treatments.

耳针：可取胰、内分泌、肾、三焦、耳迷根、神门、心、肝，每次取3～5穴，针20分钟，隔日1次，10次为1个疗程。或取胰、胆、肾、肝、缘中、屏间、交感、下屏尖为主穴，配以三焦、渴点、饥点，每次选5～6穴，隔日1次，两耳交替，10次为1个疗程。

2.5 Tuina

Push two sides along the spinal column; rub the back from the superior to the inferior; knead and

2.5 推拿康复

可推脊柱两侧，由上而下摩擦背部，揉按背俞穴，捏

press acupoints on the back; pinch toes. If eye disorders are complicated, tuina the upper Dantian, finger-press Jing Ming (BL 1) and gently knead eyelid.

捻脚趾;并发眼疾者,可按摩上丹田,点按睛明,轻揉眼胞。

Patients can often tuina on their own, for example, with abdominal breathing, tuina Cheng Jiang (CV 24), Zhong Wan (CV 12), Guan Yuan (CV 4), Qi Men (LR 14) and Shen Shu (BL 23) for 18 to 36 rounds respectively.

可嘱患者经常自我按摩承浆、中脘、关元、期门及肾俞穴,每穴按摩 18～36 周,可配合腹式呼吸进行。

2.6 Mental Rehabilitation

2.6 精神康复

Heavy stress is an important factor that triggers and aggravates this condition. Due to long-time course, various tests and worries about the treatment and prognosis, patients are often under great stress and have no confidence in recovery, feeling nervous, anxious or pessimistic. These negative emotions will worsen the condition. Therefore, patients should be guided to regulate their emotions, develop right concept of knowing and doing and cultivate positive personalities.

心理压力过高亦是诱发加重本证的重要因素,加上本病病程较长、经常接受的各类检查、多种临床治疗以及对疾病预后的担心,对病人来说往往是一种巨大的压力,甚至使其失去康复信心。病者常表现为紧张焦虑或悲观消极。而这些不良情绪反又会加重病情。因此,应注意对各患者施以情志调摄,根本上应指导患者树立正确的知行观,培养恬淡、乐观、开朗的性格。

Chapter 3 Rehabilitation for Exogenous Febrile Diseases After Recovery

第3章 中医外感热病瘥后诸症康复

Compared to western medicine, TCM is unique in rehabilitation for exogenous febrile diseases after recovery. According to TCM, people are inevitable to contract external pathogens. Severe or not, if not properly treated, pathogens will remain internally, leading to impaired healthy qi and unbalanced qi transformation. In a long term, it will give rise to other miscellaneous diseases. Therefore, in order to completely expel the pathogens and fully recover the original qi, TCM physicians pay much attention to the rehabilitation of post-heat diseases. According to the experiences of physicians in past dynasties, the pathogenesis of post-heat diseases includes remaining pathogens, depletion of qi and yin, impaired spleen and stomach, improper regulation and re-attack of external pathogens. It is mostly deficiency in nature. Therefore the rehabilitation approaches are clearing heat and eliminating pathogens, supporting healthy qi and securing root, regulating based on pattern identification, cultivating the mind and strengthening body, and keeping abreast of internal and external treatments.

外感热病瘥后诸症的康复，是中医康复学相较于西医康复学，独具特色的范畴内容。中医学认为，外感病虽轻重不一，但由于人生天地之间，难免外感，如果外感后不彻底康复，则内留余邪、正气不复、气化不衡，屡积日久则成为其他杂症重病的重要发病基础。在此认识之上，中医历来重视外感热病瘥后遗留诸症的康复，力求尽祛其邪、完复真元。综合历代认识，外感热病瘥后诸证的病机不外乎余邪残留、气阴亏虚、脾胃虚损、调摄失宜、外邪复感等几方面。其病性一般虚多实少，通常以清热除邪、扶正固本、辨证调摄、养神强身、内外并进为其康复大法。

Section 1 Cough

Cough is one of the main symptoms of lung diseases. After exogenous febrile diseases are recovered, symptoms are disappeared except for cough, which is related to qi and yin deficiency of lung and remaining pathogenic factors. If not properly treated, it will cause blood coughing, lung abscess and lung consumption.

1 Indications

After exogenous febrile diseases are recovered, patients still cough or even have short cough or blood in sputum. Other symptoms are disappeared and abnormal mental state, diet and sleep are presented, affecting work and rest.

There are three different patterns: ①heat lingering in lung: symptoms are cough without sputum, aggravating at daytime, scanty and sticky sputum, thirst with desire for water, dry throat, red complexion and anxiety, or low-grade fever, red tongue with scant liquid, fine rapid pulse; ②deficiency of qi and yin: symptoms are cough, shortness of breath, difficulty in coughing sputum, sputum with blood, dry mouth and throat, postmeridian tidal fever and reddening of the cheeks, night sweating, gradual emaciation, fatigue, red tongue, vacuous and rapid pulse; ③wind-cold lingering: symptoms are long-time cough with white sputum, stuffy nose and itching throat, aversion to cold with or without fever, red tongue tip with thin and white coating, floating and slippery pulse.

第1节 咳嗽

咳嗽为肺系疾病的主要症状之一，外感热病瘥后，诸症已退，唯咳嗽不止，多与肺之气阴亏虚及余邪未尽有关，若久延失治，容易引发咯血、肺痈、肺痨等病。

1 适宜指征

外感热病瘥后，咳嗽日久不减，甚则咳声短促或痰中带血。余症基本消失，可伴有精神、饮食及睡眠方面的异常，而影响工作和休息。

常见三种证型：①余热恋肺：证见干咳，日间较甚，痰少而黏，口干欲饮，咽燥，面红烦躁，或有低热，舌红少津，脉细数。②气阴亏损：证见咳嗽气短，咳痰不爽，或痰中带血，口干咽燥，午后潮热颧红，夜寐盗汗，日渐消瘦、神疲，舌红，脉虚数。③风寒未尽：证见外感咳嗽迁延不愈，咳吐白痰，鼻塞咽痒，畏寒或微有恶寒发热，舌边尖红，苔薄白，脉浮滑。

2 Rehabilitation Treatments

2.1 Medication

For heat lingering in lung, Sha Shen Mai Dong Tang (*Adenophora/Glehnia and Ophiopogon Decoction*) may be necessary to nourish lung-yin. Chuan Bei Mu (*Sichuan fritillaria*) and Xin Ren (*Semen Armeniacae Amarum*) can be added to moisten lung and transform phlegm. Sang Bai Pi (*Cortex Mori*) and Di Gu Pi (*Cortex Lycii*) can be added to clear and discharge lung-heat. For qi and yin deficiency, Zi Wan San (*Aster Powder*) will aid in boosting qi and nourishing yin, moistening lung and suppressing cough. Xin Ren, Sha Shen (*Radix Glehniae/Radix Adenophorae*), Kuan Dong Hua (*Flos Farfarae*) and Mai Dong (*Radix Ophiopogonis*) can be added according to the condition. Bai He Gu Jin Tang (*Modified Lily Bulb Metal-Securing Decoction*) is also available. For wind-cold lingering, modified Zhi Sou San (*Cough-stopping Powder*) may be necessary to suppress cough and transform phlegm, diffuse lung and course the exterior. If wind-cold lingering is combined with phlegm and dampness, presenting sticky and thick phlegm-drool, chest stuffness and slimy coating, add Ban Xia (*Rhizoma Pinelliae*), Hou Po (*Magnoliae Officinalis Cortex*), Fu Ling (*Poria*) to dry dampness and transform phlegm. If depressed heat is combined, presenting vexation and thirst and yellow coating, add Sang Bai Pi, Huang Qin (*Radix Scutellariae*) and Tian Hua Fen (*Radix Trichosanthis*) to clean and discharge internal heat. For lung dryness with symptoms like coughing without sputum, add Gua Lou (*Trichosanthis*), Bei Mu (*Sichuan fritillaria*) and Zhi Mu (*Rhizoma

2 康复措施

2.1 药物康复

余热恋肺者，治宜滋养肺阴兼清余热，可用沙参麦冬汤，可加川贝、杏仁润肺化痰，桑白皮、地骨皮清泄肺热。气阴亏损者，宜益气养阴、润肺止咳，可用紫苑散，可酌加杏仁、沙参、款冬花、麦冬之类，也可用百合固金汤加减。风寒未尽者，治宜止咳化痰、宜肺疏表，可用止嗽散加减，若夹痰湿而见痰涎黏稠、胸闷苔腻者，加半夏、厚朴、茯苓以燥湿化痰；若兼郁热而烦渴，苔黄者，加桑皮、黄芩、花粉清泄里热；若见肺燥而干咳无痰者，加瓜蒌、贝母、知母以润肺。

Anemarrhenae) to moisten lung.

2.2 Acupuncture

Fei Shu (BL 31), He Gu (LI 4), Qi Hai (CV 6), Zu Sanli (ST 36) may be helpful. For profuse sputum, add Feng Long (ST 40); for itching throat, add Tian Tu (CV 22); for chest stuffiness, add Nei Guan (PC 6) and Dan Zhong (CV 17); for long-time coughing with emaciation, Fei Shu (BL 31), Shen Shu (BL 23) and Pi Shu (BL 20) may be selected for warm moxibustion. Manipulations should follow the principle of balanced supplementation and drainage. If with recurrences, puncture shallowly with drainage.

2.2 针灸康复

可取肺俞、合谷、气海、足三里等穴，痰多加丰隆；咽痒加天突；胸闷加内关、膻中；久咳体瘦可温灸肺俞、肾俞、脾俞。针法宜平补平泻，若兼复感宜浅刺用泻法。

2.3 Tuina

Shao Shang (LU 11), Lie Que (LU 7), Tai Yuan (LU 9), Feng Men (BL 12), Fei Shu (BL 31) and Xuan Ji (CV 21) are selected for spot-pressing. Press Tian Tu (CV 22) for 2 minutes until soreness is felt. Tap Ding Chuan (EX-B 1) with finger tips or finger-press Feng Long (ST 40) and Zu Sanli (ST 36). Grasp the back, spot-press Fei Shu (BL 31) and knead Ming Men (GV 4). Pat the back repeatedly to make sure smooth respiration. Press and knead Dan Zhong (CV 17) to promote sputum discharge.

2.3 推拿康复

可点按少商、列缺、太渊、风门、肺俞、璇玑等穴；可按压天突穴 2 分钟，以有酸胀感为宜；也可指尖叩击定喘穴，或指按丰隆、足三里等穴；捏拿背脊部，点压肺俞，揉命门。反复拍打背部，可使呼吸通畅；按揉膻中穴，可使痰易咯出。

2.4 Diet and Daily Life

Patients should live in clean rooms with fine ventilation and fresh air. Avoid stimulation of dust, smoke and other abnormal gases. Smokers should quit smoking. Common cold will induce recurrence or aggravate cough. Keep warm and avoid cold attack. Those with long-time cough should avoid sexual intercourse to save essence.

2.4 膳食起居

居室要清洁卫生，通风良好，空气新鲜。应避免烟尘及异常气味刺激，吸烟者应戒烟。感冒会引起咳嗽复发或加重，应注意气候变化，做到防寒保暖，以免受凉外感。凡久咳不愈者，应戒房事以保精气。

Spicy, dry, fried, greasy and excessively cold food should be avoided. Eat more light and digestive food, like fresh vegetables, tangerines and pears. Those with heat caused by yin deficiency, take decoction more frequently with less volume at each. Lily bulb, lotus seed and tremella may be necessary. Those with lingering wind-cold should take warm decoction. After drinking the decoction, put on thick clothes or cover quilts. Have a hot drink or porridge to support right qi and dispel pathogens. In terms of herbal diet, Xue Li Gao (*Pear Cream*) or Sha Shen (*Radix Glehniae*) Gruel may be necessary for patients with heat lingering in lungs. Bai He (*Lily Bulb*) Gruel may be helpful for patients with deficiency of qi and yin. Zi Su (*Perilla*) Gruel may aid in treatment of lingering wind-cold.

应忌食辛辣香燥、炙烤肥腻及过于寒凉之品；宜食清淡、易于消化的食物，如新鲜蔬菜、柑橘、梨等。阴虚有热者，服汤药宜多次少饮，并可食百合、莲子、银耳等；风寒未尽者，汤药宜温服，药后宜加盖衣被，并进热饮、热粥以助正驱邪。药膳方面，余热恋肺者，可选用雪梨膏，也可食沙参粥；气阴亏损型，可选用百合粥；风寒未尽型，可用紫苏粥。

2.5 Exercises

In the morning and afternoon, take slow and relaxed exercises like walking, jogging, Tai Ji Quan, Five-animal Boxing (Wu Qin Xi), Relaxing and Calming Exercises (Song Jing Gong). The duration and intensity may be gradually increased as the body recoveries. Sunbath, air bath, forest bath and even cave bath can be performed according to the pattern identification to regulate qi and inhale fresh qi from nature to supplement insufficiency of lung and kidney.

2.5 功法锻炼

可采用轻松缓慢的活动，如散步、慢跑、太极拳、五禽戏、松静功等，每日早晨、午后进行。随着体力增加，活动时间与强度可以逐渐增加。还可辨证运用日光浴、空气浴、森林浴、洞穴浴的同时，敛息调气，摄纳自然之清气，以补肺肾之不足。

2.6 Mental Rehabilitation

Patients often feel sad. Because sorrow impairs lung, the condition will aggravates. Therefore, therapies, such as method of mutual restraining of emotions, music, entertainment and color, may be necessary to make patients feel happy and relaxed.

2.6 精神康复

情志悲郁不舒，悲则伤肺，常使病情加重。故应用情志相胜、音乐、娱乐、色彩等疗法，使病人感到欢快、舒畅、轻松。

Section 2 Low-grade Fever

第 2 节 低热

Low-grade fever is a common condition after febrile disease recovery. It refers to two conditions: one is that the body temperature is above normal but lower than 38 centigrade, the other is that patients feel a fever but with normal body temperature. After acute stage of exogenous febrile diseases, pathogens decline and high fever is gone. But because deficient healthy qi isn't regained or pathogens are still remaining, the low-grade fever is recurrent. In general, this condition is lingering and consumes essence, affecting physical, mental and even occupational capabilities.

低热，体温高于正常而低于 38 ℃，或仅自觉发热而测量体温正常，是热病瘥后常见病证。在外感热病急性期后，邪势已衰，高热也逐渐清退，但由于正虚未复，或余邪未尽，故低热反复不退。这种低热往往病程缠绵，迁延日久，耗伤精气，表现出一定程度的体力、心理以及工作能力的障碍。

1 Indications

In remission, or with long course, patients have no acute symptoms like high fever, chills, syncope and convulsion, and bleeding. Instead, they will be presented with continual recurrent low-grade fever, fatigue, poor appetite and weak pulse. Routine work will be affected due to these symptoms.

There are three patterns: ①Fever due to yin deficiency: It is a common condition at the advanced stage of warm disease with symptoms like post-meridian or night tidal fever, night sweating, insomnia and dreaminess, heat in the heart of the palms and soles, dry mouth and vexation, red tongue with scanty or no coating, fine rapid pulse. ②Fever due to qi deficiency: It is a condition following or aggravated by overexertion. Symptoms are fluctuating fever, fatigue, simultaneous sweating, shortness of

1 适宜指征

急性热病的恢复期或病程日久，已无明显的壮热、寒战以及痉厥、出血等急症表现，而以持续反复低热为主要症状，并伴见精神疲乏、食欲不振、脉虚无力等症，尚不能坚持正常工作者。

常见三种证型：①阴虚发热：多见于温病后期，证见午后或夜间潮热、盗汗、少寐多梦、手足心热、口干烦躁，舌红少苔或无苔，脉细数。②气虚发热：发热常在劳累后发作或加剧。自觉热势或低或高，神疲乏力、自汗、气短懒言、食少便溏，舌质淡、苔薄白，脉软。③余邪发热：

breath, unwillingness to speak, poor appetite and diarrhea, light-colored tongue with thin and white coating, soft pulse. ③ Fever due to remaining pathogens: It is a common condition after cold damage diseases. Symptoms are low-grade fever, or lingering fever and aversion to cold, vexation, bitter taste in the mouth and desire for vomiting, red tongue with yellow thin coating, fine rapid or string-like rapid pulse.

常见于伤寒瘥后，低热不退或发热恶寒，缠绵不解，烦躁、口苦欲呕，舌红、苔薄黄，脉细数或弦数。

2 Rehabilitation Treatments

2.1 Medications

Those with fever caused by yin deficiency can take modified Sweet Wormwood and Qing Hao Bie Jia Tang (*Turtle Shell Decoction*) or Qing Gu San (*Bone-Clearing Powder*) to enrich yin and clear heat. Those with fever due to impaired yin of lung and stomach are presented with cough with scanty phlegm or retching, and poor appetite. Sha Shen Mai Dong Tang (*Glehnia and Ophiopogon Decoction*) or Yi Wei Tang (*Stomach-Boosting Decoction*) may be helpful in enriching and nourishing lung and stomach. Those with yin deficiency of liver and kidney have symptoms like heat in the heart and even the back of palms and soles, lassitude and desire for sleep, deficient fine pulse or bound and intermittent pulse. Jia Jian Fu Mai Tang (*Modified Pulse-Restorative Decoction*) can be used to supplement genuine yin. Patients with remaining fever, phlegm, yin deficiency and stasis obstructing vessels have the symptoms of palpitation and vexation, trembling of hands and feet and torpid look. Modified San Jia San (*Triple-shell Powder*) may be necessary to transform phlegm, open orifice and free network

2 康复措施

2.1 药物康复

阴虚发热者，治宜滋阴清热，可用青蒿鳖甲汤或清骨散加减；若肺胃阴伤而余热未净，兼见干咳少痰或干呕、食欲不佳，宜用沙参麦冬汤或益胃汤滋养肺胃；肝肾阴亏而见手足心热甚于手足背、神倦欲眠、脉虚细或结代者，宜用加减复脉汤填补真阴；若阴虚兼余热夹痰、瘀滞络脉，伴见心悸烦躁、手足颤动、神情呆钝者，可用三甲散加减以化痰开瘀通络。

vessels.

For fever due to qi deficiency, modified Center-Supplementing Bu Zhong Yi Qi Tang (*Qi-Boosting Decoction*) is necessary to boost qi and fortify the spleen, eliminate fever with warmth and sweetness. If with profuse simultaneous sweating, add Mu Li (*Oyster shell*) and Fu Xiao Mai (*Tritici Fructus Levis*) to secure the exterior and constrain sweating. If with alternating cold and heat, sweating and aversion to wind, add Gui Zhi (*Cinnamomi Ramulus*) and Shao Yao (*Peony root*) to harmonize construction and defense. If qi deficiency is so severe that it affects yang and symptoms like diarrhea and cold hands and feet are presented, add Gan Jiang (*Rhizoma Zingiberis Recens*) and Rou Gui (*Cortex Cinnamomi*) to warm and transform middle-yang. If spleen deficiency is combined with dampness, add Cang Zhu (*Rhizoma Atractylodis*), Hou Po (*Magnoliae Officinalis Cortex*) and Huo Xiang (*Herba Pogostemonis*) to fortify the spleen and dispel dampness.

气虚发热者，治宜益气健脾、甘温除热，可用补中益气汤加减。若自汗多者，可加牡蛎、浮小麦固表敛汗；时冷时热、汗出恶风者，可加桂枝、芍药调和营卫；若兼见大便稀清、手足欠温者，是气虚及阳之象，可酌加干姜、肉桂温运中阳；胸脘痞闷、呕恶苔腻者，为脾虚夹湿之候，可加苍术、厚朴、藿香以健脾祛湿。

Fever due to remaining pathogens may be treated with clearing heat, support healthy qi to defend pathogens. Fever caused by poor movement of lesser yang is commonly seen and often treated with Xiao Chai Hu Tang (*Minor Bupleurum Decoction*) through disinhibiting and harmonizing. If pathogens remains and both qi and liquid are impaired, Zhu Ye Shi Gao Tang (*Lophatherum and Gypsum Decoction*) is helpful in clearing and discharging remaining heat, boosting qi and nourishing liquids.

余邪发热者，治宜清解余热、扶正御邪，其少阳枢机不利之热为多，常用小柴胡汤以疏利和解；若余邪未尽而气液两伤者，可用竹叶石膏汤以清泄余热、益气养液。

2.2 Acupuncture

Fei Shu (BL 31), Da Zhui (GV 14) and He Gu (LI 4) are main acupoints. For yin deficiency, add

2.2 针灸康复

可取肺俞、大椎、合谷为主穴，阴虚加神门、肾俞、三

Shen Men (HT 7), Shen Shu (BL 23) and Sanyin Jiao (SP 6); for qi deficiency, add Qi Hai (CV 6), Guan Yuan (CV 4) and Zu Sanli (ST 36) for acupuncture and moxibustion as well; for fever caused by remaining pathogens, add Qu Chi (LI 11) and Xing Jian (LR 2). In general, shallow puncture is used under the guidance of balanced supplementation and drainage.

阴交;气虚加气海、关元、足三里,并可艾灸;余邪未尽而发热者加曲池、行间。一般以毫针浅刺。用平补平泻法。

2.3 Tuina

Da Zhui (GV l4), Qu Chi (LI 11), He Gu (LI 4) and Sanyin Jiao (SP 6) can be selected for finger pressing. Lift and grasp Jian Jing (GB 21), pinch the corner of the nail, and knead interphalangeal joint.

2.3 推拿康复

可点按大椎、曲池、合谷、三阴交,提拿肩井,掐指甲根部,揉手指指间关节。

2.4 Diet and Daily Life

Patients should live in a quiet and clean room with fine ventilation and at moderate temperature. Avoid direct contact with wind. If with simultaneous sweating or night sweating, keep it dry and change the wet clothes timely to prevent cold attack and recurrent attack of external pathogens.

Light, nutritional and digestive food may be necessary, such as fresh vegetables, fruits, soup and porridge. Avoid greasy, fried and spicy diet. Patients with yin deficiency may take Bai He Geng (*Lily Bulb Gruel*), Jia Yu Tang (*Soft-shell Turtle Soup*), Yin Er Tang (*Tremella Soup*) and Mai Dong Zhou (*Ophiopogon Porridge*). Those with qi deficiency can have diet that can supplement and boost spleen and stomach, such as Lian Zi Zhou (*Lotus Seed Porridge*), Huang Qi Hong Zao Zhou (*Astragalus and Jujube Porridge*), Long Yan Zhou (*Longan Flesh Porridge*). Those with remaining fever can drink fruit juice, wax gourd soup, mung bean soup

2.4 膳食起居

居室应保持安静整洁、空气流通、寒温适宜,避免直接吹风。低热者常有自汗或盗汗,汗后应及时擦干,更换汗湿衣服,并应防止受凉,复感外邪。

饮食宜清淡爽口、富有营养、易于消化,宜多食新鲜蔬菜、水果、汤粥之类,忌食油腻、煎炸、辛辣之物。阴虚者可用百合羹、甲鱼汤、银耳汤、麦冬粥等;气虚者宜食补益脾胃的食品,如莲子粥、黄芪红枣粥、桂圆粥等;余热未尽者,可饮用果子汁、冬瓜汤、绿豆汤、葛粉粥等。

and Gen Fen Zhou (*Pueraria Starch Porridge*).

2.5 Exercises

In general, patients should mainly rest in bed and can also do some exercises according to the condition, such as walking indoors and then outdoors. Simple exercises can also be necessary based on the condition and constitution. They can be taken moderately and once or twice a day.

2.5 功法锻炼

瘥后发热者一般以静卧休养为主，但也应根据病人体力情况适当活动。可从室内散步开始，渐及室外，根据病情和体质可以练习做简易易体操，每日练 1～2 次，活动量以自感舒适为度，不宜过大。

2.6 Mental Rehabilitation

Low-grade fever patients often have some mental disorders and are presented with symptoms like fatigue, vexation and anxiety, worries about lingering condition. To make patients cooperate with the treatment, physicians should inform patients of the treatment process and development of disease to eliminate their worries and keep up their spirits. Music therapy may be necessary. On the basis of patients' mental status, different kinds of music can be chosen, for example, light music for those with vexation and anxiety, and exciting music for those who are in low spirits.

2.6 精神康复

低热患者常常存在一定的心理障碍，主要表现为精神疲乏、烦躁焦虑、担心病根未除，久延不愈。应向患者宣讲有关外感热病的治疗过程及演变规律，使之清除顾虑，静心调养，振作精神，配合康复治疗。可根据患者不同的心理状态，适当配合音乐疗法。如对精神烦躁焦虑者，可选择一些幽雅、恬静的乐曲；对精神疲乏萎靡者，可选择一些激昂、奔放的乐曲。

Section 3 Reduced Appetite

Reduced appetite is a condition at the later stage of heat disease or after recovery, with symptoms like no appetite for food, hunger but with inability to eat a lot and easiness to be full, lusterless complexion, emaciation, abdominal distension and bowel movement disorders. It is often caused by ex-

第 3 节　食少

食少是由于热病期间多食生冷、苦寒之品，或久病损脾，脾胃运化功能受损，脾失健运、而致胃不思纳，从而在热病后期或瘥后出现不思饮食、饥不能食、食易饱滞，常

cessive intake of cold and bitter food during the heat disease or impaired function of spleen and stomach due to chronic diseases. Spleen and stomach are roots of acquired constitution, therefore reduced appetite can significantly affect the recovery and health in the future. Active rehabilitation treatments should be given.

伴面色少华、形体消瘦、脘腹胀满、大便失调等症。脾胃为后天之本,食少严重影响疾病痊愈和今后的身体健康,故应予以积极的调理康复。

1 Indications

During heat disease in remission, those who are affected by reduced appetite and food intake and other symptoms concerning spleen and stomach are indicated. There are three common patterns: ①insufficiency of stomach yin: hunger with no appetite for food, dry mouth and throat, vexation, or low-grade fever at night, red complexion, red tongue with scanty coating, fine rapid pulse; ②remaining dampness and turbidity: no fever, vexation with no appetite for food, dizziness and blurred eyes, fatigue and lassitude, slimy coating, soggy and moderate pulse; ③deficiency of spleen and stomach: no hunger, no desire for food, abdominal distension and indigestion after diet, or desire to vomit with upwelling, diarrhea, weakness of four limbs, or even edema, light-colored tongue with white coating, weak pulse.

1 适宜指征

在热病恢复期,出现食欲减少,纳少,并伴有脾胃方面的其他症状,而影响身体康复者。常见三种证型:①胃阴不足:证见似饥而不欲食,口干咽燥,烦躁不安,或夜间低热,面微赤,舌红苔少,脉细略数。②湿浊未净:证见身热已退,烦闷不食,头晕目眩,神疲乏力,苔腻,脉濡缓。③脾虚胃弱:证见不知饥饿,不思饮食,食后腹胀不消,或泛泛欲吐,便溏,四肢乏力,甚或肢体浮肿,舌淡苔白,脉虚弱。

2 Rehabilitation Treatments

2.1 Medication

Those with insufficiency of stomach yin may be treated by nourishing yin and harmonizing stomach with Stomach-Boosting Decoction (Yi Wei Tang) or Five Juices Beverage (Wu Zhi Yin). If with severe stomach heat and desire to vomit due to counterflow of qi, patients may take Lophatherum and Gypsum

2 康复措施

2.1 药物康复

胃阴不足者,治宜养阴和胃,可用益胃汤或五汁饮;若胃热甚而气逆欲吐者,可用竹叶石膏汤清热和胃;若气液两亏而兼气短心悸、精神委顿者,可用薛氏参麦汤

Decoction (Zhu Ye Shi Gao Tang) to clear heat and harmonize stomach. With deficiency of qi and fluid, patients have symptoms like shortness of breath, palpitation and low spirits and can be treated with Xue's Ginseng and Ophiopogon Decoction (Xue Shi Shen Mai Tang) to boost qi and nourish liquid. Those with remaining dampness and turbidity may be treated by clearing the light and transforming with aromatics, flushing and eliminating remaining pathogens with modifed Xue's Five-Leaf Phragmites Decoction (Xue Shi Wu Ye Lu Gen Tang). If with deficiency of spleen and stomach, patients may take added Special Achievement Powder (Yi Gong San) or modified Ginseng, Poria and Atractylodes Powder (Shen Ling Bai Zhu San) to tonify spleen and harmonize the middle, regulate qi and transform dampness. With yang deficiency of spleen and stomach, patients have symptoms like no desire for food, yellowish complexion and vacuous and string-like pulse and can be treated by warming the middle and supplementing the deficiency with Minor Center-Fortifying Decoction (Xiao Jian Zhong Tang).

益气养液。湿浊未净者，治宜轻清芳化、涤除余邪，可用薛氏五叶芦根汤加减。脾虚胃弱者，治宜健脾和中、理气化湿，可用加味异功散或参苓白术散加减；若脾胃阳虚而见不思饮食、面色萎黄、脉虚弦者，可用小建中汤温中补虚。

2.2 Acupuncture

Zhong Wan (CV 12), Pi Shu (BL 20), Wei Shu (BL 21), Zu Sanli (ST 36) and Ran Gu (KI 2) can be selected for acupuncture based on supplementation or balanced supplementation and drainage. With qi deficiency or yang deficiency, moxibustion can be added.

2.2 针灸康复

可取中院、脾俞、胃俞、足三里、然谷等穴，针刺用补法或平补平泻法。气虚或阳虚者可加灸法。

2.3 Tuina

With patients lying on the back, physician should knead the upper abdomen first focusing on Jiu Wei (CV 15) and Zhong Wan (CV 12), and then progress downward to lower abdomen center-

2.3 推拿康复

可令患者取仰卧位，先揉上腹部，以鸠尾、中脘为重点，然后循序往下至少腹部，以脐周围之天枢、气海为重

ing on Tian Shu (ST 25) and Qi Hai (CV 6). At the same time, thump Zhong Wan (CV 12) with fingers and abdomen with palms and then rub clockwise and counterclockwise for 100 rounds respectively. After that, ask the patient to lie in prone position, roll along the bladder meridians moderately with the focus on acupoints near the 6th to 12th thoracic vertebrae. Following rolling, Pi Shu (BL 20), Wei Shu (BL 21) and Gan Shu (BL 18) are selected for mild finger pressing.

点，同时用指振法在中脘穴和掌振法在腹部振动，再用摩法顺时针和逆时针方向各摩100圈；再令患者俯卧位，沿脊往两侧膀胱经用轻柔的滚法，重点在胸椎6～12两旁腧穴，然后重点在脾俞、胃俞、肝俞用较轻手法按点。

2.4 Diet and Daily Life

Those with reduced appetite have weak stomach and spleen, so they should avoid wind and cold and prevent contraction of external pathogens. Since poor sleep affects appetite, patients should live a routine life and have enough rest. Don't stay up late. It will impair liquid and consume qi.

Diet matters to this condition. Try to use superb cooking methods to make sure the color, aroma and taste can arouse the appetite. Have more meals with less at each to promote digestion and absorption. At the same time, digestive food that can improve appetite can be added, such as Ou (*Nelumbinis Rhizomatis Nodus*) starch, Shan Zha (*Fructus Crataegi*) and fruits. Fish is nutritional and digestive and can be acceptable. Greasy or fried food, liquor and cigarette, strong tea and coffee should all be avoided. In terms of herbal diet, Mai Dong Zhou (*Ophiopogon Porridge*) is for patients with insufficiency of stomach yin; Lotus Leaf Porridge is for those with remaining dampness and turbidity; Shan Yao Bian Dou Zhou (*Rhizoma Dioscoreae and Hyacinth Bean Porridge*) is to treat those with deficiency of spleen and stomach. Shan Yao Yang Rou Zhou

2.4 膳食起居

食少者脾胃弱，故应注意避风寒、适寒温，以防挟感外邪。生活起居要有规律，睡眠和休息不足，往往影响食欲，故应保障足够的休息，切勿熬夜不眠，耗伤津气。

本病饮食调理尤为重要，尽量采用优良的烹调方法，保证饭菜的色、香、味，以激起患者的食欲，并宜少吃多餐，以利消化吸收。同时，应适当配用有助消化、增食欲的佐餐食物，如藕粉、山楂、水果等。各种鱼类营养丰富，易于消化，均可食用。忌食过于肥腻或煎炸硬固不易消化的食物，并忌烟酒、浓茶及咖啡。药膳方面，胃阴不足者，可选用麦冬粥；湿浊未净者，可选用荷叶粥；脾虚胃弱者，可选用山药扁豆粥；若脾胃阳虚者，可选用山药羊肉粥。

(*Rhizoma Dioscoreae and Mutton Porridge*) is for yang deficiency of spleen and stomach.

2.5 Exercises

Exercises can free circulation of qi and blood and improve the function of spleen and stomach. Apart from walking, jogging and Tai Ji, 30 minutes Qi Gong can be played once or twice a day, such as Relaxation Exercises (Fang Song Gong) and Breathing Exercises (Nei Yang Gong). While playing, deep abdominal breathing is used to rhythmically rub the organs in the abdomen, promoting gastrointestinal peristalsis and excretion of digestive juices. The appetite is generally improved after exercises.

2.6 Mental Rehabilitation

The condition mostly affects spleen and stomach, whose functions are closely related to emotions. Therefore, it is important to focus on mental rehabilitation. Physicians should encourage patients to worry less and be happy. To avoid mental stimulation, patients shouldn't think something over before diet. While dieting, patients should keep calm and eat in a quiet place. Don't discuss while eating. Patients may take part in some entertainment activities to amuse themselves, such as cross talk, comedy and music.

2.5 功法锻炼

功法运动可疏通气血、促进脾胃的功能。除散步、跑步、太极拳等活动外，可练习气功，一般选择放松功、内养功，每日可练1～2次，每次30分钟。练气功时，以腹式深呼吸，腹内脏器如同受到有节律的按摩，能促胃肠蠕动，使消化液增多，往往可在练功后食欲明显增加。

2.6 精神康复

本症病在脾胃，情志活动与脾胃运化功能密切相关，可直接影响食欲，故应重视精神调摄。应鼓励患者少忧愁、少烦恼，保持心境的愉快、开朗；就餐前不要思考问题，避免不良的精神刺激；用餐时要安定情绪，避免噪声，不要边吃边讨论问题。可指导患者参加欢快的娱乐活动以愉悦情致，如听相声、看喜剧、欣赏音乐等。

Section 4 Hidrosis

Hidrosis or profuse sweating, is one of the common symptoms during exogenous febrile diseases. According to the symptoms, it can be divided into simultaneous sweating, night sweating, deser-

第4节 多汗

多汗，即身体出汗过多，是外感热病过程中的常见症状之一。根据汗出的表现，中医一般分为自汗、盗汗、脱

tion sweating, and shiver sweating and yellow sweat. Among them, simultaneous sweating and night sweating are generally seen after recovery of heat diseases. After disease, unbalanced yin and yang and insecurity of the interstices lead to extravasation of sweat. As sweat and blood are of the same source and sweat is transformed by qi and blood, profuse and long-term sweating will inevitably consumes yin and yang, qi and blood of the human body. In addition, while sweating, patients are more vulnerable to external pathogens. Therefore, active rehabilitation treatment is necessary.

汗、战汗、黄汗等。热病瘥后则以自汗、盗汗为多见，由于病后体虚，阴阳失调、腠理不固，而致汗液外泄。汗血同源，汗乃气血所化生，若汗出过多过久，势必进一步耗损人体的阴阳气血；且汗之时，腠理空虚，易感外邪，故应予以积极的调理康复。

1 Indications

After heat disease, persistent simultaneous sweating and night sweating are often accompanied with varying degrees of mental, physical and sleep disorders. There are three patterns: ①insecurity due to qi deficiency: simultaneous sweating and aversion to wind that is worsened by overstrain, easy to contract external pathogens, fatigue and lassitude, lusterless complexion, thin white coating and weak pulse. ②internal heat due to yin deficiency: night sweating, insomnia due to vexation, vexing heat in the five hearts or steaming bone and tidal heat, reddening of the cheeks and dry mouth, red tongue with scanty coating, fine rapid pulse. ③deficiency of yin and yang: continuing simultaneous sweating and night sweating, emaciation, flaccidity and weakness, aversion to cold, palpitation and insomnia, white complexion and redding of the cheeks, heat in the heart of the palms and soles, light-red tongue and fine weak pulse.

1 适宜指征

热病瘥后，持续性的自汗、盗汗，并伴有不同程度的精神、体力及睡眠方面的症状表现者。常见三种证型：①气虚不固：证见自汗恶风，稍劳尤甚，容易外感，体倦乏力，面色少华，舌苔薄白，脉弱。②阴虚内热：证见夜寐盗汗，虚烦少眠，五心烦热，或骨蒸潮热，颧红口干，舌红少苔，脉细数。③阴阳两虚：证见自汗、盗汗不止，身体消瘦，肢软无力，形寒畏冷，心悸少眠，面白颧红，手足心热，舌质淡红，脉细弱。

2 Rehabilitation Treatments

2.1 Medication

Patients with insecurity due to qi deficiency should be treated by boosting qi and securing the exterior with modified Yu Ping Feng San (*Jade Wind-Barrier Powder*). For profuse sweating, add Fu Xiao Mai (*Tritici Fructus Levis*), Nuo Dao Gen (*Radix Oryzae Glutinosae*), Mu Li (*Oyster Shell*) to secure the exterior and constrain sweat; for severe qi deficiency, add Dang Shen (*Codonopsis*), Huang Jing (*Polygonatum*) and Zhi Gan Cao (Prepared *Radix Glycyrrhizae*) to secure and contain by boosting qi; for yang deficiency with cold limbs and aversion to cold, Huang Qi Jian Zhong Tang (*Astraglalus Center-Fortifying Decoction*) may be combined. For disharmony between construction and defense phases with or without external contraction, symptoms like general soreness, alternating cold and heat and slow pulse may occur and modified Gui Zhi Tang (*Cinnamon Decoction*) may be necessary to harmonize construction and defense.

Patients with internal heat due to yin deficiency should be treated by enriching yin and downbearing fire with Dang Gui Liu Huang Tang (*Chinese Angelica Six Yellows Decoction*). For profuse sweating, add Mu Li, Fu Xiao Mai and Nuo Dao Gen to constrain sweat; for severe tidal fever, add Qin Jiao (*Radix Gentianae Macrophyllae*), Yin Chai Hu (*Radix Stellariae*) and Bai Wei (*Radix Cynanchi Atrati*) to clear and discharge deficiency-heat; for yin deficiency of lung and kidney, if the fire isn't severe, modified Mai Wei Di Huang Wan (*Ophiopogon and Schisandra and Rehmannia Pill*) is necessary.

2 康复措施

2.1 药物康复

气虚不固者，治宜益气固表，可用玉屏风散加味；若汗出多者，可加浮小麦、糯稻根、牡蛎固表敛汗；气虚甚者，加党参、黄精、炙甘草益气固摄；兼阳虚而形寒畏冷者，可与黄芪建中汤合用；若兼见周身酸楚，时寒时热，脉缓；证属营卫不和或微兼外感者，则宜用桂枝汤加减调和营卫。

阴虚内热者，治宜滋阴降火，可用当归六黄汤加减；若汗出多者，加牡蛎、浮小麦、糯稻根固涩敛汗；潮热甚者，加秦艽、银柴胡、白薇清退虚热；若证属肺肾阴虚，而火热不甚者，宜用麦味地黄丸加减。

Those with deficiency of yin and yang should be treated by warming yang and boosting yin with modified Bie Jia San (*Turtle Shell Powder*). For shortage of qi and fright palpitations due to deficiency of qi and blood, Ren Shen Yang Rong Tang (*Ginseng Construction-nourishing Decoction*) is necessary to boost qi and supplement blood. For vexing heat and shortness of breath caused by deficiency of qi and yin, add Xi Yang Shen (*Radix Panacis Quinquefolii*), Sheng Di Huang (*Rehmanniae Radix*), Mai Dong (*Radix Ophiopogonis*), Huang Lian (*Rhizoma Coptidis*), Gan Cao (*Radix Glycyrrhizae*), Xiao Mai (*Wheat*), Bai He (*Lily Bulb*), Zhu Ye (*Bamboo Leaves*), Lian Zi Xin (*Lotus Plumule*) and so on.

阴阳两虚者，宜温阳益阴，可用鳖甲散加减化裁；若证属气血两虚而少气惊悸者，可用人参养营汤益气补血；若属气阴两虚而兼烦热气短者，可用西洋参、生地、麦冬、黄连、甘草、小麦、百合、竹叶、莲子心之类。

In addition, to treat night sweating, grind Wu Wei Zi (*Fructus Schisandrae Chinensis*) into powders, mix vinegar with it and then make pie-sized tablets. Apply the tablets on the navel and fix them with gauze. To treat simultaneous sweating, replace Wu Wei Zi (Fructus Schisandrae Chinensis) with He Shou Wu (Radix Polygoni Multiflori) and vinegar with water.

另外，盗汗，可用五味子研末，以醋调作饼状，贴敷脐上，外用纱布固定；自汗，可用何首乌研末，以水调敷脐上。

2.2 Acupuncture

Da Heng (SP 15), He Gu (LI 4), Yu Ji (LU 10), Fu Liu (KI 7) and Nei Ting (ST 44) can be selected for simultaneous sweating. Jianshi (PC 5), He Gu (LI 4), Yu Ji (LU 10), Fu Liu (KI 7) and Yinxi (HT 6) are necessary for night sweating. In general, manipulations should be given with supplementation method and moxibustion can also be added. For internal heat due to yin deficiency, manipulations should be guided under the principle of balanced supplementation and drainage.

2.2 针灸康复

自汗者，可取大横、合谷、鱼际、复溜、内庭等穴；盗汗者，可取间使、合谷、鱼际、复溜、阴郄等穴。一般针刺可用补法，并可加灸法；阴虚内热者用平补平泻法。

2.3 Diet and Daily Life

Those with hidrosis and weak body should live a moderate routine life. When sweating, interstices are open and vulnerable to external pathogens. Therefore, patients should avoid wind and cold attack. After sweating, wipe out the sweats and change dry clothes to keep clean and avoid cold attack.

Light, nutritional and digestive food may be necessary. Eat more fresh vegetables, fruits, soup and porridge instead of greasy, spicy food. Avoid cigarette and liquor. In terms of herbal diet, Astragalus and Jujube Porridge (Huang Qi Da Zao Zhou) is for insecurity caused by qi deficiency; Rehmannia and Spiny Jujube Porridge (Di Huang Zao Ren Zhou) is for internal heat caused by yin deficiency; Lycium Porridge (Gou Qi Zhou) is for deficiency of both yin and yang; Wheat Porridge is necessary for both simultaneous sweating and night sweating.

2.4 Exercises

Traditional exercises are conducive to improving the regulatory functions of central nervous system towards perspiration. There are various exercises such as walking, Tai Ji, Qi Gong, and gymnastic exercises for rehabilitation. Static exercises include relaxation exercises (Fang Song Gong), breathing exercises (Nei Yang Gong) and strengthening exercises (Qiang Zhuang Gong). Those with qi deficiency may strengthen breathing exercises; with yin deficiency, patients should focus on drool-swallowing exercises; those with insomnia may emphasize on will-power exercises. All the exercises should be taken step by step on the condition that patients won't feel tired or perspire.

2.3 膳食起居

多汗体虚者，应注意劳逸适度，生活有常。汗出之时，腠理空疏，很容易感受外邪，故当避风寒，以防感冒；汗出之后，应及时揩干汗水，更换汗湿的内衣，以保持清洁卫生和避免受凉。

饮食应有节制，宜清淡、营养丰富、易于消化，多食新鲜蔬菜、水果及汤粥之类，勿食过于油腻、辛辣燥热的食物，并忌烟酒。药膳方面，气虚不固者，可选用黄芪大枣粥；阴虚内热者，可选用地黄枣仁粥；阴阳两虚者，可选用枸杞粥；自汗或盗汗，均可食用小麦粥。

2.4 功法锻炼

传统功法有助于改善中枢神经系统对汗液代谢的调节功能。具体项目可因人而异，如太极拳、气功、康复体操等，静功以放松功、内养功、强壮功为宜；气虚者加强呼吸功法，阴虚者加强咽津功法，少眠者加强意守功法。活动量宜逐步增加，不应过急过大，总以不觉累、不出汗为度。

Sweat is controlled by heart, so mental status directly affects the secretion and excretion of sweat. Therefore, patients should be guided to relax and regulate their bodies and minds. Keep calm and don't be nervous, irritated and impatient. In addition, patients can also participate in some entertainment activities, such as dancing parties and music appreciation. Slow dances like ballroom dance and light music may be necessary.

2.5 精神康复

汗为心之液,受心所主。心理状态直接影响到汗液的分泌与排泄,应教育患者逐步学会身心的自我松弛和调节,遇事平心静气,避免情绪紧张、急躁和激动,以保持良好稳定的精神状态。可指导其参加健康有益的娱乐活动,如参加舞会,欣赏音乐等。跳舞宜选择慢节奏的交谊舞,音乐宜选择轻松欢快的乐曲。

Section 5 Insomnia

第5节 不寐

Insomnia, also called sleeplessness, refers to a condition that one frequently fails to get normal sleep. It is often caused by insufficiency of yin fluids and deficiency of both heart and spleen after heat diseases. It can also be induced by heart-mind internally disturbed by remaining heat and phlegm. Sleep is one of the most important approaches to regain one's spirit and mind. Therefore, long-term insomnia is bound to do harms to one's health and active rehabilitation treatments are necessary.

不寐,又称"失眠",是指以经常性不能获得正常睡眠为特征的一种病证。热病瘥后不寐多因阴液不足、心脾两虚,或余热夹痰、内扰心神所致。睡眠是人体形神得以休复的最重要途径,长期失眠势必严重影响身心健康,故应予以积极的调理康复。

1 Indications

During the recovery of heat diseases, sleeplessness is the main symptom. The condition can vary from difficulty in fall asleep, frequently waking up during sleep, unable to fall back asleep and even to sleeplessness that lasts throughout the whole night.

1 适宜指征

热病恢复期,以失眠为主要临床表现,轻者入睡困难,或寐而易醒,或时寐时醒,或醒后不能再寐,甚或整夜不能入睡,并兼见心神方

There are three common patterns: ①Deficiency of both heart and spleen: dream-disturbed sleep, palpitation and poor memory, dizziness and blurred vision, lassitude and fatigue, loss of appetite, a lusterless complexion, light-colored tongue with thin coating, fine and weak pulse. ②Hyperactivity of fire due to yin deficiency: restlessness and sleeplessness, palpitations and uneasiness, dizziness and tinnitus, poor memory, soreness in lumbar region and dream emission, vexing heat in the five hearts, dry mouth with scanty liquids, red tongue with fine rapid pulse. ③Remaining heat with phlegm: sleeplessness and heaviness of head, frequent waking up during sleep, profuse phlegm and chest oppression, aversion to food and belching, acid swallowing and nausea, vexation and bitterness in the mouth, blurred vision, greasy and yellow coating with slippery rapid pulse.

面其他症状者。常见三种证型:①心脾两虚:证见多梦易醒,心悸健忘,头晕目眩,肢倦神疲,饮食无味,面色少华,舌淡苔薄,脉细弱。②阴虚火旺:证见心烦不寐,心悸不安,头晕耳鸣,健忘,腰酸梦遗,五心烦热,口干津少,舌红,脉细数。③余热夹痰:证见不寐头重,或时寐时醒,痰多胸闷,恶食嗳气,吞酸恶心,心烦口苦,目眩,舌苔腻而黄,脉滑数。

2 Rehabilitation Treatments

2.1 Medication

Those with deficiency of both heart and spleen can be treated by supplementing and boosting heart and spleen, nourishing blood and quieting the spirit with modified Gui Pi Tang (*Spleen-Returning Decoction*). If for insufficiency of heart blood, add Shu Di Huang (*Radix Rehmanniae Preparata*), Bai Shao (*Radix Paeoniae Alba*), E Jiao (*Colla Corii Asini*) to nourish heart blood. For severe insomnia, add Wu Wei Zi (*Fructus Schisandrae Chinensis*), Bai Zi Ren (*Seman Platycladi*), He Huan Hua (*Flos Albiziae*), Ye Jiao Teng (*Caulis Polygoni Multiflori*), Long Gu (*Os draconis*) and Mu Li (*Concha Ostreae*) to nourish heart, settle heart and quiet mind. Those with

2 康复措施

2.1 药物康复

心脾两虚者,治宜补益心脾、养血安神,可以归脾汤加减;如心血不足者,可加熟地、白芍、阿胶以养心血;如不寐较重者,酌加五味子、柏子仁、合欢花、夜交藤、龙骨、牡蛎等养心镇心安神。阴虚火旺者,治宜滋阴降火、养心安神,可以黄连阿胶汤或朱砂安神丸加减。前方重在滋阴降火,适用于心烦不寐,若见面色潮红、眩晕耳鸣,可加牡蛎、龟板、磁石等重镇潜

hyperactivity of fire due to yin deficiency can be treated by enriching yin and downbearing fire, nourishing heart and quieting mind. Modified Huang Lian E Jiao Tang (*Coptis and Ass Hide Glue Decoction*) and Zhu Sha An Shen Wan (*Cinnabar Spirit-Quieting Pill*) are helpful. The former emphasizes on enriching yin and downbearing fire and applies to those with vexation and insomnia. If symptoms like tidal reddening of the face, dizziness and tinnitus arise, add Mu Li, Gui Jia (*Carapax et Plastrum Testudinis*) and Ci Shi (*Magnetitum*) to subdue yang with heavy settling herbs. The latter has similar explanation of the formula with the former one and Huang Lian (*Rhizoma Coptidis*) is the emperor herb. It is often made into pills with herbs that can nourish heart and quiet mind such as Bai Zi Ren and Zao Ren (*Semen Ziziphi Spinosi*). Those with remaining heat and phlegm may be treated by clearing heat and transforming phlegm, harmonizing the middle and quieting the mind. Huang Lian Wen Dan Tang (*Coptis Gallbladder-Warming Decoction*) added with Zhi Zi (*Fructus Gardeniae*) is helpful. If with palpitations, add Zhen Zhu Mu (*Concha Margaritifera*), Long Chi (*Dens Draconis*) and Ci Shi to settle fright and stabilize the mind. For phlegm-dampness obstruction and disharmonized stomach, Ban Xia Shu Mi Tang (*Rhizoma Pinelliae and Panici Miliacei Semen Decoction*) is added with Shen Qu (*Massa Medicata Fermentata*), Shan Zha (*Fructus Crataegi*), Lai Fu Zi (*Semen Raphani*) to disperse food and harmonize the middle jiao. If remaining heat disturbs heart, modified Zhi Zi Wu Mei Tang (*Gardeniae Fructus and Mume Fructus Decoction*) may be helpful.

阳;后方以黄连为君,方义相似,作丸便于常服,并可加入柏子仁、枣仁等养心安神。余热夹痰者,治宜清热化痰、和中安神,可以黄连温胆汤加栀子;若心悸惊惕不安者,可加珍珠母、龙齿、磁石等镇惊定志;若痰湿阻滞,胃中不和者,可合半夏秫米汤加神曲、山楂、莱菔子等以消导和中;若证属余热扰心者,可用栀子乌梅汤加减。

2.2 Acupuncture

Shen Men (HT 7), Sanyin Jiao (SP 6) and Nei Guan (PC 6) are main acupoints. For deficiency of both heart and spleen, puncture Xin Shu (BL 15), Pi Shu (BL 20) and Jueyin Shu (BL 14) with supplementation and moxibustion is also necessary. For hyperactivity of fire due to yin deficiency, puncture Gan Shu (BL 18), Jian Shi (PC 5), Tai Chong (LR 3) and Tai Xi (KI 3) with balanced supplementation and drainage. For remaining heat with phlegm, puncture Fei Shu (BL 31), Feng Long (ST 40) and Chi Ze (LU 5) with balanced supplementation and drainage.

2.2 针灸康复

可取神门、三阴交、内关等穴为主，随证选穴：心脾两虚者，加心俞、脾俞、厥阴俞，针用补法，并可加用灸法；阴虚火旺者，加肝俞、间使、太冲、太溪，针用平补平泻法；余热夹痰者，加肺俞、丰隆、尺泽，用平补平泻法。

2.3 Tuina

After pressing Yin Tang (GV 29) with fingers for half a minute, wipe along the arcus superciliaris to Tai Yang (EX-HN 5) for 5 to 6 times. Upon pressing the region around eye socket, press Er Men (TE 21), Ting Hui(GB 2) and Yi Feng (TE 17) and then knead the posterior and the anterior ear for 3 to 4 times. Following wiping forehead for 10 times, press Bai Hui (GV 20) and knead head for 4 to 5 times until the head is heated. At last, rub Yong Quan (KI 1) . For remaining heat with phlegm, press and knead Zhong Wan (CV 12), Zu Sanli (ST 36) and Feng Long (ST 40) .

2.3 推拿康复

可先点按印堂穴半分钟后，用抹法沿眉弓至太阳穴往返 5～6 次；按压眼眶周围，点压耳门、听会、翳风穴，揉耳前、耳后 3～4 次；抹前额 10 遍；点按百会，揉头部 4～5 遍，以透热为度。再擦两侧涌泉穴。余热夹痰，可按揉中脘、足三里、丰隆穴。

2.4 Diet and Daily Life

Patients should live a routine and moderate life. Alternate rest with work and avoid sexual indulgence. Develop a good habit and create a peaceful and comfortable sleep environment with moderate temperature. If it is noisy, block the external auditory canal with cotton balls and use the herbal pillow filled with He Huan Hua (Flos Albiziae).

2.4 膳食起居

应合理安排作息，注意劳逸结合，节制房事，养成良好的生活习惯。居室应温度适宜，安静舒适，避免噪声干扰和不良因素刺激，如果入睡环境嘈杂，可用脱脂棉球堵塞外耳道，并可使用合欢

Oversize and soft pajamas are necessary and it is better to lie on one's right side and not to read, talk or think before sleep. If insomnia arises at night, spend less time on afternoon nap.

花之类的药枕。睡衣宜宽畅柔软，睡姿以右侧卧为宜。睡前不宜多看书报，说话及思考问题。夜间失眠者，可酌情减免午睡。

Patients should have light diet and keep away from spicy, greasy and sweet food. Eat less at dinner. Before sleep, keep away from snacks, strong coffee, tea, cigarette and liquor to avoid abdominal distension or getting excited. In terms of herbal diet, for deficiency of both heart and spleen, Suan Zao Ren Zhou (*Ziziphi Spinosi Semen Porridge*) is available; for hyperactivity of fire due to yin deficiency, Di Huang Zao Ren Zhou (*Rehmannia and Spiny Jujube Porridge*) is helpful; for remaining heat with phlegm, Bai He Xin Ren Zhou (*Lily Bulb and Apricot Kernel Porridge*) is necessary.

饮食宜清淡，忌食辛辣、肥甘、厚味食物。晚餐不宜过饱，睡前不要吃零食、饮浓茶咖啡、吸烟喝酒，以免腹胀不适或大脑兴奋而影响入睡。药膳方面，心脾两虚者，可选用酸枣仁粥；阴虚火旺者，可选用地黄枣仁粥；余热夹痰者，可选用百合杏仁粥。

2.5 Exercises

2.5 功法锻炼

Exercises can relieve insomnia and its accompanying symptoms by regulating the function of cerebral cortex. Therefore, patients should find out appropriate and suitable exercises according to their own conditions.

功法锻炼有助于调节大脑皮质功能，消除失眠及其伴随症状。患者应视具体情况选定锻炼方法，摸索出适于本人的方式。

Before sleep, play Relaxation Exercises and take deep, long and even breath for 20 to 30 minutes each time. At the same time, repeatedly hint yourself that it's time to have a rest to exclude distracting thoughts. Breathing Exercises and Strengthening Exercises are available according to their constitutions.

临睡前可做放松功，调节呼吸而入静，使呼吸达到深、长、匀。每次可练20～30分钟。并可作些暗示睡眠的意念活动，以排除杂念。如意念“早累了，该睡觉休息了”。重复默念，以至在不知不觉中慢慢入睡。根据体质情况，也可选练内养功、强壮功等。

Simplified Tai Ji Quan is available. When pla-

太极拳可练简化太极

ying Tai Ji Quan, focus one's attention and seek tranquility through motion. It should be played once or twice a day with 20 minutes for each time. It is better to play it before sleep and stop playing when patients feel a little bit tired.

拳,练拳时要求心静神敛,动中求静,每日练 1～2 次,每次约 20 分钟,最好在临睡前练习,使形体稍感劳累为佳。

2.6 Mental Rehabilitation

Sleep is a physiological and also psychological process. There is an old saying that to treat insomnia, regulate mental status first and then eyes. Therefore, starting with mental regulation is always effective. The common approaches are explanations and empathy. Patients should be informed of the etiology, pathogenesis and nature of the disease so that they will know the condition well and then clear away the worries and be confident. Empathy refers to elimination of stimulus and inspire patients through empathy, explaining, complying and hinting according to their mental status. Learn to control emotions and keep in positive mental status.

2.6 精神康复

睡眠既是生理过程又是心理过程,自古就强调"先睡心后睡眼",所以从调摄情志着手调治不寐,每能获效。常用的方法有说理开导、移情易志等。说理开导,即给病人讲解失眠的原因、病机、性质,使患者获得这方面的知识,从而正确认识疾病,消除顾虑,增强信心。移情易志,即根据患者的心理状态,通过移情、释疑、顺意、怡悦、暗示等方式,消除其心因性刺激,并启发病人振奋精神,善于用理性支配感情,保持良好的精神状态。

Section 6 Fright Palpitation

第 6 节 惊悸

Palpitation refers to a condition that one feels uncontrollable rapid heart beat with panic or uneasiness. Clinically, it is often paroxysmal and can be induced by emotional fluctuations or overwork. The condition is often caused by internal damage due to emotional disorders. After exogenous febrile diseases, qi and blood are consumed and the heart is deprived of nourishment with or without internal dis-

惊悸,是指患者自觉心中急剧跳动、惊惕不安,甚则不能自主的一种病证。临床上多呈阵发性,每因情志波动或劳累过度而发作。本证多因七情内伤所致,而在外感热病瘥后,由于气血耗损,心失所养,或兼痰浊内扰,常

turbance of phlegm-turbidity. Therefore, fright palpitation occurs and if it is prolonged and further consumes qi, blood, yin and yang of bowels and viscera, fearful throbbing will develop, presenting as rapid heart beat aggravated with overwork. At this stage, patients have a poor condition and should be treated as early as possible.

可导致惊悸的发生，惊悸日久不愈，可进一步耗伤脏腑气血阴阳，发展成为怔忡，而表现终日心中悸动不安，稍劳尤甚，全身情况较差，故应尽早调治。

1 Indications

After heat diseases, those feeling uncontrollable rapid heart beat with fear and uneasiness and with vexation, insomnia, dreaminess and poor memory are indicated to have this condition. There are three common patterns: ① Heart-gallbladder qi deficiency: palpitations, susceptible to fear and fright, shortness of breath and fatigue, low voice, dream-disturbed sleep, light-colored tongue with thin coating and weak pulse; ②Insufficiency of yin-blood: palpitations and insomnia, dizziness and poor memory, fatigue and shortness of breath, vexation and night sweating, lusterless complexion, red tongue with scanty coating, fine or bound and intermittent pulses; ③ Internal disturbance of phlegm-turbidity: fright palpitations and vexation, insomnia, profuse phlegm and nausea, loss of appetite, or edema of four limbs, white greasy coating and string-like and slippery pulse.

1 适宜指征

热病瘥后，以自觉心中急剧跳动，惊慌不安，不能自主为主要临床表现，并可伴见心烦、失眠、多梦、健忘等心神方面症状者。常见三种证型：①心胆气虚：证见心悸易惊，胆怯怕事，气短乏力，语言低微，少寐多梦，舌淡苔薄，脉弱。②阴血不足：证见心悸少寐，眩晕健忘，神疲少气，烦躁盗汗，面色不华，舌红少苔，脉细或结代。③痰浊内扰：证见惊悸烦闷，夜寐不安，痰多泛恶，食少无味，或四肢浮肿，苔白腻，脉弦滑。

2 Rehabilitation Treatments

2.1 Medication

Those with heart-gallbladder qi deficiency should be treated by boosting qi and nourishing heart with modified Fu Shen San (*Root Poria Powder*). For heart deficiency with timidity and fright, add Long Chi (*Dens Draconis*), Hu Po (*Amber*), Ci

2 康复措施

2.1 药物康复

心胆气虚者，治宜益气养心，可用茯神散加减；若心虚胆怯而惊恐不安者，可加龙齿、琥珀、磁石、朱砂等以镇惊安神；若心之气阴亏虚

Shi (*Magnetitum*) and Zhu Sha (*Cinnabar*) to settle fright and quiet the mind. For deficiency of heart qi and heart yin, Sheng Mai San (*Pulse-Engendering Powder*) or Schisandra Decoction (Wu Wei Zi Tang) can be added to boost qi and nourish yin. Patients with devitalized heart yang can develop symptoms like chest oppression, shortness of breath and cold limbs. Modified Gui Zhi Gan Cao Long Gu Mu Li Tang (*Cinnamon Twig, Licorice, Dragon Bone, and Oyster Shell Decoction*) may be necessary to warm and supplement heart yang. Those with insufficiency of yin-blood can be given modified Tian Wang Bu Xin Dan (*Celestial Emperor Heart-Supplementing Elixir*) for enriching and nourishing yin blood. If symptoms indicating heat pattern are presented, such as vexation, dry throat and mouth, bitter taste in the mouth, Zhu Sha An Shen Wan (*Cinnabar Spirit-Quieting Pill*) may be necessary to nourish yin and clear fire. For deficiency of qi and blood, symptoms like palpitations and bound and intermittent pulses occur and Zhi Gan Cao Tang (*Honey-Fried Licorice Decoction*) is necessary to boost qi and nourish blood. For deficiency of heart and spleen, loss of appetite and fatigue are presented and modified Gui Pi Tang (*Spleen-Returning Decoction*) or Xiao Jian Zhong Tang (*Minor Center-Fortifying Decoction*) may be helpful in fortifying spleen and nourish heart. Those internally disturbed by phlegm-turbidity can be treated through transforming phlegm and quieting the heart with modified Shi Wei Wen Dan Tang (*Ten-Ingredient Gallbladder-Warming Decoction*). If patients are internally disturbed by phlegm-heat and symptoms like bitter tastes, dry mouth, yellow and greasy coating, slip-

者,可合用生脉散以益气养阴,或用五味子汤加减;若心阳不振而兼胸闷气短、形寒肢冷者,可用桂枝甘草龙骨牡蛎汤加味以温补心阳。阴血不足者,治宜滋养阴血,可用天王补心丹加减;若兼虚烦咽燥、口干、口苦等明显热象者,可用朱砂安神丸以滋阴清火;若气血两亏而见心动悸、脉结代者,可用炙甘草汤以益气养血;若心脾两虚而兼食少体倦者,可用归脾汤或小建中汤加减以健脾养心。痰浊内扰者,治宜化痰宁心,可用十味温胆汤加减;若痰热内扰而兼口苦口干,舌苔黄腻、脉滑数者,则用黄连温胆汤加减以清痰热。

pery and rapid pulses are presented, modified Huang Lian Wen Dan Tang (*Coptis Gallbladder-Warming Decoction*) may be necessary to clear phlegm-heat.

2.2 Acupuncture

Xin Shu (BL 15), Ju Que (CV 14), Shen Men (HT7); Nei Guan (PC 6) and Xi Men (PC 4) are main acupoints. For heart-gallbladder qi deficiency, add Qi Hai (CV 6), Dan Shu (BL 19) and Pi Shu (BL 20). For insufficiency of yin blood, add Pi Shu (BL 20), Xiao Chang Shu(BL 27)and Zu Sanli (ST 36). For internal disturbance of phlegm-turbidity, add Chi Ze (LU 5), Dan Zhong (CV 17) and Feng Long (ST 40) for balanced supplementation and drainage. Auricular acupoints like Heart, Brain, Shen Men and Small Intestine can be selected for ear acupuncture. Each time 2 or 3 auricular acupoints are selected for light rotation and 20 or 30 minutes' retention. Vaccariae Semen may also be applied.

2.2 针灸康复

体针一般可取心俞、巨厥、神门、内关、郄门等为主穴。随证配穴:心胆气虚者,加气海、胆俞、脾俞;阴血不足者,加脾俞、小肠俞、足三里;痰浊内扰者,加尺泽、膻中、丰隆。以毫针平补平泻。耳针可取心、脑、神门、小肠等,每次选 2～3 穴,捻转轻刺激,留针 20～30 分钟;也可用王不留行贴压法。

2.3 Tuina

For this condition, Tuina is mainly for health preservation. First press the head and face and then relax back, lumbar region and four limbs. At the same time, slowly and gently knead Nei Guan (PC 6), Shen Men (HT 7), Tong Li (HT 5) and Dan Zhong (CV 17) with fingers. Tuina the chest and precordium area with palms clockwise or from the superior to the inferior.

2.3 推拿康复

以保健按摩法为主,先按头面部,后用轻柔放松手法推拿背腰部及四肢。同时配合点揉穴位,如内关、神门、通里、膻中等穴,效果更好。点穴手法要轻缓均匀,还可用手掌在胸部及心前区,作顺时针方向或自上而下的按摩。

2.4 Diet and Daily Life

Live in a quiet place with fresh air and of moderate temperature. Keep away from noises and negative stimulus to prevent onset or aggravation of fright palpitation. Lead a routine life with ample

2.4 膳食起居

保持居处环境宁静,室内空气新鲜,温度适宜。特别要避免各种噪声及不良因素刺激,以防诱发惊悸,或使

rest and sleep. Alternate rest with work and avoid overexertion and strenuous exercises.

病情加重。生活要有规律，保证一定的休息和睡眠，注意劳逸结合，避免劳累和剧烈运动。

Diet should be nutritional and digestive. Pig heart, Da Zao(*Fructus Jujubae*), Long Yan Rou (*Arillus Longan*) and Lian Zi(*Semen Nelumbinis*) can be added. Eat more frequently with less food at each time. Don't eat too much and keep away from cigarette, liquor, strong tea, spicy, sweet and greasy food. Those with edema should have diet with low salt or even no salt. In terms of herbal diet, individuals with heart-gallbladder qi deficiency can take Ci Shi Porridge; those with insufficiency of yin blood can have Bai Zi Ren (*Seman Platycladi*) Porridge; patients internally disturbed by phlegm-turbidity can have Fu Ling (*Poria*) and Yi Yi Ren (*Coicis Semen*) Porridge.

饮食宜营养丰富，易于消化。在普通膳食基础上，可加食猪心、大枣、桂圆、莲子等，但应少量多餐，勿食过饱。忌烟、酒、浓茶、辛辣刺激及肥甘厚味。兼有水肿者，应给低盐或无盐饮食。药膳方面，心胆气虚者，可选用磁石粥；阴血不足者，可选用柏子仁粥；痰浊内扰者，可选用茯苓苡米粥。

2.5 Exercises

Appropriate exercises will do goods to physical and mental health. Based on the condition, age, habits and life style, patients can choose suitable exercises with moderate load capacity, such as walking, jogging, gymnastics, qi gong, martial arts, Five-animal Boxing (Wu Qin Xi), Tai Ji Quan and Eight Trigram Boxing (Ba Duan Jin). Relaxation Exercise should be taken twice or three times a day and for 15 to 30 minutes at each time. Through regulating mental and physical status and breathing, patients can exclude all distracting thoughts, relax the whole body and focus will-power in Dan Tian. Subjectively block fright and exclude environmental and emotional stimulus. Don't get over-excited or over-exerted in case heart load is increased. During

2.5 功法锻炼

适度的功法运动有益于身心健康。可根据患者的病情、年龄、爱好及生活条件，选定方式和负荷量。如散步、慢跑、体操、气功、武术、五禽戏、太极拳、八段锦等。气功以放松功为宜，每日练功2～3次，每次15～30分钟。运用调心、调身、调息之法，排除一切杂念，全身放松，意守丹田。以主观意念去阻断惊恐心理，排除环境和情志的不良刺激。但应注意，运动应避免情绪突然激动或过分疲劳，以免增加心

the exercises, the heart rate should be kept below 110 beats per minute in case chest oppression, rapid heart beat and shortness of breath are triggered.

2.6 Mental Rehabilitation

Fright palpitation is a condition that involves heart spirits. Patients mostly have psychological disorders like fright or fear and the condition is frequently triggered or worsened by emotional fluctuations. Therefore, it is important to regulate emotions. First of all, physicians should inform the patients of the health care knowledge about this condition so that patients will have a better understanding about it and avoid unnecessary worries and emotional fluctuations. Therefore, patients will be positively involved in rehabilitation treatments. The following approaches may be necessary based on specific conditions of individuals: ① Mutual restraining of emotions: As thoughts restrain fear, physicians should guide patients to think about the reason of fear and worry or distract patients from fear through thinking other questions according to their fear, personality and culture literacy. ② Biological feedback: By reflecting physiological changes of organs, instruments can be used to guide patients to regulate and improve organ functions. ③ Explanation: Patients with fright palpitation always worry about getting heart diseases and hope to be diagnosed. Therefore, to comfort them, cardiac tests may be necessary in excluding organic heart diseases and also in satisfying patients' psychological demands and eliminating their nervousness and fear. It is better for physicians to explain the condition to patients, especially those with organic cardiac disea-

脏负担，活动量的大小，一般以活动后心率不超过 110 次/分钟，不引起胸闷、心慌、气短等症状为度。

2.6 精神康复

本证属于心神的病变，患者大多存在惊慌和恐惧的心理障碍，且每因情志波动而诱发或加重，因而调摄情志尤为重要。首先，要向患者宣讲有关本症的卫生保健知识，使其对疾病有正确的认识，消除不必要的思想顾虑，避免情绪波动。从而保持积极而愉快的精神状态，以接受和配合康复医疗。并可因人选用如下调摄方法：①情志相胜法，“思胜恐”，根据患者不同的恐惧心理、性格特征及文化素养，既可引导病人思考其恐惧疑虑的虚无性，也可安排具体思考题目让其思索、考虑，以解除或分散其恐惧心情。②生物反馈法，采用仪器对病人的生理内脏变化情况提供强化或反馈信息，引导病人有意识地学会自我调节内脏活动，改善内脏功能，进而达到医疗作用。③释疑疗法，惊悸病人总是怀疑自己患有“心脏病”，并希望确诊。有时可以迎合这种心理，采用释疑疗法，通过心脏专科的必要

ses, with affirmation so that patients can have stabilized emotion and be confident. Patient explanation can encourage patients and do goods to rehabilitation.

检查，既可从诊断上排除心脏器质性病变，又能从心理上满足患者的要求，消除其紧张恐惧的心理。特别是医生肯定语气的解释，更有助于病人安定情绪，坚定信心，即使对心脏确有器质性病变的患者。只要医生耐心说教和解释也能提高其信心及勇气，有利于康复。

Section 7 Edema

第7节 浮肿

Edema refers to a condition characterized by cutaneous swelling. After heat disease, all symptoms are relieved but cutaneous swelling arises. After pressure, pitting is applied to a small area. For some patients, indentation persists after the release of the pressure. For other patients, the indentation does not persist. If it is severe, modern tests should be carried out. The presence of protein in urine and cytological abnormality can identify nephritis and kidney diseases, which is considered as the complication of heat diseases. The treatment of edema can apply to it. If it isn't severe and no abnormalities are presented, it is merely sequela after recovery.

浮肿，是肌肤肿胀的一种病证。热病瘥后，诸症虽已消除，但出现肌肤肿胀，有的按之凹陷不起，有的按之即起，往往日久不消。如肿势较甚，结合现代医学检查，尿液蛋白呈阳性，有细胞学异常，诊断为肾炎、肾病者，则属热病并发病证，当按内科“水肿”治；如肿势不甚，检查无明显异常者，则属瘥后遗留症范畴。

1 Indications

After heat diseases are recovered, patients will develop dropsy in face, eyelids, four limbs, abdomen and back, or even all over the body. Varying degrees of symptoms concerning mental status, diet, defecation and urination and abdomen may be ac-

1 适宜指征

热病瘥后，以头面、眼睑、四肢、腹背甚至全身浮肿为主要临床表现，可伴有不同程度的精神、饮食、二便及腹部方面的症状，但检查无

companied. But no abnormalities are identified by tests. The condition should be differentiated from qi edema (edema due to qi disorders).

明显异常者。当区分水肿和气肿。

There are three common patterns: ①Damp-heat retention: edema below the waist, distension and fullness in the epigastric and abdominal region, panting and vexation thirst, inhibited urination and ungratifying defecation, yellow and greasy coating, deep and rapid pulse; ②Qi deficiency of spleen and stomach: occasional dropsy in face or limbs, lassitude and fatigue, shortness of breath and poor appetite, light-colored tongue with scanty coating, slow and weak pulse. For yang deficiency of spleen and stomach, edema arises mainly in lower limbs and symptoms like distension and stuffiness in epigastric and abdominal areas, poor appetite and diarrhea, short voidings of scant urine, yellow complexion and cold limbs, white and slippery coating and deep and slow pulse are accompanied; ③Debilitation of kidney yang: dropsy in face and body, especially in the lower body, soreness of lumbar and knees, aversion to cold and cold limbs, decreased urine, light-colored tongue with white coating, deep and weak pulse. Long-term deficiency of kidney yang will affect yin, causing deficiency of kidney yin. Symptoms like recurrent dropsy, fatigue and reddening in the cheeks, soreness in lumbar and spermatorrhea, dry mouth and throat, vexing heat in five hearts, red tongue and fine rapid pulse will arise.

水肿常见三种证型：①湿热壅滞：热病新瘥后腰以下浮肿，脘腹胀满，喘逆烦渴，小便不利，大便不爽，苔黄腻，脉沉数。②脾胃气虚：面浮或肢肿，时肿时消，倦怠乏力，少气纳差，舌淡苔少，脉缓弱。若脾胃阳虚，则浮肿明显，以下肢为甚，并见脘腹胀闷，纳减便溏，小便短少，面黄肢冷，苔白滑，脉沉缓。③肾阳虚衰：面浮身肿，腰以下尤甚，腰膝酸软，畏寒肢冷，尿量减少，舌淡苔白，脉沉弱。若肾阳久衰，阳损及阴，也可出现以肾阴亏虚的病证，表现为浮肿反复发作，神疲颧红，腰酸遗精，口咽干燥，五心烦热，舌红，脉细数等。

There are two common patterns of qi edema: ①Qi stagnation of spleen and stomach: severe dropsy in abdomen and four limbs, unchanged color of skin, disappearance of pitting after release of pressure, distension and fullness of abdomen, oppres-

气肿常见两种证型：①脾胃气滞：浮肿以腹部和四肢明显，皮色不变，按之即起，腹大胀满，胸闷胀，喜嗳气，小便自利，苔白，脉弦。

sion and distension in the chest, belching, uninhibited urination, white coating and string-like pulse; ②Unrecovered yin deficiency: It is mostly seen in those with unrecovered yin blood after heat diseases. Symptoms are mild dropsy in four limbs, or postmeridian fever, heat in the heart of the palms and soles, red face, dry mouth and throat, fatigue, purple tongue with scant coating, vacuous and fine pulses or bound and intermittent pulses.

②阴亏未复:常见于热病伤阴后阴血未复者,症见四肢轻度浮肿,或午后发热,手足心热,面赤,口干咽燥,神倦,舌绛少苔,脉虚细或结代。

2 Rehabilitation Treatments

2.1 Medication

Those with damp-heat retention can be treated by expelling water and clearing heat with Mu Li Ze Xie San (*Oyster Shell and Rhizoma Alismatis Powder*). 5-10 g of powder may be taken each time with rice water. If damp-heat retention is mild, modified San Ren Tang (*Three Kernels Decoction*) is necessary. Patients with qi deficiency of spleen and stomach may be treated by fortifying spleen and transforming damp with modified Shen Ling Bai Zhu San (*Ginseng, Poria and Atractylodes Powder*). If it is yang deficiency of spleen and stomach with severe edema, warming spleen and disinhibiting water can be applied and modified Shi Pi Yin (*Spleen-Firming Beverage*) is necessary. Patients with debilitation of kidney yang can be treated by warming kidney and moving water with Ji Sheng Shen Qi Wan (*Life Saver Kidney Qi Pill*) combined with Zhen Wu Tang (*True Warrior Decoction*). If it is depletion of kidney yin, enriching and supplementing kidney yin and disinhibiting water may be applied. Zuo Gui Wan (*Left-Restoring (Kidney Yin) Pill*) with Fu Ling (*Poria*) and Ze Xie may be necessary.

2 康复措施

2.1 药物康复

水肿属湿热壅滞者,治宜逐水清热,可用牡蛎泽泻散,每次5~10克,以米汤调服;若为湿热郁滞轻症,可用三仁汤加减。脾胃气虚者,治宜健脾化湿,可用参苓白术散加减;若证属脾胃阳虚而浮肿较甚者,宜温脾利水,可用实脾饮加减。肾阳虚衰者,治宜温肾行水,可用济生肾气丸合真武汤化裁;若证属肾阴亏虚者,宜滋补肾阴、兼利水湿,用左归丸加茯苓、泽泻等。

For qi edema with qi stagnation of spleen and stomach, moving qi and dispersing stagnation can be applied and Kuan Zhong Tang (*Center-Loosening Decoction*) added with Mu Xiang (*Radix Aucklandiae*), Xiang Fu (*Rhizoma Cyperi*) and Qing Pi (*Pericarpium Citri Reticulatae Viride*) is necessary. Symptoms like epigastric and abdominal distention and fullness, putrid belching and vomiting, diarrhea, greasy coating and slippery pulse indicate spleen deficiency and food stagnating in middle jiao. It may be treated by drying damp and moving spleen, dispersing food and harmonizing stomach. Modified Ping Wei San (*Stomach-Calming Powder*) combined with Bao He Wan (*Harmony-Preserving Pill*) may be necessary. Those with unrecovered yin deficiency can be treated by enriching yin and nourishing fluids with Jia Jian Fu Mai Tang (*modified Pulse-Restorative Decoction*) with large dose of Gan Cao (*Radix Glycyrrhizae*).

气肿属脾胃气滞者，治宜行气消滞，可用宽中汤加木香、香附、青皮；若脘腹胀满，兼见嗳腐呕逆，或大便稀溏，苔腻脉滑，证属瘥后脾虚、食滞中焦，宜燥湿运脾、消食和胃，可用平胃散合保和丸加减。阴亏未复者，治宜滋阴养液，方用加减复脉汤重用甘草。

2.2 Acupuncture

Shui Fen (CV 9), Qi Hai (CV 6), Sanjiao Shu (BL 22), Zu Sanli (ST 36), Yin Lingquan (SP 9) are main acupoints. For yang pattern of damp-heat, add Fei Shu (BL 31) and He Gu (LI 4); for yin pattern of deficiency-cold, add Pi Shu (BL 20) and Shen Shu (BL 23) for acupuncture with supplementation and moxibustion. For swelling due to qi stagnation, add Zhong Wan (CV 12) and Tian Shu (ST 25) for acupuncture with drainage and moxibustion is also available. For edema due to yin deficiency, add Xue Hai (SP 10) and Sanyin Jiao (SP 6) for acupuncture with balanced supplementation and drainage.

2.2 针灸康复

可取水分、气海、三焦俞、足三里、阴陵泉等穴为主，辨证配穴。湿热阳证者，加肺俞、合谷；虚寒阴证者，加脾俞、肾俞，针刺用毫针补法，并可温灸；气滞肿胀者，加中脘、天枢，针刺用毫针泻法，可灸；阴亏浮肿者，加血海、三阴交，针刺用毫针平补平泻法。

2.3 Tuina

Rub lower abdomen clockwise and press and knead Zhong Wan (CV 12), Qi Hai (CV 6) and Guan Yuan (CV 4). For damp-heat, add Sanyin Jiao (SP 6), Yin Lingquan (SP 9) and Pangguang Shu (BL 28) for pressing and kneading. For spleen deficiency, Wei Shu (BL 21) and Pi Shu (BL 20) may be added for massaging. For kidney deficiency, add Shen Shu (BL 23) and Ming Men (GV 4) for pushing and rubbing. For yin deficiency, Xue Hai (SP 10), Sanyin Jiao (SP 6) and Zu Sanli (ST 36) can be added for pressing and kneading. All the manipulations should be gentle and moderate.

2.3 推拿康复

可顺时针方向摩小腹，并按揉中脘、气海、关元等穴。湿热者，加按揉三阴交、阴陵泉、膀胱俞；脾虚者，加按摩胃俞、脾俞；肾虚者，加推摩肾俞、命门；阴亏者，加按揉血海、三阴交、足三里。手法要轻柔、缓和。

2.4 Diet and Daily Life

Patients should have adequate rest and keep away from sexual activities. Common cold can worsen the disease, therefore patients should be careful for weather changes and prevent contraction of external pathogens. In the meantime, skins should be kept clean and unwounded, otherwise it can easily lead to infection, causing transmuted patterns. In general, patients with edema should take bath less frequently to avoid internal invasion of water-damp that will hinder the relief of edema.

Diet is of much importance to this condition. According to TCM, patients with edema should keep away from salt. Low-salt or no-salt diet should be given clinically based on the degree of edema. In general, patients with edema are often accompanied with gastrointestinal disorders. As spleen and stomach poorly move and transform, improper diet will impair spleen and stomach, leading to recurrence. Therefore, refined, light, nutritional and digestive diet is required and spicy, greasy and sweet diet and

2.4 膳食起居

浮肿患者要注意休息，戒房事，以防劳伤。感冒可使病情加重，应注意寒温变化，以防再感外邪。同时要保持皮肤清洁，避免皮肤破损，否则容易引起感染，发生变证。水肿患者一般不宜多沐浴，以免水湿内侵，影响水肿消退。

饮食调理尤为重要，中医历来强调水肿忌盐，临床上可依据水肿程度，分别给予低盐或无盐饮食。浮肿患者一般伴有胃肠功能障碍，脾胃运化无力，一旦饮食不慎，则损伤脾胃，使病情反复。因而要求饮食宜细软而清淡，营养丰富而易于消化，忌食辛辣、醇酒、肥甘之品。

ripe wine should be kept away. Excessive intake should be avoided especially when the condition is improved. In terms of herbal diet, edema patients with damp heat may take Mao Gen (*Rhizoma Imperatae*) and Chi Dou (*Semen Phaseoli*) Porridge. Huang Qi (*Radix Astragali seu Hedysari*), Fu Ling (*Poria*) and Yi Yi Ren (*Semen Coicis*) Porridge is effective in treating edema those with deficiency of spleen and kidney. Chen Pi (*Pericarpium Citri Reticulatae*) Porridge may be for those with qi stagnation. Duck Porridge may be helpful for patients with yin deficiency.

尤其在康复好转之际，切忌暴饮暴食。药膳方面，湿热水肿者，可选用茅根赤豆粥；脾肾虚肿者，可选用黄芪茯苓苡仁粥；气滞肿胀者，可选用橘皮粥；阴虚浮肿者，可选用老鸭粥。

2.5 Exercises

For patients with edema, appropriate exercises are conducive to circulating qi and blood and promoting qi transformation. Specific exercises, ranging from walking, jogging, qi gong to Tai Ji Quan, can be selected according to the condition. For example, for qi gong, those with strong constitution can play moving exercises. Static exercises, played while lying, sitting or standing, are necessary for those with weak constitution.

2.5 功法锻炼

浮肿患者，适当的体育活动有利于流通气血，促进气化。可因人因时分别进行散步、慢跑、气功、太极拳等项活动。气功功法应据身体情况选择，体质较好者可练动功，体质较弱者可练静养功，采用卧、坐或立式。

2.6 Mental Rehabilitation

Happiness and stable mental status can promote qi and blood circulation and function regaining of bowels and viscera. Mutual restraining of emotions, such as happiness therapy, and other entertainments are helpful. For instance, light or sprightly music can promote the metabolism of fluids and qi movement.

2.6 精神康复

患者神情舒愉稳定，可促进气血流畅、脏腑功能复常。可应用情志相胜法、娱乐方法等，以喜疗为主。如音乐疗法，可选用轻松、明快的乐曲，促进水液代谢和气机运行。

Section 8 Constipation

第 8 节 便秘

Constipation refers to a condition characterized by dry and hard stool and prolonged intervals of bowel movements, or difficult and unsmooth bowel movements. It can occur during or after the heat disease. The former condition is often caused by dryness-heat binding internally, while the latter is mainly induced by deficiency of qi, blood and fluids. In terms of pathogenesis, the former belongs to excessive pattern and the latter is deficiency pattern.

便秘是指大便秘结不通，排便时间延长，或欲大便而艰涩不畅的一种病证。它既常见于外感热病过程中，也见于热病瘥后，但前者多因燥热内结所致，后者以气血津液亏虚为主，两者病机上有虚实之别。

1 Indications

After heat disease, constipation occurs, presenting as difficult bowel movements or prolonged intervals of defecation (>4-7 days). Symptoms like abdominal distension, decreased appetite, dizziness and weakness, vexation and poor sleep can be accompanied. Anal fissure and haemorrhoids are even induced. There are three common patterns: ① Liquid depletion and intestinal dryness: dry and bound stools, dry lip and mouth, thirst with desire to drink, short voidings of scant urine, red tongue with scant coating, fine and rough pulse. If with remaining dryness-heat, symptoms like red complexion and vexation, abdominal distention or pain, dry mouth with fetid mouth odor, red tongue with yellow coating and fine rapid pulse will develop; ②Depletion of qi and blood: difficult bowel movements, lusterless complexion, dizziness and blurred vision, palpitations, or stools are neither dry nor hard but straining to defecate is needed, sweating

1 适宜指征

热病瘥后，以大便秘结为主症状，表现为排便艰难，或排便时间延长，经常 4～7 日以上排便 1 次，并可伴见腹胀，食欲减退，头昏无力，心烦少寐，甚至引起肛裂、痔疮等症者。常见三种证型：①津亏肠燥：证见大便干结，唇燥口干，咽干欲饮，小便短少，舌红苔少，脉细涩。若兼燥热未清，可见面红心烦，腹胀或痛，口干口臭，舌红苔黄，脉细数。②气血亏虚：证见大便秘结，面色无华，头晕目眩，心悸，或大便并不干硬，虽有便意，临厕努责，挣后汗出短气，便后疲乏，唇舌淡，苔薄，脉细弱。③阳虚冷秘：大便艰涩，排出困难，腹

and shortness of breath after straining to defecate, weakness after bowel movements, light-colored lips and tongue with thin coating and fine weak pulse; ③Yang deficiency: difficult bowel movement, abdominal pain with a cold sensation, cold hands and feet, or soreness and cold sensation in the lumbar region, bright white complexion, long voidings of clear urine, light-colored tongue with white coating and deep slow pulse.

微冷痛，手足欠温，或腰脊酸冷，面色㿠白，小便清长，舌淡苔白，脉沉迟。

2 Rehabilitation Treatments

2.1 Medication

Those with fluid depletion and intestinal dryness may be treated by enriching fluids and moistening intestines with Wu Ren Wan (*Five-Kernel Pill*) added with Sheng Di Huang (*Radix Rehmanniae*), Xuan Shen (*Radix Scrophulariae*) and Mai Dong (*Radix Ophiopogonis*). If abdominal distention or pain, and fetid mouth odor with yellow coating develop in patients with dryness-heat of intestines and stomach, modified Ma Zi Ren Wan (*Cannabis Fruit Pill*) can be taken to clear heat and moisten intestine. Individuals with depletion of qi and blood can be treated by boosting qi and nourishing blood, moistening the intestines and freeing the stool. Dang Gui Bu Xue Tang (*Chinese Angelica Blood-Supplementing Decoction*) combined with Shou Wu (*Radix Polygoni Multiflori*), Zhi Qiao (*Fructus Aurantii*) and Di Gu Pi (*Cortex Lycii*) may be helpful. With severe qi deficiency, patients can take Huang Qi Tang (*Astraglalus Decoction*) to boost qi and moisten intestine. With severe blood deficiency, individuals can take Run Chang Wan (*Intestine-Moistening Pill*) to nourish blood and moisten dry-

2 康复措施

2.1 药物康复

津亏肠燥者，治宜滋液润肠，可用五仁丸加生地、玄参、麦冬等；若肠胃燥热而兼见腹胀或痛，口臭苔黄者，可用麻子仁丸加减以清热润肠。气血亏虚者，宜益气养血、润肠通便，可用当归补血汤加首乌、枳壳、地骨皮等；若气虚甚者，宜用黄芪汤益气润肠，偏血虚甚者，宜用润肠丸养血润燥。阳虚冷秘者，治宜温润通便，方用济川煎，也可用半硫丸或苁蓉润肠丸等。除内服方药外，还可临时应用外导法，如蜜煎导、猪胆汁导及甘油栓、开塞露之类。

ness. For cold constipation due to yang deficiency, free the stool by warming and moistening. Ji Chuan Jian (*Ferry Brew*), Ban Liu Wan (*Pinellia and Sulfur Pill*) or Cong Rong Run Chang Wan (*Cistanche Intestine-Moistening Pill*) may be necessary. Apart from oral medication, enema is also helpful, for example, honey enema, pig's bile enema, and glycerine edema.

2.2 Acupuncture

Shu acupoint, Mu acupoint and lower uniting acupoint of large intestine meridian can be selected, such as Dachang Shu (BL 25), Tian Shu (ST 25), Zhi Gou (TE 6) and Shang Juxu (ST 37). For fluid depletion and intestinal dryness, add He Gu (LI 4) and Qu Chi (LI 11) for acupuncture with drainage or balanced supplementation and drainage; for depletion of qi and blood, add Pi Shu (BL 20) and Wei Shu (BL 21) for acupuncture with supplementation; for cold constipation due to yang deficiency, moxibust Shen Que (CV 8) and Qi Hai (CV 6).

2.2 针灸康复

可取大肠经俞、募穴及下合穴，如大肠俞、天枢、支沟、上巨虚。随证配穴：津亏肠燥者，加合谷、曲池，针用泻法或平补平泻法；气血亏虚者，加脾俞、胃俞，针用补法。阳虚冷秘者，加灸神阙、气海。

2.3 Tuina

Press and knead Zhong Wan (CV 12), Tian Shu (ST 25) and Guan Yuan (CV 4) and then rub the abdomen clockwise. Pi Shu (BL 20), Wei Shu (BL 21), Shen Shu (BL 23) and Zu Sanli (ST 36) can be selected for pressing and kneading; Cheng Shan (BL 57) and Feng Long (ST 40) for grasping. Press and rub the lumbar region until it is warmed. Tuina may be performed in the morning and in the evening and each time is for 15 to 20 minutes.

2.3 推拿康复

可按揉中脘、天枢、关元等穴，然后顺时针方向摩腹；按揉脾俞、胃俞、肾俞、足三里，拿承山、丰隆穴，按擦腰部，以透热为度。每次推拿15～20分钟，早晚各一次。

2.4 Diet and Daily Living

For patients with constipation, purgation shouldn't be applied. Instead, life styles should be changed to improve the physiological functions of

2.4 膳食起居

便秘患者，一般不要使用导泻剂，而应在生活方式上促进肠道生理性功能。应

intestines. Long-time sitting should be avoided. Develop a habit of bowel movements at fixed time and focus the attention. Don't read or think. If necessary, apply hot compress to lower abdomen to promote bowel movements. Perineum and anus should be kept clean. Wash it by warm water after bowel movements. For those with anal fissure and haemorrhoids, Huai Hua (*Sophorae Flos*), Di Yu (*Sanguisorbae Radix*) and Huang Bai (*Cortex Phellodendri*) can be boiled for fumigation and washing. Haemorrhoids ointment can be applied externally.

避免久坐少动,保持定时登厕习惯,排便时注意力要集中,不看书报,不思考问题。必要时可热敷下腹部促使排便。注意保持会阴、肛门的清洁卫生,便后用温水洗净,有肛裂、痔疮者,可用槐花、地榆、黄柏等煎水熏洗,也可外用痔疮膏。

Eat more vegetables and fruits, such as spinach, cabbage, celery, banana and peach, to take in more plant fiber and promote peristalsis. Drink warm water, especially light-salt water after getting up. Keep away from spicy food, mellow wine and excessive intake of cold food. In terms of herbal diet, those with fluid depletion and intestinal dryness can take Bai Zi Ren (*Seman Platycladi*) Porridge; for depletion of qi and blood, He Shou Wu (*Radix Polygoni Multiflori*) Porridge is necessary; for cold constipation due to yang deficiency, Rou Cong Rong (*Herba Cistanches*) and mutton Porridge is helpful.

平时应多食蔬菜、水果,如菠菜、青菜、芹菜、香蕉、桃等,以增加植物纤维,刺激肠蠕动,并喝开水,晨起可饮淡盐开水。忌食辛辣、醇酒等刺激之物,也不可过食寒凉生冷。药膳方面,津亏肠燥者,可选用柏子仁粥;气血亏虚者,可选用何首乌粥;阳虚冷秘者,可选用肉苁蓉羊肉粥。

2.5 Exercises

2.5 功法锻炼

Exercise is an effective way to manage constipation, for it can promote peristalsis and reinforce the defecation. Therapeutic gymnastics should be mainly taken, accompanied with qi gong, fast walking and jogging.

功法运动可增强胃肠蠕动,直接加强排便的动力,是调治便秘的有效方法。其中以医疗体操为主,可配合气功、快步行走及健身跑。

Therapeutic gymnastics can be taken while standing and lying on the back. Exercises like leg lifts, squats, kicks, twists and abdomen back stretch can be taken while standing. Leg flexion,

医疗体操,站位可作原地高抬腿步行、深蹲起立、踢腿、转体运动、腹背运动等;仰卧位可作屈腿运动、举腿,

leg lifting, bicycles and sit-ups are available while lying. Start every move from 16 reps and then gradually progress to 32 reps.

或踏自行车式、仰卧起坐等。每节做 2 个八拍，逐渐增至 4 个八拍。

Breathing exercise (Nei Yang Gong) is mainly for qi gong. Take deep abdominal breath for 30 to 40 minutes while in spine position. Rhythmic contraction and relaxation of diaphragm can tuina the stomach and intestine, increase the smooth muscle tensions of intestinal tract and promote peristalsis.

气功以内养功为主。练功时取仰卧位，作深腹式呼吸，每次 30～40 分钟。因膈肌有节律上下明显移动，可对胃肠起"内按摩"的作用，增加肠管平滑肌张力和促进胃肠蠕动。

Jog or walk in the morning for 15 to 20 minutes. The distance are based on the conditions of individuals. Discontinue the exercises once shortness of breath and sweating are presented. Those with weak constitution may turn to walk. It is better to take a warm bath or hip bath for 5 to 10 minutes after exercises before bowel movements.

快步行走和健步跑时间通常安排在早上进行，一般 15～20 分钟。距离的长短因人而异，以微有气急出汗为宜，体力差者可暂行散步。最好在运动后作温水浴或温水坐浴 5～10 分钟，再去排便。

2.6 Mental Rehabilitation

2.6 精神康复

Long-time and stubborn constipation can develop symptoms like dizziness and headache, somnolence or insomnia, vexation and restless. Therefore, physicians should guide patients to regulate emotions and develop the habit of defecating at fixed time. In the meantime, physicians should inform patients of the condition to eliminate their nervousness. In addition, patients can take part in some appropriate activities. For instance, appreciating music can relax and promote peristalsis.

长期而顽固的便秘，常可伴见头昏头痛、嗜睡或失眠、烦躁不安等症状。因此，康复医疗应调摄情志，做好解释工作，使患者消除紧张心理，保持精神舒畅、气机条达，并指导其学会自我调节，养成按时大便的习惯。同时，可让患者参加适当的娱乐活动，如欣赏音乐以松弛精神，促进肠管的蠕动。

Section 9 Diarrhea

第 9 节 泄泻

Diarrhea refers to a disorder featured by in-

泄泻，是指排便次数增

creased bowel movements and thin, loose, or even watery stools. Diarrhea after heat diseases are often induced by incomplete treatment of diarrhea, weak spleen and stomach caused by long-time heat diseases, or impaired spleen yang and poor transformation due to excessive intake of cold herbs. It occurs slowly and is mainly featured by thin and loose stools and manifested as chronic diarrhea.

多,便质稀薄,甚至泻出如水样的病证,以大便溏薄而势缓者为泄,大便清稀如水而直下者为泻,因两者病变性质相同,故临床上统称为泄泻。热病瘥后泄泻,多由急性泄泻治疗不彻底,以致迁延不愈或因热病日久,脾胃虚弱,或因病中过用寒凉,脾阳被伤,运化失职所致。其病势较缓,以大便溏薄而泄为主,多表现为慢性泄泻。

1 Indications

In recovery, no symptoms caused by external contractions are found and main clinical symptoms are increased bowel movements and thin loose stools. In the meantime, digestive symptoms like decreased appetite and abdominal discomfort can be accompanied. There are three common patterns: ①Deficiency of spleen and stomach: stools are sometimes loose and sometimes watery with undigested food; once taking in greasy food, bowel movements will be increased with decreased intake of food, distention and oppression of epigastric and abdominal region, sallow complexion, fatigue and lassitude, light-colored tongue with white coating and fine weak pulse; ②Remaining damp-heat: diarrhea and abdominal pain, urgent or unsmooth bowel movement, burning sensation in anus, short and yellow urine, or aggravation due to emotional disorders like anger and depression, distension and oppression in chest and hypochondriac region, belching and decreased intake of food, yellow and thin

1 适宜指征

热病恢复期,已无明显的外感症状,而以大便次数增多,粪质稀薄为主要临床表现,并伴见纳食减少、腹胀不适等消化系统症状者。常见三种证型:①脾胃虚弱:证见大便时溏时泻,水谷不化,稍进油腻之物,则大便次数增多、饮食减少,脘腹胀闷不舒,面色萎黄,体倦乏力,舌淡苔白,脉细弱。②湿热未尽:证见泄泻腹痛,泻下急迫,或泻而不爽,肛门灼热,小便短黄或每因情志郁怒而增剧,可并见胸胁胀闷不舒,嗳气食少,苔薄黄,脉弦细略数。③肾阳虚衰:证见泄泻时发时止,完谷不化,腹中冷痛,喜温喜按,或泄在黎明前,腹部作痛,肠鸣即泻,泻

coating with string-like fine rapid pulse; ③ Depletion of kidney yang: occasional onset of diarrhea with undigested food, cold sensation in abdomen relieved by warmth and pressure, or diarrhea at dawn upon abdominal pain and bowel sounds, the patients may feel better after diarrhea, cold limbs, soreness in lumbar region and knees, light-colored tongue with white coating and deep fine pulse.

后则安，形寒肢冷，腰膝酸软，舌淡苔白，脉沉细。

2 Rehabilitation Treatments

2.1 Medication

Patients with deficiency of spleen and stomach may be treated by fortifying spleen and boosting stomach with modified Shen Ling Bai Zhu San (*Ginseng, Poria and Atractylodes Powder*). For food stagnation, add Shen Qu (*Massa Medicata Fermentata*), Mai Ya (*Fructus Hordei Germinatus*), Shan Zha (*Crataegi Fructus*) to disperse food and transform stagnation. For yang deficiency of spleen and stomach with cold sensation in abdomen and cold hands and feet, modified Fu Zi Wen Zhong Tang (*Aconite Center-Warming Decoction*) may be necessary in warming the center and dispersing cold. Prolonged diarrhea with center qi falling and rectocele can be treated by boosting qi and ascending the clear, fortifying spleen and relieving diarrhea with Bu Zhong Yi Qi Tang (*Center-Supplementing Qi-Boosting Decoction*). Remaining damp-heat should be treated by clearing and resolving the remaining pathogenic factors. Ge Gen Qing Lian Tang (*Pueraria and Scutellaria Decoction*) combined with Tong Xie Yao Fang (*Pain and Diarrhea Formula*) may be applied to suppress wood by supporting earth. Fu Ling (*Poria*) and Mu Xiang (*Radix*

2 康复措施

2.1 药物康复

脾胃虚弱者，治宜健脾益胃，可用参苓白术散加减；夹食滞者，加神曲、麦芽、山楂以消食化滞；若脾胃阳虚，腹中冷痛、手足不温者，宜用附子温中汤加味以温中散寒；若久泻不愈，中气下陷，兼有脱肛者，可用补中益气汤以益气升清、健脾止泻。湿热未尽者，治宜清解余邪而扶土抑木，可用葛根芩连汤合痛泻要方，可加茯苓、木香等；若兼胃阴盛而舌尖红无苔，或中心有斑剥，可加山药、玉竹、石斛以养胃阴；肾阳虚衰者，宜温补脾肾、固肠止泻，可以四神丸酌加附子、炮姜以增强温肾健脾之力；若年老体衰，久泻不止，中气下陷，宜加人参、黄芪、白术益气健脾，或合桃花汤以固涩止泻。

Aucklandiae) can be added. For exuberant stomach yin, red tip of tongue with no coating or with peeling coating in the center will be presented. Shan Yao (*Rhizoma Dioscoreae*), Yu Zhu (*Rhizoma Polygonati Odorati*) and Shi Hu (*Herba Dendrobii*) can be added to nourish stomach yin. Those with depletion of kidney yang can be treated by warming and supplementing spleen and kidney, securing intestines and checking diarrhea with Si Shen Wan (*Four Spirits Pill*). Fu Zi (*Radix Aconiti Lateralis Preparata*) and fried ginger can be added to strengthen the function of warming kidney and fortifying spleen. If patients are aged with weak body, long-time diarrhea and center qi falling, ginseng, Huang Qi (*Radix Astragali seu Hedysari*) and Bai Zhu (*Rhizoma Atractylodis Macrocephalae*) may be helpful in boosting qi and fortifying spleen. Tao Hua Tang (*Peach Blossom Decoction*) can also be combined to secure, astrict and relieve diarrhea.

2.2 Acupuncture

Acupuncture is mainly to fortify spleen and stomach. Pi Shu (BL 20), Zhong Wan (CV 12), Zhang Men (LR 13), Tian Shu (ST 25) and Zu Sanli (ST 36) can be selected. For depletion of kidney yang, add Ming Men (GV 4) and Guan Yuan (CV 4) for acupuncture with supplementation. Moxibustion is also available. For remaining damp-heat, clearing and discharging damp-heat may be applied. Yin Lingquan (SP 9) may be added for acupuncture with drainage or balanced supplementation and drainage.

2.2 针灸康复

以健脾胃为主，可取脾俞、中脘、章门、天枢、足三里等穴。肾阳虚衰者，加配命门、关元，针用补法，可加灸；湿热未尽者，宜清泄湿热，可加配阴陵泉，针用泻法或平补平泻法。

2.3 Tuina

Zhong Wan (CV 12), Tian Shu (ST 25), Qi Hai (CV 6) and Guan Yuan (CV 4) can be selected

2.3 推拿康复

可于腹部取中脘、天枢、气海、关元等穴，用一指禅推

for pushing and rubbing with one finger. Acupoints at the back like Pi Shu (BL 20), Wei Shu (BL 21), Shen Shu (BL 23), Dachang Shu (BL 25) and Chang Qiang (GV 1) can be chosen for pressing, kneading and rubbing. To treat those with deficiency of spleen and stomach, focus on pressing and kneading Zu Sanli (ST 36) and rubbing epigastric and abdominal region. For depletion of kidney yang, transversely rub Shen Shu (BL 23), Ming Men (GV 4) and Ba Liao(BL 31—BL 34). For remaining damp-heat, press and knead Gan Shu (BL 18), Dan Shu (BL 19), Da Chang Shu(BL 25), Tai Chong (LR 3) and Xing Jian (LR 2) and obliquely rub hypochondriac region.

法、摩法；背部可取脾俞、胃俞、肾俞、大肠俞、长强等穴，运用按、揉、擦等法。脾胃虚弱者，重点按揉足三里，并摩脘腹；肾阳虚衰者，横擦肾俞、命门及八髎；湿热未尽者，按揉肝俞、胆俞、肠俞及太冲、行间，并可斜擦两胁。

Patients can perform tuina by themselves. Knead the abdomen before getting up and sleeping respectively. Centering on the navel, slowly press and knead the abdomen for more than 100 rounds alternatively with two hands. The manipulations should be given gently at first and then heavily.

患者可行自我按摩，每日早晨起床和晚上睡前，坚持揉腹。方法是两手交替缓慢按揉腹部，以肚脐为中心，每次揉 100 次左右，方向不限，注意用力由轻而重。

2.4 Diet and Daily Life

2.4 膳食起居

Living room should be kept clean and of moderate temperature to avoid cold contraction. Have adequate rest to avoid impaired spleen due to overexertion. Hot compress may be frequently applied to abdomen to relieve the symptoms. To be easily digested, diet should be light, thin and soft with less oil and fiber. Patients may have regular meals with fixed quota. To lower the burden of stomach and intestines and to promote absorption, don't take in excessive food or drink. Keep away from cold, greasy, rough and hard, and unhealthy food or food that has many scraps, or can easily generate flatus.

居室应保持清洁卫生，要注意适寒温，以防受凉感寒。注意休息，以免劳力伤脾。经常用热水袋热敷腹部，可改善症状。饮食应以清淡、稀软、少油脂、少纤维、易于消化为原则。定时定量，不暴饮暴食，以减轻胃肠负担，有利于营养吸收。忌食生冷、油腻、粗硬，及多渣、易产气、不卫生的食物。

2.5 Exercises

Exercises like walking, jogging, gymnastics, Tai Ji Quan and qi gong can strengthen the body, promote the function regaining of spleen and stomach. For example, qi Gong can be started with relaxation exercises in supine position. It may be taken twice or three times a day with 30 minutes for each time. After regaining, standing exercises or Tai Ji Qi Gong can be necessary.

2.6 Mental Rehabilitation

After diarrhea, spleen deficiency often occurs and it can affect qi circulation, causing worry and anxiety. Emotional disorders will further worsen the condition. Therefore, regulating emotions is essential to regain the functions of spleen and stomach and promote recovery. Approaches like explanation and enlightenment, mutual restraining of emotions are applied clinically. Patients can also participate in some entertainment activities, like listening to music, appreciating paintings and calligraphy and practicing chess and arts.

2.5 功法锻炼

坚持散步、跑步、广播操、太极拳及气功锻炼，可增强体质，有助于脾胃功能恢复。气功练习，开始可采用卧式放松功，每次 30 分钟，每日 2～3 次。待体力恢复后，可练站桩功、太极气功等。

2.6 精神康复

瘥后泄泻，多为脾虚，脾虚往往影响气机条畅，容易使人产生忧思和焦虑的异常情志，而这种异常情志又会进一步加重病情，应通过调摄情志，以调整脾胃功能，促进康复。临床上可采用说理开导、情志相胜等方法舒畅患者情志，也可指导参加赏心悦脾的娱乐活动，如听音乐、赏书画、习琴棋等。

Shanghai Pujiang Education Press (Former Shanghai University of Traditional Chinese Medicine Press)
1550 Haigang Haigang Avc, Shanghai, P.R.China 201306

图书在版编目(CIP)数据

中医养生康复学/马烈光主编. —上海：上海浦江教育出版社有限公司，2018.12
((英汉对照)精编实用中医文库/陈凯先，李其忠，何星海主编)
ISBN 978-7-81121-586-1

Ⅰ.①中… Ⅱ.①马… Ⅲ.①养生(中医)-康复医学-英、汉 Ⅳ.①R247.9

中国版本图书馆 CIP 数据核字(2018)第277725号

上海浦江教育出版社出版
社址：上海海港大道 1550 号上海海事大学校内　　邮政编码：201306
电话：(021)38284910(12)(发行)　38284923(总编室)　38284916(传真)
E-mail：cbs@shmtu. edu. cn　　URL：http://www. pujiangpress. cn
上海盛通时代印刷有限公司印装　上海浦江教育出版社发行
幅面尺寸：170 mm×240 mm　印张：28. 25　字数：538 千字
2018 年 12 月第 1 版　2018 年 12 月第 1 次印刷
责任编辑：黄　健　封面设计：赵宏义
定价：110. 00 元